Alex Brecher
Natalie Stein

The
BIG Book
on the
GASTRIC SLEEVE

Everything You Need To Know To Lose Weight and Live Well with the Vertical Sleeve Gastrectomy

Thank you for reading *The Big Book on the Gastric Sleeve: Everything You Need to Know to Lose Weight and Live Well with the Vertical Sleeve Gastrectomy*

We hope the book has been a valuable resource for you as you decide whether to get weight loss surgery and continue your weight loss journey with the sleeve

Need another copy? You can order them online from:

- BariatricPal.com

- Amazon

- Barnes and Noble

You can get them in print and in electronic forms for e-readers including the Kindle, iPad, Nook, Kobo and Sony. They're great gifts for other bariatric patients as well as your friends and family who want to support you in your journey.

If you liked this book, you'll also love the companion books in this series.

The Big Book on the Lap-Band: Everything You Need to Know to Lose Weight and Live Well with the Adjustable Gastric Band!

And

The Big Book on the Gastric Bypass: Everything You Need to Know to Lose Weight and Live Well with the Roux-en-Y Gastric Bypass Surgery

And coming soon…

Life after Weight Loss Surgery: Tips and Tricks for Losing Weight and Living Well

Look out for these and more weight loss surgery books from Alex Brecher and Natalie Stein to help you succeed in your weight loss journey!

Acknowledgements

The authors would like to thank everyone who made this book possible. *Surgeons*, from Alex's own bariatric surgeon to the many *knowledgeable and talented surgeons* he has worked with over the years, were instrumental in guiding the development of the book. Many of them and integrated health members also support BariatricPal.com with their membership and insights on the boards. Expertise and dedication from surgeons and integrated healthcare members drive patient success with the gastric sleeve.

The authors' *friends and family members* have continuously supported the production of this book and have made the process much easier.

The staff of BariatricPal.com keeps the boards running smoothly each day. Their skills and dedication keep old members coming back and continue to recruit new members. The staff maintains an incredible degree of courtesy and respect on the boards so that no member feels excluded or uncomfortable. This book strives to maintain this welcoming atmosphere.

This book would not have been possible without the thousands of *BariatricPal.com community members* who continue to support the forums and provide inspiration to the authors. Member moderators serve as community leaders and role models. Many members are highly participative and very engaged in the boards. The authors are grateful to all BariatricPal.com users, who represent the main target audience for this book.

In particular, the authors would like to thank each BariatricPal.com member who was kind enough to share their own personal story. They showed the true giving spirit of BariatricPal.com, and their willingness to share their stories to benefit others is indeed overwhelming. It was a pleasure to work with each of them and the book would not have been the same without them. They diligently answered the interview questions and added their own personal touches, and many of these generous members had already shared parts of their stories in previously published pieces in the BariatricPal.com member newsletters.

Finally, heartfelt thanks to the book's editor, *Melissa Se*, and illustrator, *Gary Crump*. The illustrator's clear and precise drawings are designed to help readers visualize the descriptions in the text – and in this case, each drawing truly is worth a thousand words. The publisher took the manuscript from its initial submission to an edited and formatted final form, patiently directing the authors in their first book.

We truly appreciate and thank each person who has made this book possible.

Contents

List of Figures

List of Tables

Note From the Authors

From Alex:

When I began my weight loss journey in 2003, I had no idea that it would lead to all of this. I only wanted a way to lose weight and get myself together. I had been fighting obesity my entire life, and I was desperate for a long-term solution that didn't involve starving myself, being obsessed with food, and regaining weight every time I stopped dieting. At 5 feet 8 inches tall, I hit a high of 255 pounds during college. I was able to successfully lose some weight, even a lot of weight, when I dieted, but the weight always came back when I stopped dieting.

I began seriously considering weight loss surgery because of a friend of mine. Since getting the laparoscopic adjustable gastric band (lap-band), he'd been losing weight and was looking better than I'd ever seen him. After doing a small bit of research, I decided that the lap-band could be my own ticket to controlling my eating and my weight. I got the band in 2003, and assumed that I could easily figure out what I needed to know by searching the internet when I had questions. I had thought there would be unlimited sites talking about the lap-band, providing social support and information and encouragement to all of the lap-band patients like me who were so dedicated to losing weight but needed a helping hand.

Boy, was I wrong! There weren't that many resources available, and the ones that were there weren't that useful. They didn't have the information I needed, or they didn't have a friendly, welcoming vibe that made me want to go back. I wanted a place to go to communicate with other lap-band patients. I wanted to learn from them, be able to ask my questions and receive advice and suggestions from people who'd already been exactly where I was. That's why I started LapBandTalk.com almost immediately after my surgery in 2003. I want all of the lap-band patients out there, and the people who are considering the lap-band as a tool to fight obesity, to have a place to go for the assistance and answers they need, starting from before surgery and for as long as they want to continue the lap-band lifestyle and stay healthy.

LapBandTalk.com took off beyond anything I'd ever imagined, and I realized that patients who were interested in or had gotten other weight loss surgery procedures had similar needs. I started VerticalSleeveTalk.com and other boards for different procedures. These boards, at one time under the larger umbrella name of WLS Boards (Weight Loss Surgery Boards), are now assembled as BariatricPal.com.

BariatricPal.com includes hundreds of thousands of members. Some are successfully maintaining their goal weights or are losing weight, and they attribute part of their weight loss to weight loss surgery. Other members are preparing for surgery or are trying to decide whether weight loss surgery may be right for them. I am proud of our weight loss surgery community and believe it serves a vital purpose in promoting patient success. The site is the first choice for many weight loss surgery patients, including many who use it daily, for information, encouragement, and a sense of community.

BariatricPal.com continues to grow and evolve to meet the needs VSG patients everywhere. The fully functional smartphone apps for iPhones and Androids and the app for the kindle make the site accessible at all times from anywhere that you have access to the internet. I try to be highly sensitive to members' needs and respond to them. Whether it is getting feedback from members, discussing latest sleeve and other weight loss surgery trends with surgeons, or attending the annual conference of the American Society for Metabolic and Bariatric Surgery across the country from my home, I do what I can to continually meet your needs.

Consistent with my goal of providing help to all weight loss surgery patients, I am particularly proud of the fact that full membership to BariatricPal.com is free. Not one member is paying a dime to use the site, and I have no plans to change this. Members get unlimited access to all of the services that BariatricPal.com offers, such as the discussion forums, apps, surgeon directory, ability to upload photos, personal blogs, chat rooms, and newsletters. You can read more about the site throughout the book and especially in Chapter 18, this book's final chapter.

Today, the situation on the internet has dramatically improved from when I got my lap-band procedure done in 2003. You have several hundred, if not thousands, of options for getting information and for meeting people to talk online or arrange to meet in person. Despite this, BariatricPal.com remains one of the premier sites. It is the largest, so you are sure to find people who are or were in your situation. It is non-biased, and my staff and I are very careful to keep it friendly.

So why did I feel the need for this book? It's true that you can find almost all of this information when you read the fine print online and get materials from your surgeon and hospital. But, do you really want to? This book has all of the information in one place, so it's more convenient. Plus, it's organized according to what stage you are in your weight loss journey. It goes from deciding about whether to get the gastric sleeve, through the surgery, all the way to living the sleeve lifestyle. It's available online so it's easy to access, and you can print it out a chapter at a time if you want to stick it in your purse or pocket and read it a bit at a time.

For me, weight loss surgery has been everything that I had hoped it would be. I have lost 100 pounds and kept it off for years. I am happier than I ever was. I am active and have energy, and food does not dictate my thoughts and life. I cannot be more grateful than I am toward the lap-band as a tool for weight loss, and I hope to support others who are considering weight loss surgery or who already have it to make lasting weight loss a possibility.

That is the purpose of this book. I hope you find that it is an excellent resource and guide for your own journey.

Founder
BariatricPal.com

A Note from Natalie

I was proud to play a role in helping Alex with this book. I have been increasingly involved in BariatricPal.com and working with Alex on the monthly newsletters and other behind-the-scenes work. A book for the vertical sleeve gastrectomy seemed to be a fantastic way to continue to reach out to the gastric sleeve community and provide a trustworthy and complete source of information.

As a nutritionist, I am often overwhelmed by the consequences of obesity. The physical effects, including type 2 diabetes, heart disease, arthritis and sleep apnea, are only part of it. The psychological battles, low self-esteem and social stigma, discrimination and judgment are part of daily life for an obese individual, as you well know if you suffer from obesity or are close to someone who does.

I am just as overwhelmed by how difficult it is to beat obesity. In a culture with fast food on every corner, junk food at every social event, cars to take us everywhere and busy lives without time to exercise or cook healthy meals, it's impossible to make the best health decisions all the time.

Fighting obesity is tough, and giving up can seem easier. However giving up can be devastating. For many people, weight loss surgery has been the only successful treatment for obesity in their whole lives, or at least in decades. If you are among the people who have tried every diet under the sun, without success, and you are ready to make a permanent and dramatic lifestyle change, you might be a good candidate for the gastric sleeve.

When we first began the process of writing this book, there was no other comprehensive book dedicated solely to the sleeve. The vertical sleeve gastrectomy is a relatively new stand-alone surgery for weight loss, and there isn't much information about it yet. Patients who have the sleeve or are considering it don't have a lot of sources of trustworthy and useful information. You can find plenty of information on weight loss surgery in general if you're willing to do some digging, but you shouldn't have to search hard.

We wanted to put everything together in a single book to make it easier for you find information. Unfortunately, some sleeve patients don't do all of the background research that they should before deciding to get the sleeve or undergoing surgery. It is heartbreaking to learn of sleeve patients who jumped into the surgery without having realistic expectations about weight loss or lifestyle changes. Just as sad is when weight loss surgery patients *think* they're doing everything right, but aren't losing the weight they wanted because they don't have the correct information about what to eat and how to make healthy lifestyle changes.

By the time Alex asked me if I would work with him on this book, I was already starting to "meet" (in a virtual sense – online!) a large number of wonderful members through my experiences working with and writing for BariatricPal.com. These sleeve patients impressed me in several ways. I admire their dedication to their weight loss despite the hardships they faced. I respect that each of them has a personal story that brought them to the vertical sleeve gastrectomy, and I appreciate the common ground that all sleeve patients share.

Most of all, what struck me about so many of the BariatricPal.com members that I talked to, and continues to amaze me, is their generosity. They express gratitude for BariatricPal.com and members who have helped them along the way, and would like nothing more than to give back to the weight loss surgery community. They love to help others who are beginning their sleeve journeys, just like they were helped.

You will see bits and pieces of some of their stories throughout this book. This is just a small sample of the warm and caring people that I have met so far. I am sincerely grateful to those of you who have been kind enough to share your stories for this book. I know that you will touch thousands of lives.

I hope, in some small way, that this book is inspirational and informative for anyone interested in the vertical sleeve and living a healthy lifestyle.

Natalie Stein

MS, MPH
Author

Prologue

Are you sick and tired of struggling with obesity? If you've been obese for years and have tried every weight loss diet without lasting success, weight loss surgery may be the right choice for you. *"The Big Book on the Gastric Sleeve: Everything You Need to Lose Weight and Live Well with the Vertical Sleeve Gastrectomy"* is your complete guide to the vertical sleeve gastric, or gastric sleeve.

Like so many other patients who have struggled with obesity for many years, you may find that the gastric sleeve is the tool you need to eat well and finally lose weight for good. This book guides you through each step of the journey, from deciding to get the sleeve, finding a surgeon and paying for surgery, to recovering from surgery, following the sleeve diet and losing weight and maintaining your weight loss for life.

"The Big Book on the Gastric Sleeve: Everything You Need to Lose Weight and Live Well with the Vertical Sleeve Gastrectomy" treats you with the respect you deserve and provides facts and analysis in simple and easy to understand language. It discusses everything related to obesity, weight loss, the gastric sleeve and the sleeve diet so that you can make the best decisions for yourself. The book also helps you by being a source of advice and motivation, too. It has stories from real-life sleeve patients, told in their words.

When you're ready to learn all about losing weight and living well with the vertical sleeve gastrectomy, grab your copy of the book and get reading!

Overview and Benefits of Each Chapter

Chapter 1: Obesity – A Costly Epidemic

This chapter talks about the obesity epidemic and provides a reminder of the dangers of obesity. Obesity contributes to type 2 diabetes, heart disease, stroke, sleep apnea and osteoarthritis. It can make you depressed, and you might already be familiar with social stigma, such as people looking down on you, that comes with obesity. Yet, one-third of Americans are obese and another third are overweight. Our lifestyles and our environment make losing weight hard. Each day, we face fast food, junk food, not enough opportunities for exercise and too much time sitting around. How much is obesity affecting you? Read chapter one and find out for yourself!

Chapter 2: Weight Loss Options

Why is weight loss so difficult when it sounds so simple? Eat less and exercise more, and you should lose weight, right? It's not so easy, though. This chapter takes a look at your options for losing weight and why they don't work for most people, or why they may have not have worked for you before.

- Diets don't usually work in the long-term if you don't make them true lifestyle changes; you'll gain the weight right back if you try extreme diets such as low-carb diets or diets that only let you eat boxed meals or shakes.
- Exercise programs are healthy, but they don't usually burn off enough calories to motivate you to continue them.
- Weight loss drugs can be dangerous and are not necessarily effective.

Weight loss surgery, or bariatric surgery, is an alternative option for losing weight and keeping it off. The major types in the United States are:

- Vertical sleeve gastrectomy
- Roux-en-Y gastric bypass
- Sleeve plication (or curvature plication)
- Laparoscopic adjustable gastric band (brand name: Lap-Band)

This chapter discusses each of these approaches to weight loss so you can consider more seriously whether weight loss surgery, possibly the vertical sleeve gastrectomy, may be the right choice for you.

Chapter 3: Vertical Sleeve Gastrectomy 101

You may have considered the vertical gastrectomy as an obesity treatment, but do you know exactly what it is and how it works? This chapter describes the vertical sleeve gastrectomy procedure and how it can help you lose weight if you follow the sleeve diet. During surgery, the surgeon removes the majority of your stomach pouch and forms the remainder of the stomach into a tube-shaped sleeve. The surgery is usually laparoscopic, or minimally invasive, but it can be open. This chapter explains both of these options. When you swallow, food travels down your throat, through the sleeve and into your intestines. The gastric sleeve helps you feel full faster so you're less likely to eat as much. The vertical sleeve gastrectomy is permanent and irreversible, so you need to follow the sleeve diet for life.

Chapter 4: Potential Benefits of the VSG

Did you know that the vertical gastric sleeve has a much smaller pouch than your original stomach? It can hold only about 15 percent of the amount of food that your original stomach could hold. You're likely to eat less and lose weight when you have the gastric sleeve because of the smaller amount of food and because the vertical sleeve gastrectomy changes your hormones to make you less hungry. This chapter talks about how much weight you can expect to lose with the sleeve if you follow the sleeve lifestyle goes smoothly. It also explains some of the other benefits of losing weight with the sleeve, such as feeling better and getting off of some of your medications.

Chapter 5:VSG: Risks and Considerations

Any surgical procedure has risks, and this chapter presents them to you so that you can make an informed decision about whether you think the vertical sleeve gastrectomy is worthwhile for you. Infections and bleeding are the most common risks of surgery. Pain can be severe as you recover from surgery. Serious complications requiring a second surgery are rare. Nausea, vomiting and gastrointestinal discomfort are possible, but are often preventable if you follow your surgeon's diet and other instructions carefully. Chapter 5 makes sure that you're going into the sleeve gastrectomy with all the information you need.

Chapter 6: Are You a Good Candidate for the Sleeve?

If you've read the chapters this far, you will know about the sleeve procedure, how the sleeve can help you lose weight and what the risks are. Now, it's time to start thinking about whether you're a good candidate to get the vertical sleeve gastrectomy. Chapter 6 introduces the eligibility criteria for obese patients who want the gastric sleeve, as well as exclusion criteria – or contraindications (medical conditions) that may prevent you from getting the sleeve. This chapter also talks about some special conditions, such as pregnancy, revisional weight loss surgery patients and adolescents. By the end of this chapter, you'll have a much better idea about whether the vertical sleeve gastrectomy is for you.

Chapter 7: Tips when Planning for the Sleeve

After deciding to get the sleeve, it's time to plan your surgery. This chapter suggests sources for expanding your knowledge about the surgery. Selecting a surgeon is an important step in your journey, and this chapter gives you tips on finding a surgeon who's qualified and a good fit for your personality. We also introduce the other members of the healthcare team, such as a mental health professional and dietitian. These health professionals will be working with you for years. Finally, the chapter discusses some characteristics to look for when you're deciding where to get your surgery done. While it's not as cozy as a smaller clinic, a bariatric center in a large hospital has many advantages.

Chapter 8: Insurance, Self-Pay and Medical Tourism

Financing your surgery can be challenging, but you have multiple options. This chapter walks you through finding out whether your insurance coverage includes the sleeve gastrectomy and the steps of getting your pre-approval letter. Finance plans can help you cover the surgery if you don't have health insurance coverage and you can't afford to pay the entire cost in cash. Since other nations often offer vertical sleeve gastrectomies at lower overall costs than in the U.S., each year thousands of patients go to Mexico or Venezuela for their vertical sleeve gastrectomies. This chapter provides advice and tips for medical tourism.

Chapter 9: Pre-Surgery Preparations

You've chosen a surgeon and figured out financing, and you're getting excited! What's next? Relax, take a deep breath and dig into Chapter 9! As you prepare for surgery, you'll meet with your surgeon for medical tests and to discuss your concerns. You'll get a psychological evaluation, and a dietitian may work with you on a pre-surgery diet as well as some plans for your post-surgery gastric sleeve diet.

Chapter 10: Final Preparation for the Sleeve Surgery

Chapter 10 goes over some of the pre-surgery details, such as getting time off work and making sure your kitchen is well-stocked. The chapter provides lists of what to take to the hospital and what to leave at home. If you're going abroad for your vertical sleeve gastrectomy, check out the checklist of important things to take care of as surgery approaches! This chapter has you covered through checking into the hospital and going in for your procedure.

Chapter 11: Recovering from Surgery

Congratulations! You're now a sleeve patient for life! Taking precautions during this important period in your gastric sleeve journey can make your weight loss easier and faster down the road. Chapter 11 talks about what to expect during the rest of your time in the hospital. We also give you some useful tips for speeding your recovery when you get home. During this period, you'll gradually return to your normal activities and to work.

Chapter 12: Post-Op Care

Since the gastric sleeve is a lifelong procedure, your post-op care goes from the end of surgery through the rest of your life. The more seriously you take your post-surgery care, the more likely you are to avoid complications and have weight loss success with the sleeve. Your post-op, or aftercare, program usually includes:

- Your post-surgery surgeon appointments
- Medical tests that you may have
- Other healthcare appointments in your post-surgery care program
- Support group meetings and other sources of support
- Staying positive and persistent during this time

Chapter 13: Recovery and Your Post-Surgery Diet

Food is central to weight loss and health, but you can't jump right into the full gastric sleeve diet right after surgery. The first four to six weeks after surgery are for focusing on recovery, not on weight loss. Eating the right foods now can help you prevent complications later. Chapter 13 goes through your diet during the first several weeks after surgery. During this time, stick carefully to the allowed foods and get in the habit of measuring portions. Drink plenty of water throughout the day but not at meals. This chapter has food lists for each phase plus suggested meal plans and other tips to get you through these first several weeks. Chapter 13 covers the first three out of these four phases of your post-surgery diet progression:

- Liquid diet
- Pureed diet
- Soft foods diet
- Regular sleeve diet

Chapter 14: Losing Weight with the Sleeve Diet

You get to start the solid foods diet after you successfully complete the semi-solid phase. The solid foods phase is designed to be your long-term diet; it'll help you lose weight and maintain your weight for as long as you choose to follow it. This chapter will let you stick to your sleeve diet with confidence. You'll see lists of foods and their serving sizes for each food group plus suggested meal plans and tips for following the sleeve diet. We'll teach you how to make your own meal plans so you can eat the foods you prefer and change up your diet to prevent boredom.

Chapter 15: The Sleeve Diet, Weight Loss and Your Health

You can eat most foods on the gastric sleeve diet, but you'll do best if you focus on high-protein and nutrient-dense foods. We'll show you how! This chapter tells you about water, protein, carbohydrates, fats, vitamins and minerals – all the nutrients you need to stay healthy! High-protein and nutrient-dense choices are critical for preventing deficiencies, so we'll tell you what you need to know. You'll also get to learn about nutrition labels so you choose healthy foods. It'll become natural if you practice it constantly!

Chapter 16: Getting and Staying in Shape with Exercise

Physical activity, or exercise, helps you burn calories and control your weight, and this chapter has a list of common activities and the calories you can burn doing them. Regular exercise has other benefits, too. It reduces your risk for the obesity-related chronic diseases discussed in Chapter 1 and improves your mood. You can start, after getting your surgeon's approval, with light exercise, such as slow walking or water aerobics. Then progress as you are comfortable. In the chapter, you can find recommendations for amount and types of exercise and ways to fit it in when you're short on time. Of course, sticking to an exercise program is even harder than starting one – and there are tons of tips in the chapter so that you are able to stick to your program – and enjoy it! Chapter 16 talks about:

- Why exercise is good for your weight and health
- Recommended amounts of exercise
- How a complete beginner can safely and gradually start a physical activity program when you still have a lot of weight to lose
- How to make your program more advanced as you progress
- How to stick to your exercise program for the long term

Chapter 17: What to Expect in the First Year after VSG

The changes during the first year can be overwhelming – unless you're prepared for them! Chapter 17 gives you a nice overview of the changes to expect – keeping in mind, of course, that each individual's gastric sleeve experience is slightly different. During the first year on the sleeve diet, you can expect significant weight loss and changes in your body. You'll probably feel better about yourself and notice that others treat you differently as you lose weight. This chapter helps you recognize symptoms of sleeve complications so you know whether to call your surgeon. Chapter 17 also provides tips on staying motivated. Cosmetic surgery to remove extra skin is something that you may want to consider as you lose weight, and the chapter outlines the most common options.

Chapter 18: Build a Strong Support System

The last chapter discussed some of the changes to expect after your vertical sleeve gastrectomy. With so many changes, you'll need a lot of support. Chapter 18 helps you build a fail-proof support system. This chapter will talk about the sources of support that may be available to you. These include:

- Yourself
- Your family and friends
- Members of your medical team
- Other bariatric surgery patients from your support group meetings and online communities.

Chapter 19: Online Support and BariatricPal.com

There's always more to learn. You can read "The Big Book on the Gastric Sleeve: Everything You Need to Lose Weight and Live Well with the Vertical Sleeve Gastrectomy," call your surgeon and talk to all of the members of your support groups, and you'll never know every detail about the gastric sleeve that you'll be wondering about eventually. That's where online resources come in; there's a nearly infinite array of sites that can answer your questions.

BariatricPal.com is an online community with more than 100,000 members, many of whom have been in your shoes and can provide advice from personal experience. Members are encouraging, too, so you can feel comfortable there. Membership is free and features include regular newsletters, a profile page with space for your photos and a blog, a surgeon directory with member ratings and reviews and a live chat room.

Ready to get started? Read on…

1

Obesity—A
Costly Epidemic

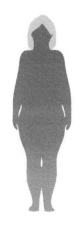

You can choose not to be obese.

Do you want to hear that again?

You can choose not to be obese.

For many reasons, you may not think that obesity is your choice. You've been struggling with your weight for years, and possibly for your whole life. You have tried every diet on the planet; none has worked for more than a few weeks or months. You have health problems or worry about developing them. The whole nation and people all over the western world are getting fatter. Everything seems stacked against you, and this thought might cross your mind often.

"What's the point? Why even bother to try?"

But you can't fool us, and you can't fool yourself. Deep down, you still have a glimmer of hope. We know you're still fighting to be healthy because you're reading this book. Is the vertical sleeve gastrectomy weight loss surgery the right choice for you? It could very well be. Thousands of patients worldwide have had the vertical sleeve gastrectomy, which is a relatively new and increasingly popular procedure. Many of them can tell you that it changed their lives and can change yours.

But let's start at the beginning—*obesity*. This chapter will cover the following topics:

- The obesity epidemic in the U.S.
- Harmful effects of obesity
- Causes of obesity in society.
- Your own causes of obesity.
- Your motivation for losing weight.
- Defining obesity with the BMI.

Obesity: Truly an Epidemic

The dictionary defines an "epidemic" as a disease "affecting a disproportionately large number of individuals within a population."[1] Based on this definition, obesity is an epidemic in the United States and many countries around the world.

An Epidemic Is a Disease

Obesity is a disease because it makes us sick. As this chapter will explain, obesity causes chronic illnesses, such as type 2 diabetes and heart disease. It can lead to painful conditions, such as osteoarthritis, and mental illness, such as depression. After tobacco use, obesity is the second leading underlying cause of death in the U.S.

An Epidemic Is Widespread

The Centers for Disease Control and Prevention report that more than one out of every three American adults is obese.[2] Another third of the adult population is overweight, which means that they are at risk for becoming obese. This leaves less than one-third of the entire American adult population at a "normal" weight. In fact, obesity is so widespread in the U.S. that there are more obese people than so-called "normal-weight" people!

Obesity isn't just an American problem. More than 500 million people worldwide are obese; 1.4 billion are overweight or obese.[3] In fact, the World Health Organization lists obesity and overweight as one of the top risk factors for death in the world.[4]

Economic Costs of Obesity

Obesity is expensive. Even worse, the costs of obesity are growing as fast as the rates of obesity. In 1998, less than 20% of adults in the U.S. were obese; that year, total medical costs related to obesity were $78.5 billion in medical costs.[5] By 2008, the rate of obesity was significantly higher; more than one-third of Americans were obese. Medical costs related to obesity were $147 billion.[6] And in 2010, medical costs hit $190 billion.

Medicare and Medicaid Pay Some of the Cost of Obesity

Medicare and Medicaid pay about half of the medical costs caused by obesity. Medicare is the health insurance program for adults over age 65, people with disabilities, people with end-stage renal disease (or chronic kidney failure) and people with a low income who may not be able to afford another health insurance plan or health care. It is run by the national government. Medicaid is the health insurance program for low-income adults and children and individuals with disabilities. It is a federal program that is run slightly differently in each state.

Medicare is funded by the U.S. federal government, and Medicaid is funded by both the federal government and by individual state governments. Because about half of obesity-related medical costs are paid for by Medicare and Medicaid, everyone's tax dollars are paying for nearly $100 billion per year of the medical costs of obesity. To put it another way, the total costs of these healthcare insurance programs for the needy would be 10% less if obesity did not exist.

Who Else Pays for Obesity?

If Medicare and Medicaid pay for about half of the nation's obesity bill, who covers the rest? The payers are individuals, such as you, and private healthcare insurance companies. Compared to an employee who is at a healthy weight, someone who is mildly obese (we'll get to the exact definitions in a minute) can cost an employer-sponsored insurance plan about an extra $1,850 per year. A more obese individual can cost a healthcare coverage plan about $3,086 extra per year, while a very obese person can cost an extra $5,530 per year compared to someone who is not obese.

Why Is Obesity So Expensive?

You may be wondering why we keep talking about the "medical" costs of obesity. What other costs are there? Health economists divide the costs of obesity into two main categories:

medical and non-medical.

More than 20%, or one out of every five dollars, spent on health care in the United States is spent on treatment for a medical problem that is caused by obesity. In addition, there are non-medical costs associated with obesity. The non-medical costs are more difficult to calculate than medical costs, but they make obesity an even more expensive disease.

Medical Costs of Obesity

Medical costs, or direct medical costs, are easy to visualize. These costs are what you or your insurance company pay when you or your dependent needs medical treatment because of a health problem caused by obesity. Just to give you an idea, here are a few examples of possible medical costs from obesity.

- Blood sugar testing supplies to monitor type 2 diabetes that was caused by obesity
- Extra visits to a primary care physician to monitor changes in weight and vital signs, such as blood pressure or blood cholesterol levels
- Visits to medical specialists that are required due to any obesity-related health situation, each of which can cost hundreds of dollars before even counting the cost of tests and medical equipment. You might need:
  - Endocrinologists to monitor hormones if you have diabetes
  - Pulmonologists, or lung doctors, if you have trouble breathing
  - Sleep doctors if you have sleep apnea

Non-Medical Costs of Obesity

You may not think of the non-medical costs when you think about obesity, but these costs are substantial. They come from work-related problems and from a variety of unexpected sources.

Obesity mainly hurts the economy because of lower overall productivity at work. Absenteeism, or days missed from work, is a huge problem related to obesity. A man who is obese takes 5.9 sick days per year more than a non-obese man, and an average obese woman takes 9.4 extra sick days per year compared to a healthy-weight woman. Absenteeism from obesity really hurts companies and the economy at the local, state, and national levels; on average, it costs $1,000 to $1,200 per obese person per year.

Even while at work, obese individuals may not be as productive. You yourself may be familiar with feeling tired and having more trouble getting through the day. You're lazy or avoiding effort. More likely, obesity makes you tired by interfering with your sleep and reducing your daytime energy levels.

Obesity has additional costs that aren't from medical costs. We said that the non-medical costs of obesity weren't that easy to list, and we weren't joking. One unexpected cost is the cost of fuel. Gas mileage goes down and costs $4 billion extra per year because of obese drivers and passengers. Airplane passengers pay $5 billion extra per year in additional fuel because the heavier weights of the average passenger.[7] On the ground, 39 million gallons of additional gasoline are required annually for each extra pound that the average driver weighs.[8] Even more tragic is that obese individuals are less likely to buckle up, making accidents more devastating. You yourself might regularly skip the seatbelt because it's too small for you.

Additional prices of obesity come from making society somewhat more accommodating for obese people, although if you're obese, you'll probably testify that the system isn't perfect! Some costs of obesity that you might not have thought about are the costs of making "bariatric chairs" or "bariatric toilets" available in public places at a cost of more than $1,000 each.

Obesity Is on the Rise

The rate of obesity was relatively constant for many years, but it has sharply increased in recent decades. The rate of obesity worldwide has more than doubled since 1980.[9] The same is true in the U.S.; 15% of American adults were obese in 1980, while 34% of adults were obese by 2007-2008.[10]

The number of states with high obesity rates is increasing each year, too. The National Center for Health Statistics (NCHS) is part of the Centers for Disease Control and Prevention (CDC). This agency is responsible for keeping records of the nation's health. The NCHS monitors the number of people who are obese each year.

We can summarize this information in *Table 1* so that you can easily see the relationship between obesity rates and medical costs. As Americans become more obese, medical costs also increase.

Year	% of Americans Who Were Obese	Number of States With Obesity Greater Than 30%	Annual Medical Costs Related to Obesity
1998	20%	0	$78.5 billion
2008	33.9%	6	$147 billion
2010	34%	13	$190 billion

Table 1: Relationship between obesity rates and medical costs

Health Effects of Obesity

Let's go back to the first part of the definition of an "epidemic:" It's a disease. In the U.S., obesity is the second leading cause of death after tobacco. Obesity causes more than 300,000 deaths per year in the U.S. alone.[11] The life expectancy of severely obese individuals is more than 10 years less than that of non-obese individuals.

Obesity increases your risk for each of the following conditions that are described. You may already have them, or your doctor may have told you that you are at high risk for them. These diseases and conditions are so numerous that they may seem like a laundry list of diseases and conditions. The problem is that each one of them is real, and one or more of them can impact your life or already is a factor in your life.

Are These Diseases Really Preventable?

The following diseases and conditions are so common and so harmful that it may be hard to believe that they're mostly preventable, and that if you are obese, you can greatly reduce your risk of developing these diseases by losing excess body weight. Plus, if you are obese and you already have these conditions, losing weight can help you reverse some of these conditions, and reduce your risk of complications from others.

BariatricPal.com is a friendly community that is full of real-life examples of people who have gotten healthier by losing weight after having a vertical sleeve gastrectomy. You might want to check out the discussion forums to learn about other people's experiences and ask your own questions.

Type 2 Diabetes

Diabetes mellitus, or diabetes, is the seventh leading cause of death in the U.S., and the underlying cause of many deaths due to other diseases. In 2010, more than 20 million Americans knew that they had diabetes, and another five million were likely living with undiagnosed diabetes, according to the Centers for Disease Control and Prevention.[12] More than 90 percent of people with diabetes have type 2 diabetes. The most stunning part about these facts is that type 2 diabetes is related to obesity.[13]

What Is Diabetes Mellitus?

Diabetes occurs when your body can't control your blood sugar, or blood glucose. If you have diabetes, your blood sugar levels are higher than they should be most of the time. A high-carbohydrate or high-calorie meal can make your blood glucose levels go even higher. High blood sugar is called "hyperglycemia," or, literally, "high blood sugar." People with diabetes have hyperglycemic most of the time, but can occasionally get "hypoglycemia," or low blood sugar. That happens when your blood glucose levels drop fast and uncontrollably. You might feel weak or even faint. This dangerous condition is called "hypoglycemia," or, literally, "low blood sugar."

Why does this happen? What changes occur when you get diabetes so that your body can no longer control your blood sugar levels?

First, let's go over what happens when you are healthy. When you eat and digest carbohydrates, enzymes in your saliva, stomach and small intestine break them down into increasingly smaller units. Eventually, these small units are released into your bloodstream as glucose, which itself is a carbohydrate.

> **Tip**
>
> For more information about types of carbohydrates, their food sources, and their role in nutrition, see Chapter 15, "The Sleeve Diet, Weight Loss and Your Health."

Most of the cells in your body use glucose for energy. They take the glucose from your blood and use it for energy, so your blood glucose levels go back to their normal, fasting state. Most of the cells in your body, including your muscle, liver and fat cells, depend on insulin to help them carry in glucose from your blood. In type 2 diabetes, you develop *insulin resistance*. This means that even when insulin is there, your cells don't really recognize it any more. Your cells are not insulin sensitive any more, and they cannot remove glucose from your blood.

This means that glucose stays in your blood, and you have hypoglycemia.

Type 1 versus Type 2 Diabetes

Have you ever wondered about the difference between type 1 and type 2 diabetes? They both consist of trouble controlling your blood sugar levels, but they have different causes. Type 1 diabetes is often described as a lack of insulin, while type 2 diabetes is often described as insulin resistance.

Type 1 diabetes has a much stronger genetic component. Your genes are predisposed, or pre-programmed, to be ready to develop type 1 diabetes. You can't do much to avoid it. Type 1 diabetes develops quickly. It usually occurs in children or adolescents when they get sick with a normal illness, such as a cold. The illness triggers their immune systems to turn against their own pancreas and destroy their insulin-producing beta cells. Without insulin, most of the cells in body can't take glucose from the blood, so blood sugar levels stay high. This type of diabetes is sometimes known as "insulin-dependent diabetes," because patients need regular insulin injections for the rest of their lives.

Type 2 diabetes develops slowly. It's often linked to weight gain or obesity. When you consistently eat extra calories – which is true when you're gaining weight – you're consistently breaking down a lot of food into sugar. This sugar goes into your blood. It's a lot to demand of your body to keep your blood sugar levels down when you are constantly placing too much sugar in your body.

At first, your body can keep up with this demand by making and secreting more insulin from your pancreas. For a while, this extra insulin is enough to let the glucose in your blood enter your cells and your blood sugar back to normal levels. This works okay for a while, but then you start to develop insulin resistance. You may have heard of this; it's just what it sounds like. Your cells are no longer very sensitive to insulin; they are resistant. That means that you need more and more insulin to get the same amount of glucose into your cells and maintain the same blood sugar levels as before.

When you need more and more insulin, you get "hyperinsulinemia," or abnormally high levels of insulin in your blood. Finally, your pancreas can no longer keep up with the high demand for insulin, and your blood sugar levels start to rise. This is a condition called prediabetes, and it can develop into diabetes as your blood sugar levels continue to rise.

Complications of High Blood Sugar Levels and Diabetes

Are high blood sugar levels really that important? YES! Glucose in your blood can stick to your blood vessels and other body cells and cause damage. High blood glucose levels can cause a lot of damage. These are some of the most common complications of uncontrolled diabetes.

- *Heart disease*: Damaged blood vessels are a sign of heart disease. When your blood vessels have glucose stuck to them, they don't function as well. This prevents healthy blood flow to the heart, and you can have a heart attack. Diabetes is also bad for your heart because it increases your risk for high cholesterol levels.

- *Chronic kidney disease*: Your kidneys act as filters for your blood so that waste products can leave your body. The small vessels and nephrons in your kidneys progressively become impaired when you have high blood glucose levels, and you may develop chronic kidney disease. This can lead to needing dialysis multiple times a week.

- *Infections*: When your circulation is slower or restricted because your blood vessels don't work well, your blood does not clear out toxins as well. You can get more infections from minor injuries. You can also get more respiratory infections, such as colds and the flu. Diabetes can weaken your immune system.

- *Peripheral neuropathy*: This condition is also caused by damaged blood vessels from diabetes. You have trouble getting your blood to your legs and feet, and may feel numbness or tingling.

- *Amputations*: The result of infections and peripheral neuropathy can be amputations. When you have an infection in your foot and can't feel it or heal it well, the infection may get so bad that you need to have an amputation. In fact, diabetes is the leading cause of amputations in the U.S.

- *Blindness*: Blood vessels in your eyes can get damaged when glucose attaches to them, so you may eventually become blind. An early symptom is blurry vision that progressively gets worse.

Diagnosing Diabetes

- *Fasting Blood Sugar:* Your doctor might use a fasting blood sugar test to diagnose diabetes. This test is standard when you go to the lab in the morning before breakfast. *Table 2* shows how the results are interpreted.

Category	Value
Normal	Less than 100 mg/dL
Impaired fasting glucose (IFT, or prediabetes)	100-125 mg/dl
Diabetes	Greater than 126 mg/dL

Table 2: Interpreting Blood Sugar Tests

- *Oral Glucose Tolerance Test:* Your doctor might also prescribe an oral glucose tolerance test, or OGTT, to diagnose type 2 diabetes. In the test, you drink a solution of 75 grams of glucose dissolved in water.[14] Because glucose is a kind of sugar, this drink is very, very sweet. To give you an idea of how sweet it is, it has 300 calories from sugar—or twice as much as the amount in a can of soda! These are the cut-off values for diagnosing type 2 diabetes from an oral glucose tolerance test.

Time With Respect to Drinking Glucose Water	Normal Value (a Higher Value Is an Indicator of Type 2 Diabetes
Fasting (before drinking)	60 to 95 mg/dl
1 hour after drinking	Less than 200 mg/dl
2 hours after drinking	Less than 140 mg/dl

Table 3: Cut-off values for diagnosing type 2 diabetes from an oral glucose tolerance test

- **A1c, or glycated hemoglobin**, is a test that your doctor has probably ordered for you if you have diabetes. The value measures how well you have controlled your blood sugar over the past three months.[15] It's expressed in terms of percent of red blood cells that have glucose attached to them because of high blood sugar levels. A normal value is less than 6%, and your goal might be less than 7% if you have diabetes. Higher values are more likely to lead to complications of diabetes.

Heart Disease — Heart disease, or cardiovascular disease, is the leading cause of death in the U.S. The 'term heart disease' actually includes several different diseases.

- *Atherosclerosis* is a hardening of the arteries because of the buildup of plaque. It can prevent you from getting enough blood to your arms, legs, heart, or brain.
- *Congestive heart failure* happens when your heart is too weak to pump enough blood around your body, so you may be tired and out of breath all the time.
- *Coronary heart disease* happens when your blood vessels narrow so that not enough blood gets to your heart.[16]

Each kind of heart disease can lead to a fatal or disabling heart attack or stroke. A heart attack is when blood flow to your body is blocked because of a blood clot or narrowed arteries. A stroke happens when the blood supply to your brain is cut off so your brain cells start to die from lack of oxygen.

Heart disease is strongly linked to obesity.

- You are much more likely to get heart disease if you are obese.
- You are more likely to get heart disease if you have type 2 diabetes, which is often caused by obesity.
- Obesity makes your heart work harder to pump blood.

Dyslipidemia, or High Cholesterol — Dyslipidemia is a major risk factor for heart disease, and obesity is a major cause. "Dyslipidemia" means abnormal levels of cholesterol and triglycerides in your blood. "Dys" means "abnormal," "lipid" refers to a kind of fat, such as cholesterol and triglycerides, and "emia" refers to your blood.

A lipid panel, or "cholesterol test," is a simple blood test that is used to measure your blood lipid levels. You probably get your lipid panel done regularly when you go for a physical at your doctor's office. These are the components of a lipid test and normal results:[17]

- Total cholesterol should be under 200 mg/dL.
- HDL cholesterol should be between 40 and 60 mg/dL, and a higher number is even better. HDL cholesterol is your "good" cholesterol because it helps clear away bad fats from your body.
- LDL cholesterol should be under 130 mg/dL. LDL cholesterol is your "bad" cholesterol because it can stick in your arteries and cause atherosclerosis from plaque build-up.
- Triglycerides should be under 150 mg/dL. Similar to LDL cholesterol, triglycerides can lead to atherosclerosis.

You have dyslipidemia if any of your values are unhealthy. Dyslipidemia is linked to obesity.

- Obesity increases total cholesterol, LDL cholesterol, and triglycerides
- Obesity lowers HDL cholesterol.[18]
- Weight gain leads to dyslipidemia.

Hypertension (High Blood Pressure) — Obesity can increase your risk for high blood pressure, or hypertension.[19] More than one-third of U.S. adults have high blood pressure, and many more have prehypertension, or above-normal blood pressure that can soon become hypertension.[20] Your blood pressure is the force of your blood against the walls of your blood vessels, which include your arteries, veins, smaller arterioles and venules, and tiny capillaries.

Most people get their blood pressure measured each time they visit the doctor. Usually, a nurse takes your blood pressure when you check in for your appointment. The nurse has you sit down and places a cuff around your forearm. He or she inflates the cuff until you feel it tighten around your arm. Then the nurse slowly releases the cuff and listens for two sounds. You get your blood pressure results in two familiar values, which might appear as 150/100.

This fraction is the systolic blood pressure number over your diastolic blood pressure. Here is what each of those really means.

- *Systolic blood pressure*: This is the higher blood pressure value of the two. It is measured when your heart is in systole. That means your heart is contracting to pump blood throughout your body, and occurs once per heart-beat.
- *Diastolic blood pressure*: This is the lower blood pressure value of the two. It is measured when your heart is in diastole, or relaxation. The blood is not being pumped

as forcefully through your blood vessels. Each period of diastole occurs when your heart relaxes in between beats. You get one systolic measure (heart contraction) per heartbeat, and one diastolic measure (heart relaxation) in between heart beats. So, if your pulse is 70, you have 70 systolic periods and 70 diastolic periods per minute.

These are the different categories for blood pressure, as defined by the National Heart, Lung and Blood Institute.[21] Your blood pressure is normal only if *both* your systolic and diastolic blood pressures are normal; that is, if your blood pressure is 120/80 or below. If even one of your values is outside of the normal range, you have prehypertension, stage 1 hypertension, or stage 2 hypertension.

Stage	Systolic		Diastolic
Normal	Less than 120	And	Less than 80
Prehypertension	120-139	Or	80-89
Stage 1 Hypertension	140-159	Or	90-99
Stage 2 Hypertension	160 or higher	Or	100 or higher

Table 4: Blood Pressure Range

Obesity can lead to some of the factors that raise blood pressure. For example, obesity can increase your risk for atherosclerosis, or narrow, more rigid blood vessels. Obesity can also increase your pulse rate. Atherosclerosis and a higher pulse rate can both increase blood pressure.

You've probably heard about the link between sodium, or salt, and high blood pressure. Your blood pressure can increase if you eat too much salt. Salt leads to water retention, so the amount of water in your blood increases and you get more force against your blood vessel walls – or higher blood pressure. Your diet might be high in sodium if you eat a lot of processed and fast foods. A single crispy chicken sandwich from a fast food restaurant can easily have over half the maximum amount of sodium you should have in a day.

Blood pressure has a well-deserved nickname as "the silent killer". You don't feel any symptoms, but it can be fatal. High blood pressure increases your risk for heart disease, which, as you know, is the leading cause of death in the U.S. Hypertension can cause strokes, the fourth leading cause of death, and kidney disease, which is the ninth leading cause of death.[22]

Arthritis — You might think of arthritis as an old person's disease that can't be prevented. It's true that arthritis is often to blame for the aching joints that many older adults suffer from, but it's also true that arthritis affects many younger people, too. In addition, many cases of arthritis have nothing to do with aging – instead, they're caused by obesity. Arthritis can lead to stiffness, swelling and pain in any of your joints, such as those of your fingers, toes, elbows, knees, and ankles.

Osteoarthritis — Osteoarthritis is the most common kind of arthritis, and 27 million Americans have it, according to the National Institute of Arthritis and Musculoskeletal and

Skin Disorders (NIAMS).[23] One way to think about osteoarthritis is wear-and-tear on your joints. These factors can cause arthritis because they're associated with wear and tear.

- Older age – because you've using your joints for a longer time
- Overuse from exercise – which is why baseball pitchers might get arthritis in their shoulders, and tennis players develop it in their elbows – you've probably heard of "tennis elbow!"
- Obesity – because your joints are supporting far more weight than they are designed to support

Gout — Gout is another kind of arthritis that can be caused by obesity, and six million Americans have it. This form of arthritis is caused by uric acid building up in your joints, especially a joint in your toe or another single joint.[24] You are more likely to develop gout if you are obese, do not exercise much, or frequently follow fad diets that are designed for fast weight loss.

You are more likely to get *osteoarthritis* and *gout* if you are obese. If you already have these conditions and are obese, losing weight can help. Why? There are a few reasons.

- The first reason is pretty simple. Extra body weight places extra stress on your joints. Whenever you walk, stand, or move, your joints have to support your extra body weight. Over time, this can break down the natural supportive cushioning in your joints and cause the pain and swelling of osteoarthritis.
- The second reason involves chronic inflammation. Arthritis is an inflammatory disease, and obese individuals have more chronic inflammation. Chronic inflammation is different from acute inflammation, which is your body's normal, healthy response to an injury. An example of acute inflammation is when you get a swollen finger as your body tries to heal itself after you jam it into a wall. Chronic inflammation is a risk factor for many chronic diseases, including heart disease and diabetes, as well as arthritis. Losing weight can lower your levels of chronic inflammation help prevent or treat osteoarthritis.
- The third reason why losing weight can reduce joint pain is that gout is caused by too much uric acid. Your body produces uric acid as a normal part of metabolism when you break down and rebuild your healthy tissues, such as muscles, bones, and fat. When you have a lot of body tissue, which happens when you are overweight, your body produces more uric acid because of a higher amount of metabolism. This causes uric acid to build up in your joints.

Obstructive Sleep Apnea — When you have obstructive sleep apnea, you stop breathing for seconds or even minutes while you are sleeping. Usually, you stop each episode by snorting or coughing yourself awake. The cycle can repeat itself five to 30 times per hour throughout the night. As you can imagine, you never get a good night's sleep or feel rested when you wake up in the morning. Sleep apnea makes you tired nearly constantly during the day so you have no energy and can't focus. Another problem with sleep apnea is that it increases your risk of having a heart attack or stroke. Even scarier, you could die in your sleep when you stop breathing.

More than half of the people with sleep apnea are overweight, according to the National Heart, Lung and Blood Institute.[25] Larger throat muscles from being obese block the airways in your throat as you sleep. If you have sleep apnea, your doctor may have told you to use a continuous positive airway pressure, or CPAP, machine overnight to keep your airways open.

Sleep apnea is not just an effect of obesity. It can also contribute to obesity as part of a vicious cycle. You are more likely to gain weight when you have sleep apnea, and being overweight makes your sleep apnea worse. Losing weight can cure sleep apnea so you don't have to worry about having a heart attack during the night or using your CPAP machine anymore.

Psychological Disorders — *Clinical depression* is more likely in obese individuals. You may feel helpless about your weight and carry that helplessness over to other parts of your life. Other symptoms of depression include:

- Feeling tired
- Not being able to unable to care much about anything
- Not wanting to talk to people
- Feeling unable to or unwilling to get up and face the day

Social stigmatization is another of the unfortunate consequences of obesity. You've probably run across more than one person who judges you based on your weight. Many unpleasant people automatically decide that you are stupid or lazy simply because they don't like the way you look. They may do this intentionally or subconsciously, without realizing it, but it hurts you either way.

Poor body image and *low self-esteem* are other common effects of obesity, according to the National Institutes of Health.[26] Even though you are a wonderful person with so many unique and valuable qualities, you yourself may not even realize it. All you see are your faults. These feelings of low self-worth can make you binge eat or eat emotionally when you are alone.

Obesity and Quality of Life

It's no fun being the fat kid, the jolly uncle, or the social outcast. Obesity doesn't just make your physical health worse. Obesity lowers your quality of life in ways that can't be diagnosed by your doctor. Obesity can make your life flat-out miserable. Maybe it has made your own life miserable for years.

Obesity has effects that you have to deal with every single day. Recent years or your whole life may be a collection of memories of embarrassing moments. Maybe each day is devoted to your attempts to avoid reminders that you are obese. You may spend your time pretending that you don't want to participate in fun things with your friends and family or making up excuses for why you can't make it to a business meeting. But what are your real reasons for avoiding these occasions? You know that you won't be able to fit into the movie theater seats, that you can't wear a nice dress to the party or that your work colleagues won't bother to take you seriously. How do you know? You know from years of experience.

An average day may consist of being the good-natured butt of jokes. These jokes cut you deeply, but you feel obligated to laugh at them because the only thing worse than being the good-natured fat friend is to be the fat social recluse. In the best case, the fat jokes come from strangers; in the worst case, they come from your friends who still haven't figured out how much they hurt.

Each day you face people who make you feel bad for being obese. Some people are "kind" enough to "ignore" your looks—they tend to hold eye contact or look anywhere but at you to avoid the appearance of staring at your body. Other people are less considerate, and even self-righteous. They make it clear that they think they are better than you and that you are obese because, somehow, you *want* to be. These are the people who are quite comfortable ordering dessert for themselves and asking you whether, "you really feel that you should be eating that bite of pasta, because, well, you don't look like you need it."

You know these and numerous other examples, so there's no point in hashing them out all over again. Let's get on to the important parts—what causes obesity, why are you obese and, most important, what are you going to do about it?

Obesity and BMI

Most of us use and hear the term "obesity" all the time, and we have a pretty good idea of what it means. It describes extra body fat that can harm your health and make you uncomfortable in your daily life. But it's important to know that there are different levels of obesity and to know where you fall along the continuum.

Calculating the BMI

Doctors measure obesity by calculating a number called your body mass index, or BMI. Your BMI is a ratio of your weight to the square of your height. This is the formula using pounds and inches.

$$\frac{\textbf{Weight (pounds) x 703}}{\textbf{Height (inches)}^2}$$

Don't worry if you're not a numbers person. You don't have to calculate your BMI yourself! You can take a look at the BMI table (*Table 5*) to check your BMI. Find your height in feet and inches along the left-hand side of the table. Trace that row to the right until you get to your weight. Then, trace that column upward until you see your BMI in the top row of the table.

		Normal Weight: BMI 18.5 to 24.9						Overweight: BMI 26 to 30						
	BMI →	18.5	19	20	21	22	23	24	25	26	27	28	29	30
Height														
Feet	**Inches**													
4	10	89	91	96	100	105	110	115	120	124	129	134	139	144
4	11	92	94	99	104	109	114	119	124	129	134	139	144	149
5	0	95	97	102	108	113	118	123	128	133	138	143	149	154
5	1	98	101	106	111	116	122	127	132	138	143	148	153	159
5	2	101	104	109	115	120	126	131	137	142	148	153	159	164
5	3	104	107	113	119	124	130	135	141	147	152	158	164	169
5	4	108	111	117	122	128	134	140	146	151	157	163	169	175
5	5	111	114	120	126	132	138	144	150	156	162	168	174	180
5	6	115	118	124	130	136	143	149	155	161	167	173	180	186
5	7	118	121	128	134	140	147	153	160	166	172	179	185	192
5	8	122	125	132	138	145	151	158	164	171	178	184	191	197
5	9	125	129	135	142	149	156	163	169	176	183	190	196	203
5	10	129	132	139	146	153	160	167	174	181	188	195	202	209
5	11	133	136	143	151	158	165	172	179	186	194	201	208	215
6	0	136	140	147	155	162	170	177	184	192	199	206	214	221
6	1	140	144	152	159	167	174	182	190	197	205	212	220	227
6	2	144	148	156	164	171	179	187	195	203	210	218	226	234
6	3	148	152	160	168	176	184	192	200	208	216	224	232	240
6	4	152	156	164	173	181	189	197	205	214	222	230	238	246
6	5	156	160	169	177	186	194	202	211	219	228	236	245	253
6	6	160	164	173	182	190	199	208	216	225	234	242	251	260

Obese: BMI 30 to 39.9										
BMI →		31	32	33	34	35	36	37	38	39	40
Height											
Feet	Inches										
4	10	148	153	158	163	167	172	177	182	187	191
4	11	154	158	163	168	173	178	183	188	193	198
5	0	159	164	169	174	179	184	189	195	200	205
5	1	164	169	175	180	185	191	196	201	206	212
5	2	170	175	180	186	191	197	202	208	213	219
5	3	175	181	186	192	198	203	209	215	220	226
5	4	181	186	192	198	204	210	216	221	227	233
5	5	186	192	198	204	210	216	222	228	234	240
5	6	192	198	204	211	217	223	229	235	242	248
5	7	198	204	211	217	223	230	236	243	249	255
5	8	204	210	217	224	230	237	243	250	257	263
5	9	210	217	223	230	237	244	251	257	264	271
5	10	216	223	230	237	244	251	258	265	272	279
5	11	222	229	237	244	251	258	265	272	280	287
6	0	229	236	243	251	258	265	273	280	288	295
6	1	235	243	250	258	265	273	280	288	296	303
6	2	241	249	257	265	273	280	288	296	304	312
6	3	248	256	264	272	280	288	296	304	312	320
6	4	255	263	271	279	288	296	304	312	320	329
6	5	261	270	278	287	295	304	312	320	329	337
6	6	268	277	286	294	303	312	320	329	338	346

Morbid Obese: BMI Over 40												
BMI →		41	42	43	44	45	46	47	48	49	50
Height												
Feet	Inches											
4	10	196	201	206	211	215	220	225	230	234	239
4	11	203	208	213	218	223	228	233	238	243	248
5	0	210	215	220	225	230	236	241	246	251	256
5	1	217	222	228	233	238	243	249	254	259	265
5	2	224	230	235	241	246	252	257	262	268	273
5	3	231	237	243	248	254	260	265	271	277	282
5	4	239	245	251	256	262	268	274	280	285	291
5	5	246	252	258	264	270	276	282	288	294	300
5	6	254	260	266	273	279	285	291	297	304	310
5	7	262	268	275	281	287	294	300	307	313	319
5	8	270	276	283	289	296	303	309	316	322	329
5	9	278	284	291	298	305	312	318	325	332	339
5	10	286	293	300	307	314	321	328	335	342	349
5	11	294	301	308	316	323	330	337	344	351	359
6	0	302	310	317	324	332	339	347	354	361	369
6	1	311	318	326	334	341	349	356	364	371	379
6	2	319	327	335	343	351	358	366	374	382	389
6	3	328	336	344	352	360	368	376	384	392	400
6	4	337	345	353	362	370	378	386	394	403	411
6	5	346	354	363	371	380	388	396	405	413	422
6	6	355	363	372	381	389	398	407	415	424	433

Height Feet	Inches	BMI → 51	52	52	54	55	56	57	58	59	60
4	10	244	249	254	258	263	268	273	278	282	287
4	11	253	257	262	267	272	277	282	287	292	297
5	0	261	266	271	277	282	287	292	297	302	307
5	1	270	275	281	286	291	296	302	307	312	318
5	2	279	284	290	295	301	306	312	317	323	328
5	3	288	294	299	305	311	316	322	327	333	339
5	4	297	303	309	315	320	326	332	338	344	350
5	5	307	313	319	325	331	337	343	349	355	361
5	6	316	322	328	335	341	347	353	359	366	372
5	7	326	332	338	345	351	358	364	370	377	383
5	8	335	342	349	355	362	368	375	381	388	395
5	9	345	352	359	366	372	379	386	393	400	406
5	10	355	362	369	376	383	390	397	404	411	418
5	11	366	373	380	387	394	402	409	416	423	430
6	0	376	383	391	398	406	413	420	428	435	442
6	1	387	394	402	409	417	425	432	440	447	455
6	2	397	405	413	421	428	436	444	452	460	467
6	3	408	416	424	432	440	448	456	464	472	480
6	4	419	427	435	444	452	460	468	477	485	493
6	5	430	439	447	455	464	472	481	489	498	506
6	6	441	450	459	467	476	485	493	502	511	519

Height		BMI → 61	62	63	64	65	66	67	68	69	70
Feet	Inches										
4	10	292	297	301	306	311	316	321	325	330	335
4	11	302	307	312	317	322	327	332	337	342	347
5	0	312	317	323	328	333	338	343	348	353	358
5	1	323	328	333	339	344	349	355	360	365	371
5	2	334	339	344	350	355	361	366	372	377	383
5	3	344	350	356	361	367	373	378	384	390	395
5	4	355	361	367	373	379	385	390	396	402	408
5	5	367	373	379	385	391	397	403	409	415	421
5	6	378	384	390	397	403	409	415	421	428	434
5	7	390	396	402	409	415	421	428	434	441	447
5	8	401	408	414	421	428	434	441	447	454	460
5	9	413	420	427	433	440	447	454	461	467	474
5	10	425	432	439	446	453	460	467	474	481	488
5	11	437	445	452	459	466	473	480	488	495	502
6	0	450	457	465	472	479	487	494	501	509	516
6	1	462	470	478	485	493	500	508	515	523	531
6	2	475	483	491	499	506	514	522	530	537	545
6	3	488	496	504	512	520	528	536	544	552	560
6	4	501	509	518	526	534	542	550	559	567	575
6	5	514	523	531	540	548	557	565	574	582	590
6	6	528	537	545	554	563	571	580	588	597	606

Table 5: BMI Table

Another way to get your BMI is with an online calculator or mobile smartphone app. The National Heart, Lung, and Blood Institute provides a calculator and app for free. Just enter your height and weight, and you'll see your BMI: *http://www.nhlbisupport.com/bmi/*.

What is your BMI?

Interpreting BMI: Normal Weight, Overweight and Obesity

So now, what does the number mean? The BMI divisions are as follows:

- ≤ 18.5 Underweight
- 18.5–24.9: Normal Weight
- 25–29.9: Overweight
- 30-39.9: Obesity
- ≥ 40: Morbid Obesity
- ≥: Superobesity

For most people, the healthiest BMI is between 18.5 and 24.9. Looking at the BMI table, this means that a woman who is 5'1" (five feet and one inch) tall is healthiest at a weight between about 100 and 132 pounds, while a 5'9" man is healthiest between 128 and 169 pounds. In our example, the woman would be overweight between 132 and of158 pounds, and the man is overweight between 169 and 209 pounds. You are at a slight risk for obesity-related health problems when you're overweight. Being in the overweight BMI category also puts you at risk for becoming obese.

The examples provide practice in using the BMI table more easily to avoid confusion. Continuing with our example, the woman is obese between 158 and 211 pounds and morbidly obese above 211 pounds. The man is obese above 209 pounds, and morbidly obese above 270 pounds. Most people with morbid obesity have significant risk factors for health problems that can lead to diseases and disabilities if they haven't already.

Ways to Use BMI

We're spending so much time on BMI because it will continue to come up throughout the book and your weight loss journey. These are a few of the ways that you'll use it.

- BMI helps determine eligibility for the vertical gastric sleeve or another weight loss surgery. We'll go over this in just a moment.
- BMI helps you set healthy long-term weight loss goals. It doesn't make sense for a short person and tall person to both say they want to end up at the same weight. BMI helps each person set goals that are realistic and can help you live a longer and healthier life.
- BMI helps you measure your weight loss progress. As you lose weight, you'll probably want to keep yourself motivated by seeing how your weight loss compares to other sleeve patients' progress at the same post-surgery time-points. Again, it doesn't make sense for you to compare your own weight loss in pounds to someone else's weight loss if they're taller or shorter than you.
- If you're a supporter of a gastric sleeve patient, the BMI helps you understand what your loved one is going through. You can use BMI to put yourself in their shoes to realize their starting weight and how well they are doing throughout their journey. Because you may be seeing some pretty dramatic changes in their appearance, the BMI helps you think clearly about the healthy changes they are making.

Superobesity: The Upper Levels of BMI

Extreme obesity, or super obesity, can be defined as having a BMI of 50 or greater. This BMI puts you at higher risk for obesity-related diseases than obese individuals with a lower BMI. Bariatric surgery, or weight loss surgery, is becoming more common as a treatment for extreme obesity. When it's done on the right patients, weight loss surgery can lower the risk of death and severe health problems related to obesity.[27]

The vertical sleeve gastrectomy is one option for bariatric surgery. It seems to be lower-risk for extremely obese patients than some of the other kinds of weight loss surgery. It's a pretty new technique, but so far surgeons are generally reporting positive results. The remaining chapters of this book focus on weight loss surgery and particularly on the VSG.

What Causes Obesity?

Even before reading this, you knew that for one reason or another, obesity is bad. Everybody knows that at some level. For each of us, it may be embarrassing, uncomfortable, debilitating, or life-threatening. We know that we should not become obese, and if we are, we know we should lose weight. And we even know the secret to weight loss—eat less and exercise more.

But of course losing weight isn't so simple. If it were, we would do it—and even better, nobody would have gotten obese in the first place.

So what happened?

Calorie or Energy Balance

First, let's review the basics of weight gain. It's all about calorie balance, or energy balance. This is the balance between the calories you eat and the calories you burn, or expend. You gain weight if you eat too many calories and don't burn enough calories, and you lose weight if you take in fewer calories and burn more. You gain a pound if you eat an extra 3,500 calories, and you lose a pound if you burn off an extra 3,500 calories.

Normal Regulation of Energy Balance

Humans are pretty smart. Our brains are wired monitor our food intake and energy balance. When we need energy, we feel hungry and know that it's time to eat. When we've eaten the right amount of food, we feel full and know that it's time to stop eating. Then we get hungry again at the next snack or meal time. Our brains even encourage us to move – that's why you feel a little more alert and energetic during the day when you've been moving around for a while compared to in the early morning, when you first wake up after lying still for hours.

Energy balance, or calorie balance, is a pretty simple concept. Plus, our own physiology is designed to keep us in balance. The system has worked for thousands of

> **Tip**
>
> In Chapter 16, "Getting and Staying in Shape with Exercise," we'll go over some reasons why you might think you don't like exercise...and how you can learn to love it. We'll also talk about starting an exercise program at any weight and staying safe while exercising.

Calorie Expenditure: How You Burn Calories

Your calorie expenditure is the amount of calories you burn. It comes from:

- Your basal metabolism
- Your physical activity
- The thermic effect of food

Your basal metabolic rate, or BMR, is also called your metabolic rate or metabolism for short. It's the number of calories you burn in a day without doing much of anything. You are always using some energy to stay alive. Your body needs to breathe, pump blood, maintain acid-base balance and send signals throughout your nervous system. Your BMR is higher if you are a male, if you are a young adult compared to an older adult and if you are taller. It can be about 1,000 to 2,500 calories per day, so the range is pretty big. You can use an online calculator to estimate your BMR fairly accurately.

An obese person has a slightly higher BMR than a normal-weight person of the same gender, height and age, but not much higher. That's because fat tissue doesn't do much compared to muscle. Fat doesn't have high energy, or calorie, requirements.

Physical activity is another name for exercise. It includes your "purposeful activity," or movements that you make that are extra and beyond your normal movements. A few examples of physical activity are walking, dancing, gardening, playing sports, and swimming. Physical activity is the most variable component of the calories you burn. You can burn hundreds of extra calories per day if you are very active, but you will burn almost no calories from physical activity if you are sedentary, or sit around a lot. You can really affect your weight loss by increasing your physical activity.

Many obese people say that they don't like to exercise, and this can turn into a vicious cycle. Maybe you don't like to exercise because you're obese and movement feels difficult, awkward, painful, or embarrassing. When you don't exercise, gaining weight is even more of a threat because you're not burning very many calories each day.

years, but it's not working now. You can tell that it's not working because obesity rates have doubled in the past few decades. Now, one-third of American adults are obese, and 42 percent are expected to be obese by the year 2030.

Dealing With Obesity

What has gone wrong in the course of only a few short decades? Our genes haven't changed much; it takes thousands or millions of years for the gene pool to change. What *has* changed is our lifestyle. These are some of the reasons why we overeat and don't exercise enough – leading to obesity.

Food Is Everywhere

Food used to be something you'd eat at meals. Meals used to be occasions when you'd sit down at the table and eat home-cooked food. Now, Americans eat meals and snacks not only at the table, but also while driving, working, studying, and socializing. Food is everywhere, and a lot of it isn't home-cooked or healthy. In fact, Americans now spend nearly half of their food dollars outside the home, compared to one-third in 1970.[28]

Fast food is available on every corner, and you don't even have to get out of your car to get it if you go to drive-through restaurants. Convenience stores and gas stations sell high-calorie snacks, and vending machines with high-sugar and high-fat snacks and high-calorie drinks are everywhere. They're in schools, workplaces and even places that are supposed to be healthy, such as hospitals and fitness centers. Parties, meetings, and family gatherings tend to revolve around food, and saying "no" is considered rude. Avoiding food is nearly impossible no matter how hard you try.

Processed Foods Are Less Filling

Throughout history, humans ate fruits, vegetables, nuts, whole grains, and meats. These are unprocessed foods that tend to make you full before you eat too many calories from them. That's because they're high in fiber and protein. These foods fill you up fast and keep you feeling full for longer after a meal so you don't want to eat again too soon.

Today, we eat less fresh food and more processed foods. Food processing has led to the sad fact that in recent years, we've eaten more refined grains, added sugars, saturated fats than before. It's very easy to gain weight when you eat refined pasta, prepared foods such as burgers and pizza, sweets, such as cake and ice cream, and fried foods, such as French fries and doughnuts. You can eat tons of calories from these foods without even realizing it because they're high in calories but not very filling.

Portions Are Bigger

You tend to eat more when you're served a bigger portion. That means you'll take in more calories and be more likely to gain weight – without even realizing that you ate more![29] Portion sizes have increased drastically within the past several years, just as obesity rates have increased.

Eating less fresh food and more restaurant food doesn't just lead to lower nutrient intake. It's also linked to larger portion sizes and overeating. Most restaurants serve about twice what you really should be eating – or often even more than double.[30] Sadly enough, the first reaction, when the food comes, is rarely based on how good or bad it looks. Our first reaction is usually based on the serving size. We're pleased when we get a heaping plate of food, and disappointed when the meal is smaller than expected.

We've been trained to think that "bigger" means "better." This dangerous mentality has carried over to irresistibly cheap value meals with high-calorie beverages, appetizers, sides, and desserts that we absolutely do not need. And, of course, there's the famous "all-you-can-eat," which can easily turn into a sort of frantic frenzy to make sure it's worth the money – at the cost of your weight, health, and dignity Source[31]

Calorie Expenditure: How You Burn Calories

Portion Distortion: Soft Drinks

Soft drinks and pasta both provide great examples of portion distortion.

Sugar-Sweetened (Non-Diet) Soft Drinks

An official serving of a beverage is eight ounces, or one cup. This has 100 calories and about 7 teaspoons of sugar. A can of cola, which seems miniscule by today's standards, contains 150 calories and 10 teaspoons of sugar.

A "single-serving" bottle of soda, as you might get in a vending machine, officially has 2.5 servings – but let's be serious. Nobody saves a bottle of a soft drink from a vending machine for 2.5 days; you drink it in a few hours, and get 250 calories and 16 teaspoons of sugar.

Then we get to the real villains. There's the 32-ounce fountain drink, which theoretically counts as four servings and has 400 calories and 27 teaspoons of sugar. The amount of calories you can get from soft drinks is literally unlimited – because many places allow unlimited refills.

If you drink an extra bottle of soda each day, you will gain one pound every two weeks, or 26 pounds per year.

Pasta

An official serving size of pasta is one ounce of dry pasta, which makes about ½ cup of cooked pasta and has 100 calories. You can have it with ½ cup of tomato sauce, 1 cup of vegetables and 3 ounces of grilled chicken for 300 calories.

When you order pasta in a restaurant, you're more likely to get six ounces of pasta. Along with a generous portion of high-fat meatball sauce and parmesan cheese, the total for this meal is over 1,000 calories before talking about sides such as breadsticks.

Food Can Be Addictive

Junk food is literally addictive. Eating sugar and other unhealthy foods can cause changes in your hormones and brain chemistry that make you crave more junk food. When you get addicted, the part of your brain begging you to eat more is louder than the part of your brain telling you that you've had enougwwh calories. The more we get, the more we want.

Fast food is especially addictive because it is high in sugar and fat; it tastes good, and is comforting. [32] Plus,

Tip

See Chapter 16, "Getting and Staying in Shape with Exercise," for ideas on small changes that increase your calorie burn, making time for physical activity, and fun ways to exercise in any climate or neighborhood.

reminders to eat it are everywhere on the streets and in advertising. It's a physical addiction that causes withdrawal symptoms. You may get the jitters or feel anxious when you *don't* get your usual fix.

Another aspect of an addition to fast food is a psychological dependence on it. Food is always on your mind. You may be hungry all of the time or be looking forward to your evening fix of brownies, ice cream or pizza—whatever high-fat, high-sugar food satisfies that craving. Another symptom of psychological dependence on junk food is emotional eating, whether it's to reduce stress, cheer you up, numb your feelings, or even celebrate a happy event.

Too Much Sitting

Humans are built to move—after all, our ancestors were hunters and gatherers. But we don't move much anymore. Most of us lead a sedentary lifestyle, with hours of sitting every day and not many calories burned from physical activity. We have cars, remote controls, elevators, and online shopping portals. We go to the grocery store or a restaurant instead of running after our meat, gathering berries, or farming the land.

Not Enough Exercise

Exercise isn't built into our daily lives the way it used to be when people hunted or farmed. For most of us, exercise is something that we have to set aside time to do, and it's so difficult with a busy schedule. Sometimes it seems there's no fun exercise to do, or something else gets in the way so exercise gets pushed aside.

Take a moment or two, if you haven't already, to think about your own reasons for being obese. Do you live in a neighborhood with more opportunities to buy fast food meals instead of fruits and vegetables? Do you always clean your plate, no matter how much is on it, because your mother told you about starving children in Africa? Do you always order- and eat- the value menu because it's cheap and convenient? Do you eat hundreds of extra calories at night because you're bored or lonely, or maybe simply because it tastes good? Write down your reasons at the worksheet at the end of this chapter.

Obesity and You: The "I in Epidemic"

Yes, obesity is an epidemic. Yes, a lot of things are stacked up against you because our environment is obesogenic – it encourages you to become obese by eating too much and not getting enough exercise. But despite this, you have responsibility for yourself. Your body is your own, and it's time for you to take control.

And you can. No matter how many times you've tried before, you can still try again and make this time a success.

In this section, you'll identify some of your own personal reasons for wanting to lose weight so that you can be motivated and ready to put in the dedication that you'll need if you're going to succeed with the sleeve.

What's Your Personal Reason?

So far, most of the information in this chapter isn't entirely new to you. You could probably already recite the obesity statistics by heart before even picking up this book; if not, you probably at least knew the patterns. You already knew about calories, healthy eating, exercising, and too much fast food. You could probably already point to a few things in your life that could change and help you lose weight.

But those aren't what brought you to this book. You're not here to save a million lives, and you're not here because you're an angry taxpayer protesting the annual cost of obesity in this country. You're not here to learn about why there's a hamburger restaurant on every corner or how the average American lifestyle is different now than hundreds of years ago.

You're here for you, so what is *your own* reason for wanting to lose weight? You're not just concerned about the millions of obese patients, the list of obesity-related diseases, and national health care costs. You're concerned about yourself, as you should be. Think about your own, personal reasons for losing weight. Everyone has a few. Some of the common ones are:

- You want to live long enough to see your son get married or your granddaughter graduate from high school.
- You don't want to live with diabetes, like your mother did, and die as young as she did.
- You want to be able to go clothes shopping with your friends—and buy things in the same stores they do.
- You want to fit into your car without moving the seat back and removing the seat-back cushion and squashing your stomach against the steering wheel.
- You want to be able to order in a restaurant without hearing, even if nobody says it out loud, "should you really be eating that?"

Take some time to go over your reasons for losing weight. Write them down on the form at the end of this chapter, and keep your list handy. The only way you'll ever be successful is if you're motivated so that when the going gets tough, you'll be able to remind yourself why you're trying so hard and what the prize will be.

Sometimes, you have a bunch of reasons for wanting to lose weight, but one particular incident, what I call the "Ah-Ha! Moment," is the final straw. It's what pushes you to go from yo-yo dieting and thinking about a lifestyle change to making the final decision that *I will lose weight.*

These are a few stories of Ah-Ha! Moments that we've heard:

- "I just wanted to look normal so that I could walk down the street and look into store windows without people staring or looking away."
- "One day I realized that my obesity was making me take up two seats on the bus so that older people didn't even have a place to sit."

- "The day we found out our first child was a boy; I had images of playing catch and hitting fly balls outdoors with my son in a few years. Then I realized my obesity wouldn't let me be active, and I might not even be around to see him play ball."
- "I looked in the mirror and saw my mother. At age 45, I looked just like she did at age 45. She was obese like me, and she died of diabetes five years later. I didn't want to die, so I knew I had to do something. The gastric sleeve worked for me."

It's Time for You to Take Control

Maybe you've put on a brave face every day for years because that's all you know how to do, because you're resigned to being obese, because diets haven't worked for you. Maybe you've never told anyone or even admitted to yourself how miserable you really are because… well, why? Because you're afraid of what will happen? Because you don't know what to do about it? It's time to get going.

You're Worth It

One of the barriers to losing weight is…yourself. If you're not careful, you may fall into the trap of being your own worst enemy. You may feel sorry for yourself, or you might feel as though you don't deserve to succeed in weight loss. Or you might just feel like giving up because it seems as though you've tried and failed at every possible weight loss attempt.

No More Excuses

These are just excuses. The truth is that you deserve happiness, health, and a healthy weight. Living a healthy life will take time and effort, and you are worth it. And you can have it. Everyone can find a weight loss method that works for them. Your method may not be the same as your neighbor's, but in the end, you can both achieve the results you want by following the best method for you.

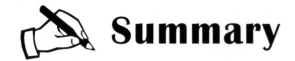

Summary

This chapter provided an introduction to obesity. If you couldn't before, now you can name specific reasons why obesity is such a problem. It's expensive; it increases the risk of many chronic diseases, and it kills hundreds of thousands of Americans each year. The personal costs of obesity have probably been plaguing you for years, not only in the form of health problems, but also in your daily life. Your obesity may make you ashamed, interfere with work or other activities that you want to do, or cause people to treat you with disrespect.

This chapter covered a lot of reasons why so many Americans are obese. Many of them, such as too many fast food restaurants and lack of physical activity in daily life, are out of your control. Still, you can take charge of your weight as long as you find and follow a method that is right for you.

If you are wondering what that method is, then move to the next chapter to find out. The next chapter will explore different approaches to weight loss and describe the different options for weight loss surgery. Maybe the vertical sleeve gastrectomy is the right choice for you.

Your Turn: Set Your Goal and Name Your Reasons

Write your current weight here. ....

Using the BMI tables in the chapter or a BMI calculator, find out what weight you would need to be at to have a BMI of 25, which is a normal-weight BMI. You'll need to know your height for this. Your weight at a BMI of 25 is your goal weight. Write your goal weight here. ....

Subtract your goal weight from your current weight. ....

…That's the amount of weight you need to lose to get to your goal weight.

Now, write down the reasons you want to hit your goal weight. Examples include having better health, being able to be more energetic around your kids, being more comfortable in your daily life and fitting into your dream outfit. ....

Finally, write down a personal, secret reason to lose weight. It's a reason that you've never told anyone, and maybe have never let yourself think about too much. It could be something such as showing up your mother who put you on a diet when you were 10 years old because she thought you were chubby. ....

1 Epidemic. Merriam-Webster. Web site. http://www.merriam-webster.com/dictionary/epidemic. Accessed November 9, 2012.

2 Centers for Disease Control and Prevention: Overweight and Obesity http://www.cdc.gov/obesity/index.html. Updated 2012, November 6. Accessed November 9, 2012.

3 Obesity and Overweight. Fact Sheet No. 311. World Health Organization. Web site. http://www.who.int/mediacentre/factsheets/fs311/en/index.html. 2012, May. Accessed November 9, 2012.

4 Global Health Risks. World Health Organization. http://www.who.int/healthinfo/global_burden_disease/global_health_risks/en/index.html. 2009, December. Accessed November 9, 2012.

5 Finkelstein E, Trogdon JG, Cohen JW, Dietz W. Annual medical spending attributable to obesity: payer-and service-specific estimates. Health Affairs. 2009;28(5):w822-w831.

6 Reuters. Study: obesity adds $190 billion in health costs. MSNBC. Web site. http://today.msnbc.msn.com/id/47211549/ns/today-today_health/t/study-obesity-adds-billion-health-costs. 2012. Accessed June 15, 2012.

7 Reuters. Study: obesity adds $190 billion in health costs. MSNBC. Web site. http://today.msnbc.msn.com/id/47211549/ns/today-today_health/t/study-obesity-adds-billion-health-costs. 2012. Accessed June 15, 2012.

8 Barth L. U.S. obesity problem impacts automobile safety and fuel economy. Consumer Reports. Web site. http://news.consumerreports.org/cars/2010/08/-us-obesity-problem-impacts-automobile-safety-and-fuel-economy-.html. 2010, August 12. Accessed November 9, 2012.

9 Obesity and Overweight. Fact Sheet No. 311. World Health Organization. Web site. http://www.who.int/mediacentre/factsheets/fs311/en/index.html. 2012, May. Accessed November 9, 2012.

10 Ogden CL, Carroll MD. Prevalence of overweight, obesity and extreme obesity amon adults: United States, trends 1960-1962 through 2007-2008. NCHS E-Stat, Centers for Disease Control and Prevention. Web site. http://www.cdc.gov/nchs/data/hestat/obesity_adult_07_08/obesity_adult_07_08.htm. Updated 2011, June 6. Accessed November 9, 2012.

11 Allison DB, Fontaine KR, Manson JE, Stevens J, Vanitallie TB. Annual deaths attributable to obesity in the United States. JAMA. 1999;282(16)1530-8.

12 Diabetes data and trends. Centers for Disease Control and Prevention. http://apps.nccd.cdc.gov/DDTSTRS/default.aspx. 2010. Accessed November 9, 2012.

13 Diabetes overview. National Diabetes Information Clearinghouse. Web site. http://diabetes.niddk.nih.gov/dm/pubs/overview/. 2012, April 4. Accessed November 9, 2012.

14 Dugdale DC, Zieve D. Glucose tolerance test. Medline Plus, National Library of Medicine. Web site. http://www.nlm.nih.gov/medlineplus/ency/article/003466.htm. Updated 2012, June 2. Accessed November 11, 2012.

15 Topiwala S, Dugdale DC, Zieve D. HbA1c. Medline Plus, National Library of Medicine. Web site. http://www.nlm.nih.gov/medlineplus/ency/article/003640.htm. Updated 2012, April 29. Accessed November 11, 2012.

16 Conditions. American Heart Assocation. Web site. http://www.heart.org/HEARTORG/Conditions/Conditions_UCM_001087_SubHomePage.jsp. Accessed November 2012.

17 Dugdale DC, Zieve D. Coronary risk profile. Medline Plus. http://www.nlm.nih.gov/medlineplus/ency/article/003491.htm. Updated 2012, June 3. Accessed November 11, 2012.

18 Adult Treatment Panel III. (2001). Executive summary of the third report of the National Cholesterol Education Program (NCEP) expert panel on detection, evaluation, and treatment of high blood cholesterol in adults (Adult Treatment Panel III). National Institutes of Health. Retrieved from http://www.mayoclinic.com/health/hdl-cholesterol/CL00030/NSECTIONGROUP=2

19 High blood pressure and kidney disease. National Heart, Lung and Blood Institute. Web site. http://kidney.niddk.nih.gov/kudiseases/pubs/highblood/. Updated 2010, September 2. Accessed November 11, 2012.

20 High blood pressure. Centers for Disease Control and Prevention. Web site. http://www.cdc.gov/bloodpressure/. Updated 2012, September 6. Accessed November 11, 2012.

21 What is high blood pressure? National Heart, Lung and Blood Institute. Web site http://www.nhlbi.nih.gov/health/health-topics/topics/hbp/. 2012, July 12. Accessed November 11, 2012.

22 Leading causes of death, 2009. FastStats, Centers for Disease Control and Prevention. Web site. http://www.cdc.gov/nchs/fastats/lcod.htm. Updated 2012, October 19. Accessed November 11, 2012.

23 Handout on health: osteoarthritis. National Institute of Arthritis and Musculoskeletal and Skin Diseases, National Institutes of Health. Web site. http://www.niams.nih.gov/Health_Info/Osteoarthritis/default.asp. 2010. Accessed November 11, 2012.

24 Questions and answers about gout. National Institute of Arthritis and Musculoskeletal and Skin Diseases, National Institutes of Health. Web site. http://www.niams.nih.gov/Health_Info/Gout/default.asp. 2010. Accessed November 11, 2012.

25 What is Sleep Apnea? National Heart, Lung and Blood Institute. Web site. http://www.nhlbi.nih.gov/health/health-topics/topics/sleepapnea/. 2012, July 10. Accessed November 11, 2012.

26 Obesity Education Initiative. Clinical guidelines on the identification, evaluation and treatment of overweight and obesity in adults: the evidence report. National Heart, Lung and Blood Institute, National Institutes of Health. NIH No. 98-4083.1998.

27 Christou NV, Sampalis JS, Liberman M, Look D, Auger S, McLean APH, MacLean LD. Surgery decreases ong-term mortality, morbidity and health care use in morbidly obese patients. Ann Surg. 2004;240(3):416-424.

28 Young LR, Nestle M. The contribution of expanding portion sizes to US obesity epidemic. Am J Public Health. 2002;92(2):246-249.

29 Diliberti N, Bordi PL, Conklin MT, Roe LS, Rolls BJ. Increased portion size eads to increased energy intake in a restaurant meal. Obes Res. 2004;12(3):562-8.

30 Condrasky M, Ledikwe JH, Flood JE, Rolls BJ. Chefs' opinions of portion sizes. Obesity (Silver Spring). 2007;15(8):2086-2094.

31 Condrasky M, Ledikwe JH, Flood JE, Rolls BJ. Chefs' opinions of portion sizes. Obesity (Silver Spring). 2007;15(8):2086-2094.

32 Garber, A.K., & Lustig, R.H. Is fast food addictive? Current Drug Abuse Reviews. 2011; 4(3):146-62.

2
Weight Loss Options

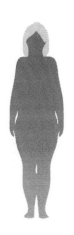

Why is losing weight so difficult? The science behind losing weight is simple. You just have to create a calorie deficit, which means eating fewer calories than you use. It really is that simple, so why is it so difficult to lose weight? This chapter will explain why losing weight is such a challenge. To do that, we'll go over each of the possible options for weight loss, how they work, and their potential benefits and problems.

These are the options:

- *Diet:* You can change your diet so that you're eating fewer calories.
- *Exercise:* You can be more active so that you're burning more calories.
- *Weight loss drugs:* These may decrease your appetite so that you eat fewer calories, speed up your metabolism so that you burn more calories, or interfere with digestion so that you do not absorb all of the calories from your food.
- *Weight Loss Surgery*: This is a weight loss tool that has helped hundreds of thousands of very obese people lose weight, and it may be able to help you. There are many different types of weight loss surgery. This chapter will explain the most common options, and then the rest of the book will focus on the vertical sleeve gastrectomy.

By the end of the chapter, you'll have a good idea of your options for losing weight, and you'll be able to think carefully about whether you might be a good candidate for weight loss surgery and the gastric sleeve.

The Truth Behind Diets

We're willing to bet that you've tried countless diets that haven't worked for you. That's why you're considering weight loss surgery. You're not alone. More than 95 percent of diets fail eventually.[1] They may help you lose a little bit of weight or even get you to your goal weight, but they don't help you keep the weight off.

Common Types of Diets

There are many, many approaches to dieting, and you may have tried many of them. Each weight loss diet restricts calories in some way. That's true for any weight loss diet that helps you lose body fat. We're not talking about crash diets that help you lose 10 pounds in a couple of days. When you lose weight that fast, you're just losing water weight and maybe some lean muscle, but not much body fat.

Table 6 shows just a few of the common approaches to dieting, how they help you cut calories, and their pros and cons.

Approach	How Calories are Reduced	Benefits	Disadvantages
Calorie Counting Diets	You count your calories and stay within your daily limit. A "regular" low-calorie diet has at least 1,200 calories per day, and some medically supervised very low-calorie diets have even fewer.	• It's straightforward, and it makes sense: calories in versus calories out. • You don't have to cut out specific foods or food groups as long as you stay within your calorie limits.	• It's a hassle. You have to add up each calorie that you eat. • You don't always know the number of calories in a food.
Prepackaged Meals (e.g., Nutrisystem and Jenny Craig)2	Portion control: you only eat the meals and snacks that are delivered in your weekly shipment, plus a few approved snacks throughout the day.	• You don't have to cook fancy meals. • You don't have to measure portions from multi-serving packages or from large recipes. • You get to "eat the whole bag" because each bag (or carton) has only one serving.	• It's expensive. • You don't necessarily learn the skills you need to select your own healthy foods and proper portions. • You can get tired of the options.
Low-Carbohydrate Diets and Sugar-Free Diets	You cut out nearly all carbohydrates, which are sources of calories. If you normally eat potatoes, pasta, bread, desserts, fruit, beans and cereal, a low-carb diet is almost certain to reduce your total calorie intake, even though you're eating meat, cheese, and nuts. A variation of a low-carbohydrate diet is a diet without added sugars or refined grains, so you avoid pasta, desserts, and white bread.	• They can keep you from being tempted by trouble foods if you're one of those people who can't stop at one serving. • They can be easier to follow because the emphasis on food types rather than portions. • They discourage some unhealthy refined foods, such as sweets.	• They can cause nutrient deficits. • They can be high in saturated fat from meat and cheese. • They discourage some healthy carbohydrates, such as whole grains, beans, and fruit. • They can get boring and cause you to quit. • You're likely to regain the weight when you go off the diet.
Low-Fat Diets	This is a traditional diet approach. Fat has more calories per gram than protein and carbohydrates, so cutting out fat helps you cut out a lot of calories.	• It encourages fruits, vegetables, whole grains, beans, fat-free dairy products, and lean proteins. • It leaves you with a wide variety of options. • It discourages fatty junk food, such as fried foods, pizza, doughnuts, and hamburgers.	• Low-fat, high-carbohydrate diets can be bad for your blood sugar and cholesterol. • It can be boring and unsatisfying. • It doesn't distinguish between healthy and unhealthy carbohydrates and fats.

Approach	How Calories are Reduced	Benefits	Disadvantages
Single Food-Focused Diets	These unhealthy diets help you lose weight because you cut out most types of foods. Examples include cookie diets, which might include a few cookies plus a single daily meal, the grapefruit diet, which consists of large quantities of grapefruit to fill you up, and the cabbage diet, which has you eating low-calorie cabbage and vegetable soup with some beef or chicken.	• They're simple. • You don't have to count.	• It's not nutritious. • It can be dangerous. • You won't lose weight in the long-term.
Meal Replacement Diets	These diets are similar to food-focused diets. You might have a diet bar or shake to replace two or even three of your regular meals.	• It's convenient and easy. You don't have to cook. • They can satisfy your sweet tooth if you like standard chocolate-flavored bars and shakes.	• They're boring. • They're made up of highly processed foods. • You don't get to learn portion control or healthy eating habits. • You may be hungry from eating bars instead of meals.

Table 6: Common approaches to dieting, how they help you lose weight, and some of their benefits and limitations.

Why Don't Diets Work?

Some people are able to lose weight and keep it off with diet, but most people aren't. If you're reading this book, you probably didn't have much success with diets. Why hasn't dieting worked for you? These are a few common reasons why diets fail, and you may recognize them as part of your own story.

They're Temporary -- You follow the diet to the letter, achieve your goal weight, and then "go off your diet." Guess what? As soon as you start to go back to your "regular" eating habits, you go back to your "regular" weight. A successful eating plan for maintaining a

> **Tip**
>
> See Chapter 15, "The Sleeve Diet, Weight Loss and Your Health," for meal planning help and information on characteristics of healthy diets to control your calories and meet your nutritional needs.

healthy weight needs to be a lifestyle change, not a short-term program. Success with the vertical sleeve depends on eating well for life.

You Feel Deprived and Quit -- A lot of diets forbid your favorite foods, but you still want them. You might break your low-carbohydrate diet because you crave pasta, go off a low-sugar diet because you love apple pie, go off a prepared meals diet because you have friends over for dinner or break a low-fat diet because you want a piece of pizza. Or you may want to go out to eat with friends at a restaurant, but you can't find anything that's allowed on your diet. Eventually, you may go off your diet because the benefits don't seem worth the cost.

The All or Nothing Trap -- Some people have an all-or-nothing approach. They feel that giving in to a single French fry makes the day and the diet a failure, and therefore it's pointless to continue. These people might reason that as long as they had a forbidden fry, they might as well have the whole order…and a cheeseburger and milkshake, too.

You're Still Hungry -- You might not be doing well at diets because they don't fill you up. You might eat the right amount of calories to lose weight or maintain your weight, but you're still hungry, so you eat some more. This is actually more likely to happen in obese people than in normal-weight people. The brains of skinny people might get the "stop eating" signals from their stomachs fast. You might not be so lucky, so your brain doesn't know to "stop eating" until you've eaten more calories than you really need. Bariatric surgery can make you feel full faster, and the vertical sleeve gastrectomy might reduce your overall hunger levels.

Diets are great in theory, but they don't seem to work in practice. There are a number of reasons why diets don't work for most people, and you may have faced all of them. There's still hope, though, and failing at a diet or many diets — does *not* make you a failure or condemn you to lifelong obesity.

Why Exercise on Its Own Isn't Effective

What about exercise? Like dieting, exercising is another approach to weight loss that seems foolproof—and is, in theory but not in practice.

How it Works: Theory behind Exercising to Lose Weight

You can look at tables or use calculators to estimate the calories you can burn per hour of physical activity. Someone who weighs 240 pounds can burn 305 calories per hour walking at a speed of two miles per hour, and you can increase that to nearly 470 calories in an hour by walking at three and a half miles an hour. All you would have to do to lose one to two pounds per week is walk an hour in the morning and an hour in the evening.

Some of these numbers seem pretty impressive, right? They are, until reality hits. It's almost impossible to lose weight just by exercising. These are some of the reasons why.

It's Hard to Burn a Lot of Calories with Exercise

The calories you burn from exercise might be a lot lower than you'd expected. You may find that you're not physically able to walk as fast as you're hoping for, or for as long. Even if you can, you may not enjoy it or might not have time for it, which means you probably won't be doing it every day. You might start off expecting to burn 1,000 calories a day, for a weight loss of two pounds per week, by walking briskly for two hours per day. You might find out that you're only able to manage one hour of slow walking on five days each week—or about the amount of exercise to lose half a pound per week.

Bad Food Choices Usually Outweigh Exercise

It's tough to burn enough calories to balance out bad food choices. The calories that you can burn during physical activity are not that high compared to calories you can eat within minutes. This table can give you an idea of how much you'd have to exercise to burn off the calories from certain food choices — and that's just to *balance* them out, not to *lose weight*!

Table 7: Is It Worth It? Take a look at these foods, their calorie counts, and the amount you'd have to exercise to burn off these foods. The bottom line is that you need to exercise a lot to burn off the calories from these foods.

To Balance	You'd have to burn	A 200-pound person can burn the calories by:
Small beef burrito	420 calories	Playing tennis for an hour.
Slice of large pepperoni pizza	300 calories	Biking moderately for an hour.
1 buffalo wing with 1 ounce dipping sauce	270 calories	Walking for an hour.
1 large chocolate chip cookie	210 calories	Playing tennis for 30 minutes.
1 large slice triple chocolate cheesecake	830 calories	Jogging for an hour.

Table 7: Is It Worth It?

Sticking to an Exercise Program Is Challenging

You've probably tried an exercise program once or a thousand times before. You start out enthusiastically, but within days, weeks or even months, you start to fade. It may be because you're unmotivated because you're not seeing results. It can also be because you're bored. Obesity may make your boredom worse by limiting the variety of activities you *can* do or *want* to do. Some activities may be painful, too hard, or simply embarrassing because you feel conspicuous or awkward in your body. So exercise isn't a reliable obesity cure.

Don't get the wrong impression here. Exercise is wonderful and necessary for health. It makes your heart healthier, improves your insulin sensitivity, helps you think better, and reduces stress. But, exercise on its own is not a complete successful weight loss program.

> **Tip**
>
> Chapter 1, "Obesity – A Costly Epidemic," and type 2 diabetes. Chapter 16, "Getting and Staying in Shape with Exercise," has a discussion of the benefits of exercise, how many calories different activities can burn and how to design an exercise program.

Weight Loss Drugs—Not the Solution

Everyone wants a cure-all medication because it seems so easy…just pop a pill and watch your problems disappear. Wouldn't it be nice if a pill could "cure" obesity in the same way painkillers make your headaches and muscle cramps go away? Unfortunately, it's not that easy. Scientists have been searching for obesity drugs for years, and they haven't yet found the perfect formula.

How Weight Loss Drugs Work

As mentioned at the beginning of this chapter, there are a few different ways that weight loss drugs can work:

- *Appetite suppressants*: These drugs suppress your appetite so that you don't eat as much. They work by increasing the amount of serotonin and catecholamines in your brain. These chemicals are neurotransmitters that help you feel full and satisfied.

- *Metabolism boosters*: They can increase your metabolism, so that you burn more calories. Similar to caffeine, they may work by increasing your heart rate and breathing rate.

- *Nutrient Absorption*: They can reduce the amount of nutrients from food so that you don't absorb all of the calories that you are eating. They may grab onto the fat in your food so that you can't absorb it from your stomach or small intestine.

> **Tip**
>
> Chapter 1, Obesity – A Costly Epidemic reviews the metabolic rate, or your metabolism. Chapter 6, "Are you a Good Candidate for the Sleeve?" has guidance for navigating your insurance policy and financing weight loss surgery.

Which Weight Loss Drugs Are Available?

Table 8 lists some of the weight loss drugs available that the FDA has approved to be marketed as weight loss drugs.[3]

Drug	How it Works	FDA Approval	Side Effects
Orlistat	Decrease nutrient absorption (blocks fat)	Approved for use up to 1 year in adults and children over age 12 years; Xenical is prescription; Alli is over-the-counter (OTC)	Need to restrict dietary fat intake to avoid severe diarrhea; may lead to vitamin and mineral deficiencies; cramping
Phentermine ("fen-fen")	Appetite suppressant	Approved for use up to 12 weeks in adults; OTC	Raises blood pressure and heart rate; nervousness; insomnia
Diethylpropion (Tenuate)	Appetite suppressant	Approved for use up to 12 weeks in adults; OTC	Raises blood pressure and heart rate
Lorcaserin (Lorqess) (prescription)	Appetite suppressant	Approved for use up to one year; prescription	May cause birth defects
Qsymia (formerly known as Qnexa) (phentermine and topiramate)	Appetite suppressant	Approved as prescription drug by FDA in July of 2012[4]	Increased pulse and blood pressure, dizziness, constipation, birth defects, dry mouth

Drug	How it Works	FDA Approval	Side Effects
Phendimetrazine	Appetite suppressant	Approved for use up to 12 weeks in adults; OTC	Nervousness and insomnia
Belviq (lorcaserin hydrochloride)	Appetite suppressant	Approved in June 2012 as prescription drug[5]	Headaches, nausea, dizziness, heart complications

Table 8: FDA Approved Weight Loss Drugs

There are a few other drugs available that may help you lose weight, but the FDA has not yet approved them to be labeled as weight loss drugs. The FDA does not believe that there is enough evidence to prove that they are effective. *Table 9* provides some examples of medications that may help you lose weight.

Drug (Generic Name)	Main (FDA-approved) Purpose	Side Effects
Topiramate	Prevent seizures	Numbness, changes in taste
Metformin	Diabetes: control blood sugar	Dry mouth, metallic taste, nausea, weakness
Zonisamide	Prevent seizures	Fatigue, nausea, headache, dry mouth, dizziness
Bupropion	Depression treatment	Dry mouth, sleeplessness

Table 9: Examples of medications that may help you lose weight (not FDA approved)

This is how the weight loss drug market currently stands. Weight loss drugs aren't likely to provide a long-term solution to your obesity.

- There aren't many options.
- They can cause side effects and complications.
- Their results aren't that impressive if you have a lot of weight to lose. You can expect to lose about 10 to 15 pounds in 12 weeks, or about three months, if you take weight loss drugs and follow the recommended diet.
- Weight loss might not last. The limit for using many of these drugs is 12 weeks to a year, and you probably won't hit your goal weight during that time. After that, your hunger will increase and your metabolism will decrease back to their pre-drug levels.

Consider Weight Loss Surgery

Diets nearly always fail; physical activity alone isn't enough to get you to your goal weight, and a safe and effective weight loss medication doesn't yet exist. Many people have found weight loss surgery, also called bariatric surgery, to be the only option for losing significant amounts of weight and, even more important, keeping it off.

Myths and Realities of Weight Loss Surgery

Most people don't know much about weight loss surgery. Maybe you don't know much about it either, or you didn't until you started considering it. *Table 10* identifies some common myths surrounding weight loss surgery and explains the truth about each.

Myth	Reality
All weight loss surgery is the same.	There are many different kinds of weight loss surgery, as you'll see in the next section. There's roux-en-Y gastric bypass, duodenal switch, adjustable laparoscopic gastric banding, and vertical sleeve gastroplasty, just to name a few.
Bariatric surgery is a complicated and unusual medical procedure.	Hundreds of thousands of bariatric surgeries are performed each year. Surgery usually takes 1 to 2 hours. Many weight loss surgery patients leave the hospital within days, and patients return to work within weeks. Many surgeries now are laparoscopic, or minimally invasive, with a few small incisions.
You will only be interacting with your surgeon.	Your entire medical team is important. In addition to your surgeon, your weight loss surgery team includes a dietitian, nurses, and mental health professionals. You'll work closely with your team before and after your surgery.
Bariatric surgery is the easy way out for lazy people.	Losing weight is hard work, whether or not you have weight loss surgery. Most surgeons only accept patients who have tried many diets and have been unable to keep the weight off. The surgery is a tool to help you eat less, but it only does part of the work. You do the rest.
You'll never eat normal food again.	Within days after surgery, you transition to solid foods. Eventually, most patients can eat any kind of food. Some patients may need to avoid sugary foods if they cause diarrhea. The key is to limit your portion sizes.
Weight loss surgery causes long-term health complications.	Serious complications from bariatric surgery performed in a reputable clinic are very rare, although they can happen. Some kinds of bariatric surgery can lead to nutrient deficiencies. You may need to take dietary supplements.
Weight loss surgery is a quick option for losing weight.	Successful weight loss with bariatric surgery is a lifetime commitment. You'll need to follow the healthy diet that your dietitian recommends. It may take years to achieve your goal weight, and you should follow your new diet for life.
No insurance plans cover weight loss surgery.	Some insurance plans cover all or part of weight loss surgery if you meet certain criteria and approach your surgery and financial payments as required by your plan.

Table 10: Weight loss surgery-Myths Vs. Reality

How Does Weight Loss Surgery Work?

There are two main ways that a weight loss surgery can help you lose weight: restriction and malabsorption.[6] In addition, some bariatric surgeries reduce your hunger.

Restrictive Weight Loss Surgery

All bariatric surgeries include restrictive components to limit your food intake. The way they work is by making your stomach smaller. Your stomach is like a food storage container. When it fills up at the end of the meal, it sends signals to your brain that you are full. When your stomach is smaller as the result of a restrictive weight loss procedure, it fills up faster and sends the signal to your brain. You feel full sooner, before you have eaten as much food as you would have eaten before surgery.

Examples of restrictive weight loss surgeries include:

- Vertical banded gastroplasty (VBG)
- Vertical sleeve gastrectomy (VSG), laparoscopic sleeve gastrectomy (LSG), or gastric sleeve. This book focuses on the sleeve.
- Sleeve plication, or laparoscopic greater curvature plication
- Roux-en-Y gastric bypass (RYGB)
- Adjustable gastric banding (AGB) and laparoscopic adjustable gastric banding (LAGB).

Malabsorptive Weight Loss Surgery

Some surgeries are both restrictive and malabsorptive. Malabsorptive procedures reduce the absorption of calories and nutrients from food to help you lose weight. The surgeon alters your gastrointestinal tract to exclude part of the small intestine. The small intestine is where a lot of absorption occurs, so skipping over it lets your body absorb fewer nutrients and calories into your body.

Examples of malabsorptive weight loss surgeries include:

- Roux-en-Y gastric bypass (RYGB)
- Biliopancreatic bypass diversion (with or without duodenal switch) (BPD-DS). This surgery is a two-step process, and the VSG is the first step.

Reducing Your Hunger

Some kinds of weight loss surgery may reduce your hunger and increase your feelings of fullness. The procedures affect different hormones in your body that are involved in hunger.[7] After the surgery, some patients report less hunger and fewer cravings for high-sugar foods. The VSG is a surgery that reduces levels of at least one of your hunger hormones. Upcoming chapters will discuss that in more detail.

Learning the Facts before Deciding on Weight Loss Surgery

The number of annual surgeries in the U.S. has skyrocketed since 1990, when 16,000 patients underwent some type of weight loss surgery. By 2003, 103,000 patients had bariatric surgery; and in 2008, there were 220,000 weight loss surgeries.[8] Along with the increase in number of surgeries performed, evidence is continuously coming to light about the safety and effectiveness of weight loss surgery.

> **Tip**
>
> Chapter 1, "Obesity—A Costly Epidemic," we'll go over specific criteria for qualifying for gastric sleeve surgery in Chapter 3, "Vertical Sleeve Gastrectomy 101"

Not every obese individual is necessarily a good candidate for weight loss surgery. You need to meet certain criteria first. In most cases, you have to have a BMI of 40 or have a BMI over 35 and a health condition due to your obesity. You also need to have documentation that you've tried diets before and they haven't worked for you. Most of all, you need to be ready to make the lifestyle changes that are required for success with weight loss surgery.

You may also need to postpone your weight loss surgery or consider other options if any of these descriptions are true for you:

- You are pregnant or are planning to become pregnant within the next year.
- You have a severe medical condition that can be made worse with surgery.
- You abuse alcohol or drugs.
- You are unwilling to commit to a lifetime of careful food choices.

Open versus Laparoscopic Surgery

Two main surgery categories are laparoscopic and open. Most weight loss surgeries today are laparoscopic instead of open. You and your surgeon will decide which is best for you, so you might want to learn a little bit about each one. This section describes each of them briefly, and the rest of the book will continue to mention laparoscopic and open surgeries.

Open Surgery - is what probably comes into your mind when you think about surgery. The surgeon makes an incision, or cut, into your abdomen to get access to your stomach and the rest of your gastrointestinal tract. After finishing the bariatric procedure, the surgeon sews up the incision.

Laparoscopic Surgery is a technique that lets the surgeon make smaller incisions than in open surgery. It is classified as a minimally invasive surgical procedure. Your surgeon makes a few small incisions in your abdomen and inserts a camera (the laparoscope) and the surgery instruments. Then the surgeon uses a camera to visualize your insides and the surgical tools on a screen. The surgeon controls the thin surgical tools instruments by remote control. Laparoscopic surgery is safer and has fewer complications than open surgery. Many bariatric surgeries today are laparoscopic.

Risks of Weight Loss Surgery

Bariatric surgery patients face risks and complications from the surgical procedure and from the after-effects.

All kinds of surgery carry some risks. Weight loss surgery carries these same risks, but in general, weight loss surgery is safer than other kinds of surgery.

- *Embolism, or blood clot.* Within the days following surgery, your risk of blood clots increases and you could have a stroke or heart attack.

- *Infection.* Surgery requires one or more incisions, and you can be infected any time you have broken skin or an open wound. Furthermore, obesity increases your risk of infections. Obese patients have a 10 percent rate of infections compared to a two percent risk for normal weight patients. You can reduce your risk by choosing a doctor at a clinic that you trust and following your surgeon's instructions for keeping your incision(s) protected and clean.

> **Tip**
>
> Chapter 5, "VSG: Risks and Considerations," has tips on choosing a surgeon and clinic to reduce your risk of complications from your weight loss surgery.

- *Death.* Death is always a risk when going into surgery, but weight loss surgery is relatively safe compared to other kinds of surgery. Fewer than one in 200 patients die from weight loss surgery.

Because you can lose weight at a relatively fast rate after weight loss surgery, bariatric surgery also increases your risk for some other conditions. You have a higher risk of developing gallstones if you have weight loss surgery, and your surgeon may remove your gallbladder during your surgery. Your gallbladder helps digest fat, but it is not a necessary organ, and you can digest fat without it, too.

Some weight loss surgery patients become depressed after surgery, even when they are losing weight as expected and hoped. This may be because you have underlying issues that were not caused by your weight. It's also possible that depression is your reaction to how differently people treat you when you lose weight. The risk of depression makes it even more important for you to see a psychologist before getting approved for the surgery. Your after-care team should also be very careful to monitor you for signs of depression and get you help if you need it.

How Your Body Gets Nutrients from Food

Weight loss surgery alters your digestive tract. To understand these changes and how they can help you lose weight, it's helpful to understand normal metabolism, or how your body gets nutrients from food when you eat.

Digestion and absorption are necessary parts of metabolism because you can't just put entire foods directly into your body's cells. First, you have to *digest* food. This includes breaking it down into smaller components, such as fractions of larger fats and carbohydrates, and proteins, and releasing other nutrients, such as vitamins and minerals. Next, your body needs to *absorb* the nutrients, or get them out of the GI tract and into your body. A basic idea of how food is digested helps explain how type of weight loss surgery works. This discussion won't get too technical, so don't worry if you're not an expert in physiology and anatomy.

The gastrointestinal tract, or GI tract, is the series of tubes and compartments that food travels through as it goes from your mouth to your colon (*See Figure 1*).[9] During the passage, nutrients are absorbed into your body. The remainder of the food becomes waste and is excreted as feces and urine. This is a list of the parts of the digestive tract and a description of what happens as food passes through each one.[10]

- *Mouth*: Chewing grinds food into smaller pieces and mixes it with saliva so you don't choke when you swallow. Saliva also has a minor role in starting to break down some of the starches, or carbohydrates, in your food.

- *Esophagus:* Food enters the esophagus, or throat, when you swallow. Not much digestion happens in the esophagus; it is mainly just a tube that pushes food from mouth from your stomach.

- *Stomach:* The stomach is an expandable pouch that stores food from your meal. Hydrochloric acid in the stomach breaks food down into smaller particles. The stomach mixes your food with digestive juices to continue the digestive process. Carbohydrates and proteins are largely broken down in the stomach. The stomach slowly empties the partially digested food into your small intestine. Your stomach is very important in sending hunger and fullness signals to your brain. A full stomach tells your brain that it's time to stop eating, and an empty stomach tells your brain that you're hungry. Bariatric surgeries, such as the vertical sleeve gastrectomy, that make the stomach smaller can reduce hunger and make you feel full sooner.

- *Small intestine:* The small intestine is so important to nutrition because this is where most of your nutrients are absorbed. That means that they go from your GI tract across the wall of the small intestine, and into your bloodstream. Proteins, carbohydrates, fats, vitamins, and minerals all get absorbed from the small intestine. Food enters the small intestine at the portion called the duodenum, which is the portion closest to the stomach. The next portion of the small intestine is called the jejunum, and the last part, just before the large intestine, is the ileum.

- *Large intestine:* Most of the "food," or material, that gets to the colon consists of waste products that will be excreted. Some of the dietary fiber that you have eaten is fermented by healthy bacteria in your large intestine. Not much nutrient absorption occurs from your large intestine.

- *Rectum and anus*: Waste products leave your body as feces.

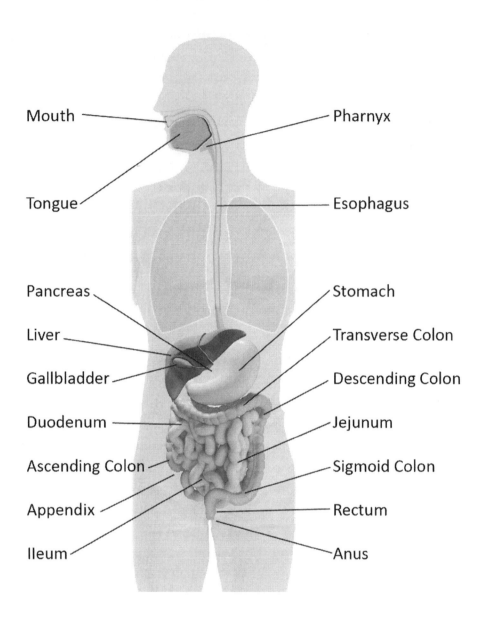

Figure 1: The Digestive System

Food enters your GI tract by entering your mouth when you eat or drink. You put food into your mouth, and it moves through your gastrointestinal tract as you absorb the nutrients and the waste is excreted through the anus.

Digestive Juices – Various organs produce digestive juices that mix with your foods and help break them down into nutrients that your body can use.

- *Stomach*: Your stomach produces stomach acid, or hydrochloric acid, which breaks down food. It also produces enzymes to help digest carbohydrates and proteins.
- *Pancreas:* Enzymes from your pancreas break down carbohydrates, proteins, and fats.
- *Liver*: Your liver secretes bile, which helps digest fat.
- *Gallbladder*: The gallbladder stores bile until you eat a meal with fat or cholesterol. Your gallbladder is not an essential organ, and sometimes it is removed during weight loss surgery to avoid the risk of getting gallstones when you lose weight fast.

Hormones Related to Digestion and Hunger – Your body produces hormones that trigger digestion and also affect your levels of hunger and fullness.

- *Ghrelin:* Ghrelin is known as the hunger hormone. This hormone is produced and released by your stomach when it is empty. Ghrelin goes to your brain and stimulates your brain to tell your body that you are hungry. Some obese individuals have higher levels of ghrelin than normal-weight people.
- *Gastrin, secretin, and CCK*: These hormones sense the presence of food, and signal your organs to produce and secrete digestive juices when you eat.
- *Peptide YY*: This hormone comes from your GI tract and tells your brain that you are full after eating.

Tip

See Chapter 1, "Obesity – A Costly Epidemic," for a discussion of the role of insulin in carbohydrate metabolism and its relationship to diabetes. Chapter 3, "Vertical Sleeve Gastrectomy 101," discusses how the VSG might affect these hormones and help you lose weight.

Types of Weight Loss Surgery (Bariatric Surgery)

As the list of myths pointed out, many people think that there's only one kind of weight loss surgery. You may have thought so too, before you started thinking about it. When you start doing some research, you quickly discover the numerous options for bariatric surgery. In fact, the number of different options can be overwhelming. This quick run-down can help clarify the major types of weight loss surgery.

The four most common in the U.S. are adjustable gastric band, roux-en-Y gastric bypass, vertical sleeve gastrectomy, and biliopancreatic diversion with duodenal switch.[11] You might also hear about the vertical banded gastroplasty, which is becoming less common, and sleeve plication, which is relatively new. So far, the sleeve plication appears to be as effective as the

Where Can I Get More Information?

Everyone can use some good advice when making a decision as important as weight loss surgery. Understanding each of the different kinds of weight loss surgery and their pros and cons can be confusing. If you're considering bariatric surgery, BariatricPal.com is an excellent resource. You can communicate with a friendly and welcoming community of vertical sleeve gastrectomy patients, experts, and surgeons.

other surgeries, but there's not much data yet. The next section summarizes these procedures and some benefits and drawbacks.

The book focuses on the vertical sleeve gastrectomy, and we'll talk about it in detail the next chapter and throughout the rest of the book. In this chapter, we'll just introduce it briefly along with the other kinds of weight loss surgery.

Vertical Banded Gastroplasty: Restrictive

Vertical banded gastroplasty, or VBG, is also known as stomach stapling. It is a restrictive type of bariatric surgery. The patient feels full sooner and is unable to eat as much food. Immediately after surgery, the stomach pouch holds only one tablespoon, or one-half ounce, of food.

This bariatric procedure dates back to 1982, when Dr. Edward Mason from the University of Iowa developed it. Laparoscopic vertical banded gastroplasty has been introduced since then, but 90 percent of vertical banded gastroplasty surgeries in the U.S. are still open surgeries, which have a higher risk of complications than laparoscopic procedures.

The surgery takes one to two hours and requires general anesthesia.[12] The laparoscopic vertical banded gastroplasty takes two to four hours. You may need to stay in the hospital for up to five days. Once inside the abdomen, the surgeon makes a cut in the stomach wall starting from a few inches below the esophagus. The surgeon staples the stomach closed so that the small usable pouch is only about 10 to 15 percent of its original size. The surgeon inserts a band, which seals off the large part of your stomach from the small pouch. The large pouch is no longer usable.

Common short-term risks within the days and weeks after vertical gastroplasty include nausea and vomiting, injury to the spleen, and an incisional hernia. You may also get dehiscence, which is when your staples are displaced or loosened so that the cut in your stomach lining is opened. Over the long term, you may experience continued nausea, heartburn, and depression. Vertical banded gastroplasty is less effective than other forms of weight loss surgery, with less than a 50 percent rate of maintaining weight loss after 10 years. Because of its dangers and poor weight loss results, the VBG is not very common any more.

Vertical Sleeve Gastrectomy: Restrictive

Vertical sleeve gastrectomy is also known as a sleeve gastrectomy, the gastric sleeve and a greater curvature gastrectomy.[13] Your stomach size is reduced to 15 percent of the original size so that it fills up faster and you feel full faster. The VSG was originally done as the first step of a two-surgery procedure known as the biliopancreatic diversion with jejunal switch bypass. When surgeons saw how effective the VSG could be, they started to do the gastric sleeve as its own weight loss surgery. It is often done laparoscopically in the U.S.

The vertical sleeve gastrectomy usually takes one to two hours. You'll be in the hospital for two to seven days. A vertical sleeve gastrectomy is similar to a vertical band gastrectomy, but instead of folding over the stomach, as in the VBG, the surgeon actually *removes* 80 to 85 percent of your stomach in the VSG. The surgeon uses the remaining portion of your stomach to make a tube-shaped sleeve that goes from the esophagus to your small intestine. Finally, the surgeon stitches closed the sleeve in your stomach and uses a sealant to prevent leaks.

After the procedure, the size of your sleeve is only 15 to 20 percent of the original size of your stomach. The sleeve gastrectomy is a restrictive procedure because small sleeve fills up quickly when you eat so that your brain realizes that you are full. It doesn't interfere much with nutrient absorption. Another way that the vertical sleeve gastrectomy works is a result of the actual removal from your body of 80 to 85 percent of your stomach. Your stomach produces a hormone called ghrelin, which sends signals to your brain to make you feel hungry. When your stomach size is reduced, the amount of ghrelin in your body is reduced, so you don't have as many hunger signals.

Along with the normal risks of surgery, specific risks of vertical sleeve gastrectomy include internal injury to your organs during surgery and leaking from the staples. If you get scarring inside your abdomen as you heal, the scar tissue can eventually block your bowel, or colon or large intestine, and cause constipation in the future. You may develop gastritis, or inflammation and pain in your stomach, ulcers and heartburn. If you eat too much food at once, you will probably end up vomiting.

Vertical sleeve gastrectomy is a relatively safe surgery, especially for very obese patients who need a two-step process instead of undergoing gastric bypass all at once. You can lose most of your excess weight within two or three years with a vertical sleeve gastrectomy, but the procedure itself may not be enough for all patients. Some individuals with a vertical sleeve gastrectomy eventually choose to have their surgeries converted into a biliopancreatic diversion with duodenal switch (BPD-DS).

The remainder of this book focuses on the gastric sleeve, and we will cover each portion of it in more detail later.

Sleeve Plication: Restrictive

Sleeve plication is also known as laparoscopic greater curvature plication or gastric imbrication. This relatively new technique is similar to vertical sleeve gastrectomy, but no part of your stomach is actually removed.[14] Instead, the part that will not be used is sutured shut. The sleeve plication is usually performed on patients with a BMI of less than 50. Your surgeon might recommend a vertical sleeve gastrectomy if your BMI is over 50.

For a laparoscopic greater curvature plication, the surgeon makes small incisions into your abdomen to place the instruments. The surgeon uses a line from below your esophagus to above your small intestine. The large pouch of your stomach is sutured, or folded in, along that line, so it can't be used anymore. The usable pouch of your stomach will be about 15 percent of its original size, and the rest of your stomach is folder over and held shut. The procedure takes two to four hours.

Some of the benefits compared to the vertical sleeve gastrectomy are a shorter hospital stay and less of a risk of nutritional deficiencies. Plus, there's no insertion of an object into your body – you don't have a ring or tube or staples in your body. This means that there's no risk of things getting loose. Some of the possible complications of sleeve plication are an inability to digest food properly and swelling of the stomach from the procedure. It may also cause gastroesophageal reflux disease, or GERD, which you may feel as heartburn. GERD increases your risk of developing esophageal cancer. Also, it's not widely used in patients with a BMI over 50.

Laparoscopic Adjustable Gastric Banding: Restrictive

Adjustable gastric banding is the least invasive type of weight loss surgery because it does not alter your body physiology. This is the only bariatric procedure that is both adjustable and reversible. The LAP-BAND® system, made by Allergan,[15] and REALIZE™ adjustable gastric band, made by Ethicon Endo-Surgery,[16] are FDA-approved medical devices for the treatment of obesity. The lap-band can be used in lower-BMI patients and has been approved for patients with a BMI as low as 35.

A typical laparoscopic adjustable gastric banding procedure takes 30 to 60 minutes, and you may go home on the same day. Some patients spend a night or more in the hospital. [17] The surgeon makes three to five cuts in your abdomen to insert the laparoscope and other instruments. The gastric band is a silicon tube that goes around the upper part of your stomach and divides it into a small upper pouch and a large lower pouch. The upper pouch is about 15 percent of the size of the original stomach and the lower pouch is 85 percent. When you eat, food goes into the upper pouch, called the stoma. The gastric band is tight enough around the stomach to keep the food from passing quickly into the lower stomach. The stoma fills up fast so you feel full soon.

The lap-band has a lower rate of complications than some other weight loss surgeries. For example, compared to roux-en-Y gastric bypass and biliopancreatic diversion with a duodenal switch (discussed below), the lap-band has less than half the rate of mild complications, such as nausea, and less than one-tenth the rate of serious complications, such as organ injuries.[18] Most lap-band patients do have some form of mild complications, such as vomiting, diarrhea, or gastroesophageal reflux.

The surgeon can adjust the band by filling it with saline solution, or salt water, to make it tighter. That makes it more restrictive. You may need it deflated to increase the size of your stomach during times when you need more nutrients, such as during pregnancy. The lap-band does not cause dumping syndrome or lead to nutrient deficiencies.

It may take three or four adjustments for the surgeon to be able to inflate the band to the exact right pressure to restrict food intake enough to help you lose weight, but not so tight that you vomit a lot. Another drawback is that the lap-band can be displaced and require another surgery to reposition or replace the band. The lap-band helps you lose weight more slowly than the other kinds of weight loss surgery. It may take you three or more years to get to your goal weight while following a strict diet. Of course, all of the weight loss surgeries require you to pay attention to your diet.

Roux-en-Y Gastric Bypass: Restrictive and Malabsorptive

Roux-en-Y surgery may be the most well-known form of the set of weight loss surgeries known as gastric bypass.[19] The surgery shrinks size of your stomach to restrict food intake and changes your digestive tract so that you absorb fewer nutrients from food. After the surgery, your stomach pouch is the size of a walnut and the bottom of your stomach is attached to the jejunum of your small intestine.

The roux-en-Y surgical procedure takes two to four hours. It can be open or laparoscopic. Similar to the restrictive procedures discussed above, the surgeon closes off most of the stomach with staples or a band, leaving just a small pouch. Then, the surgeon attaches the bottom of the small pouch to the jejunum, or middle of the small intestine, rather than to the ileum. It takes three to five weeks to fully recover from roux-en-Y and get back to your usual activities.

Right after surgery, your stomach pouch will be able to hold one to two ounces of food, or about 15 to 20 percent of your former stomach capacity. That's the restrictive part of roux-en-Y. The "gastric bypass" results from the small stomach emptying into the jejunum, therefore "bypassing" the majority of your original stomach.

The malabsorptive part of the surgery comes from the "roux-en-Y" part. The term describes the final anatomical appearance of your surgery. Your gastric pouch is called the roux limb, and the "Y" shape is formed by the three arms coming together at a junction. The three arms are:

- Your small stomach pouch that holds food
- Your large stomach pouch that secretes digestive juices
- The jejunum of your small intestine that receives food from the small pouch

Roux-en-Y can help you lose more than half to three-quarters of your excess body weight within one to two years. The surgery also helps to resolve diabetes or reduce its severity. Roux-en-Y patients have increased levels of CCK, which is one of the hormones that helps you digest food and tells your brain that you're full. Gastric bypass tends to increase the hormone peptide YY, which is another hormone that tells your brain that you're full.

The roux-en-Y reduces nutrient absorption by making food avoid your duodenum, which is where a lot of nutrient absorption usually takes place. That helps you lose weight, but it can also cause nutritional deficiencies if you do not take supplements. You will need to be monitored by a dietitian or doctor for the rest of your life to make sure you don't get anemia, osteoporosis, or vitamin deficiencies. Roux-en-Y gastric bypass can be a good choice for individuals who tend to overindulge in sweets because you can't eat them after the surgery. Eating sweets after gastric bypass can lead to dumping syndrome, with symptoms of cramping, nausea, and diarrhea, can happen if you eat sweets because the sugars do not get digested properly because your food leaves your stomach faster.

Biliopancreatic Diversion with Duodenal Switch: Restrictive and Malabsorptive

Biliopancreatic diversion with duodenal switch, or BPD-DS, has a very long name, but it's quite descriptive. This surgery is a form of gastric bypass surgery, but it's less common than roux-en-Y. In a biliopancreatic diversion with duodenal switch, your stomach pouch becomes smaller and nutrient absorption decreases because food bypasses part of the small intestine and because your digestive juices are rerouted.

This surgery is more extensive than laparoscopic roux-en-Y gastric bypass or simple restrictive weight loss surgeries. It is a two-step process, and the first step is a vertical sleeve gastrectomy. However, compared to the VSG, the portion of your stomach that is removed is smaller, and the portion that remains is bigger. The remaining stomach portion stays at about half of your original stomach size, compared to only 15 percent of the original size in the other procedures. The BPD-DS can be done in super-obese patients. The first step, the VSG, is a lower-risk procedure that lets patients lose some weight before undergoing the second surgery, the diversion and switch.

In the second surgery, your small intestine is divided into two parts. One part, the *alimentary limb*, gets connected to the bottom of your stomach. The rest of your small intestine, now called the *biliopancreatic limb*, is attached to the bile duct. Food travels down the alimentary limb into your colon without being absorbed in the biliopancreatic limb. Digestive juices are free to flow from your biliopancreatic limb to your alimentary limb. This means food is digested (broken down), but not absorbed (taken into your body). This is how the BPD-DS causes nutrient malabsorption.

The biliopancreatic diversion with duodenal switch is one of the bariatric surgeries with the most rapid weight loss in the first year or two. It's also likely to have good results for long-term weight loss and prevention of weight regain. And, this procedure is good for patients with an initial BMI of more than 55 because it works so well. The biliopancreatic diversion with duodenal switch helps to prevent dumping syndrome, or diarrhea, because of the digestive juices that come through the biliopancreatic limb and digest your food.

The biliopancreatic diversion with duodenal switch has some drawbacks, though. It may lead to chronic diarrhea. There is also a high risk of chronic malnutrition because of the reduced absorption of nutrients. An iron deficiency causes anemia, and calcium deficiency causes osteoporosis, or the increased risk of fractures, especially in your hips, back, and wrists. Dumping syndrome can occur in BPD-DS, especially if you have high-sugar foods.

Summary of Types of Weight Loss Surgery

Table 11 summarizes the different kinds of weight loss surgeries described above. It may be a handy resource to review as you read this book. It'll help you compare the sleeve to the other surgeries at a glance.

Name (and alternate names)	Description	Notes
Vertical Banded Gastroplasty (Stomach Stapling)	The surgeon divides the stomach into two parts by using staples so that you cannot eat as much. Your pouch is 10 to 15% of its original size.	This surgery can be done open or laparoscopically. It's less effective than other types of bariatric surgery. Risks include nausea, vomiting, and dehiscence, or displacement of staples.
Vertical Sleeve Gastrectomy (Gastric Reduction, Gastric Sleeve, the Sleeve)	The surgeon reduces your stomach to 15% of its original size by surgically removing the rest of your stomach.	This surgery helps reduce food intake by restricting your stomach size and reducing levels of a hunger-increasing hormone called ghrelin. The Sleeve was originally part of a two-step procedure for biliopancreatic diversion with duodenal switch gastric bypass, but has been effective on its own. It can cause bleeding and gastritis.
Sleeve Plication	Sleeve plication is similar to a vertical sleeve gastrectomy because it reduces your stomach size to about 15% of its original size. However, your stomach is sewn shut, not removed.	This relatively new type of weight loss surgery has results comparable to gastric bypass, but it is safer and has fewer side effects. Because your stomach is sutured and not removed, there is less chance of nutrient malabsorption and internal bleeding than with the gastric sleeve, but it's less well-studied.
(Laparoscopic) Adjustable Gastric Banding	The adjustable gastric band goes around the tube from your throat to your stomach. The surgeon inflates the tube with saline solution to narrow it and reduce your food intake.	Adjustable gastric banding is a restrictive procedure that doesn't cause nutrient deficiencies. This approach is the only weight loss surgery approach that is both adjustable and reversible. It is FDA-approved as an obesity treatment. It may be best choice for some lower-BMI patients.
Roux-en-Y Gastric Bypass (gastric bypass)	This surgery reduces your stomach size to about one ounce. The surgeon then connects your stomach to the jejunum of your small intestine. Roux-en-Y gastric bypass can be a laparoscopic or open procedure.	Roux-en-Y is restrictive and malabsorptive. Patients lose about 70% of excess body weight within the first year. This surgery is known for its resolution of diabetes, and it alters your hormone levels for a result of reduced hunger. It raises the risk for nutrient deficiencies.

Name (and alternate names)	Description	Notes
Biliopancreatic Diversion with Duodenal Switch Gastric Bypass	This surgery is a two-step process. The first step is the vertical sleeve gastrectomy, which reduces stomach size. The second step reroutes your digestive tract so food goes from your small stomach to your lower small intestine. The rerouting procedure also alters the effects of digestive juices, such as bile.	The approach works in three ways. It reduces stomach size (restrictive); it reduces nutrient absorption by avoiding the small intestine; and it interferes with absorption by altering bile and other digestive juices. It can lead to anemia and osteoporosis because of reduced absorption of iron and calcium.

Table 11: Summary of Types of Weight Loss Surgery

✍ Summary

This chapter introduced some of the different approaches to weight loss. We talked about why weight loss surgery may be the only realistic option for effective, long-term weight loss for you.

☞ For many people, dieting does not work because it is temporary and can lead to yo-yo diets.

☞ Exercise is healthy and a great way to support additional methods for losing weight, but you probably can't burn enough calories to lose weight very fast from exercise without other weight loss methods.

☞ Weight loss drugs seem appealing, but you may not lose weight very fast with them. Plus, many weight loss medications are only approved for short-term use, between 12 weeks and one year, and they have side effects that can be serious.

☞ Weight loss, or bariatric, surgery can be a good tool to help you lose weight. Procedures can be restrictive, to shrink the size of your stomach, and malabsorptive, to reduce the absorption of nutrients from food. Weight loss surgeries have the same risks as any surgical procedures. Additional complications depend on which surgery you choose, and may include nausea, internal bleeding, leaks and nutritional deficiencies.

Your Turn: What Have You Already Done to Try to Lose Weight?

List the diets and weight loss pills that you've tried over the years.

....

....

....

Describe your weight loss results. Include how much you typically lost, how long the diet lasted, and when you started to regain the weight.

....

....

....

Why haven't the diets worked for you? Your answer might be because you were too hungry, too bored, unmotivated to continue, or unable to afford them or take the time to prepare the right foods.

....

....

....

After reading this chapter, do you think weight loss surgery is the right choice for you? YES/NO

If you think weight loss surgery is right for you, do you understand that weight loss surgery is only a tool? YES/NO

Do you understand that your own diet decisions will determine your weight loss success after bariatric surgery? YES/NO

Finally, are you ready at this point in your life to commit to lasting weight loss and a lifestyle change that will require a lot of effort? YES/NO

If no, what is holding you back?

....

....

1   Phelan S, Hill JO, Lang W, Dibello J, Wing RR. Recovery from relapse among successful weight maintainers. American Journal of Clinical Nutrition. 2003;78(6):1079-1084.

2   This book is not affiliated with Nutrisystem or Jenny Craig, which are branded companies.

3   Weight-Control Information Network. Prescription medications for the treatment of obesity. National Institute of Diabetes and Digestive Kidney Diseases. Web site. http://win.niddk.nih.gov/publications/prescription.htm. Updated 2010, December. Retrieved December 7, 2012.

4   FDA approves weight management drug Qsymia. Food and Drug Administration. Web site. http://www.fda.gov/NewsEvents/Newsroom/PressAnnouncements/ucm312468.htm. 2012, July 17. Accessed November 14, 2012.

5   Food and Drug Administration. FDA approves Belviq to treat some overweight or obese adults. Web site. http://www.fda.gov/NewsEvents/Newsroom/PressAnnouncements/ucm309993.htm. 2012, June 27. Accessed December 7, 2012.

6   Bennet JMH, Mehta S, Rhodes M. Surgery for morbid obesity. Postgraduate Medical Journal. 2007;83(975):8-15.

7   Rao RS. Bariatric surgery and the central nervous system. Obes surg. 2012;22(6):967-78.

8   Weight-Control Information Network. Longitudinal assessment of bariatric surgery. National Institute of Diabetes and Digestive Kidney Diseases. NIH No. 04-5573. 2010. http://win.niddk.nih.gov/publications/labs.htm.

9   National Digestive Diseases Clearinghouse. Your digestive system and how it works. NIH 08-2681. http://digestive.niddk.nih.gov/ddiseases/pubs/yrdd/. 2012.

10 Truesdell D. Digestion and absorption. The Gale Group, MacMillan Reference. Healthline. Web site. http://www.healthline.com/galecontent/digestion-and-absorption. Published 2004. Accessed November 15, 2012.

11 Weight-Control Information Network. Bariatric surgery for morbid obesity. National Institute of Diabetes and Digestive Kidney Diseases. NIH Publication No. 08–4006. http://win.niddk.nih.gov/publications/gastric.htm. 2011. June. Accessed December 7, 2012.

12 Frey, R. Vertical banded gastroplasty. Healthline. Web site. http://www.healthline.com/galecontent/vertical-banded-gastroplasty. 2004. Accessed December 7, 2012.

13 Nall R. Vertical sleeve gastrectomy. Healthline. Web site. http://www.healthline.com/adamcontent/vertical-sleeve-gastrectomy#1. 2012, July 25. Accessed November 16, 2012.

14 Gebelli JP, de Gordejuela AGR, Badia AC, Medayo LS, Morton AV, Noguera CM. Laparoscopic gastric plication: a new surgery for the treatment of morbid obesity. Cirugia Espana. 2011;89(6):356-61.

15 FDA expands use of banding system for weight loss. Food and Drug Administration. Web site. http://www.fda.gov/NewsEvents/Newsroom/PressAnnouncements/ucm245617.htm. 2011, February 16. Accessed November 16, 2012.

16 Realize Band-P070009. Food and Drug Administration. Web site. http://www.fda.gov/NewsEvents/Newsroom/PressAnnouncements/ucm245617.htm. 2007, September 28. Accessed November 16, 2012.

17 Nall R. Laparoscopic adjustable banding. Healthline. Web site. Retrieved from http://www.healthline.com/adamcontent/laparoscopic-gastric-banding. 2012, July 25. Accessed November 16, 2012.

18 Parikh MS, Laker S, Weiner M, Hajiseyedjavadi O, Ren CJ. Objective comparison of complications resulting from laparoscopic adjustable banding. Journal of the American College of Surgeons. 2006;202(2):252-61.

19 Laberge M. Gastric bypass. Healthline. Website. http://www.healthline.com/galecontent/gastric-bypass. 2004. Accessed November 16, 2012.

3

Vertical Sleeve Gastrectomy 101

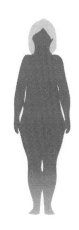

In the last chapter, we talked about why losing weight is so hard and some of the ways that you may have already tried to lose weight. You've almost certainly tried a bunch of diets and even seen some success with them – that is, you were successful for a while! Then you hit your goal weight, went off the diet, and gained the weight back, or you gave up on the diet before hitting your goal weight because the diet was too hard to follow. The story's the same with exercise and drugs. They just didn't work for you.

So where does that leave you? The chapter ended with a discussion of weight loss surgery, or bariatric surgery. Bariatric surgery may:

- Help you lose weight
- Help you keep it off
- Improve your health profile
- Be more successful in the long run than diets, exercise and/or weight loss drugs

In particular, we introduced the gastric sleeve, or vertical sleeve gastrectomy, or VSG. It's:

- An increasingly popular option for weight loss surgery
- A permanent change to your body
- A restrictive procedure designed to help you eat less
- Likely to be about as successful as other weight loss surgeries

Keep reading if you're still considering the VSG or you've already decided to get it! This chapter will tell you what you need to know about it. The chapter will answer questions such as:

- What is the sleeve?
- How was it developed?
- How does the surgery work?

By the end of the chapter, you'll have a clear picture of the sleeve. This'll take you a step closer to making a decision on whether or not you're still interested in getting the sleeve.

Learning About Vertical Sleeve Gastrectomy (VSG)

We introduced the VSG in Chapter 2, "Weight Loss Options." The concept is pretty simple. Basically, the surgeon takes out the majority of your stomach. The portion of your stomach that's left is much smaller than your original stomach. The idea is that the smaller stomach makes you feel full faster, you won't be able to eat as much, and you'll lose weight.

Source: [1]

Development of the Laparoscopic Vertical Sleeve Gastrectomy

Bariatric surgery has been around since 1954. Since then, weight loss surgery has become more common and safer, and more options are available.[2] Where did the idea of the VSG come from? How much has it progressed since the beginning? Here's a short history of the sleeve.

Gastrectomy as Step 1 of a Two-Step Bariatric Procedure

The gastrectomy was originally used as the first part of a two-step procedure called the biliopancreatic diversion with duodenal switch (BPD-DS). It's introduced in Chapter 2, and it involves removal of part of the stomach (gastrectomy) followed by resectioning and repositioning of the bile duct as well as redirecting food away from the small intestine.[3]

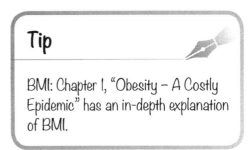

Tip

BMI: Chapter 1, "Obesity – A Costly Epidemic" has an in-depth explanation of BMI.

The BPD-DS has some benefits: it decreases nutrient absorption to help you lose weight and makes you feel full faster so you eat less.[4] But, it's a pretty long complicated surgery and is especially risky for the most morbidly obese of patients, such as those with a BMI greater than 50. For these patients, surgeons did the gastrectomy and waited a few weeks or months until the patient lost enough weight for the BPD-DS to be safer. Then the patient would undergo the second surgery, this time the actual BPD-DS.

So, until the early 1990s, the gastrectomy was mainly used as the first part of the more complicated BPD-DS.[5]

The Sleeve Gastrectomy as a Stand-Alone Surgery

But then, surgeons noticed something very interesting. Patients were doing just fine with the VSG. They were losing weight – and continuing to lose weight, even if they didn't get the BPD-DS as they had originally planned. As long as they stuck to their prescribed diet plans, patients were able to hit their weight loss goals just by having a gastrectomy – or just by having a portion of their stomachs removed.[6] That was great news! It meant that patients didn't have to undergo the BPD-DS with all of its risks.

Magenstrasse and Mill: The What?!

Actually, the terms make perfect sense if you speak German and you're a physiologist. Magenstrasse literally means, "street of the stomach," and it describes the tube that food goes through to get from the esophagus to the small intestine. In the vertical sleeve gastrectomy, the Magenstrasse is like the sleeve that is created out of the remainder of your stomach. The Mill refers to the "antral mill," which is named that way because it helps grind up bigger chunks of food.

The BPD-DS is an open procedure with all of the risks of a full surgery. And, rearranging the body's physiology with alterations in the small intestine and bile duct is a scary proposition. Any responsible surgeon or savvy patient would be thrilled at the prospect of being able to treat obesity without needing the BPD-DS. And that's exactly what they found with the VSG. The VSG is a safer procedure, especially for very morbidly obese patients, than the BPD-DS.

Bariatric Surgery without Foreign Materials

Magenstrasse and Mill: Dr. Johnston, Dr. Carmichael, Dr. Sue-Ling, and colleagues in Leeds, United Kingdom, developed the Magenstrasse and Mill gastrectomy. The goal was to have an option for effective weight loss that was simple and did not require surgeons to implant foreign materials, such as bands and reservoirs, into the body.[7] It was simpler and safer than extensive procedures such as the BPD-DS, and it helped morbidly obese patients to lose weight.[8] Many morbidly obese patients who got the Millenstrasse and Mill operation done had better insulin sensitivity, or improvements in their diabetes and blood sugar control, than before their operations.[9]

Further Developments in the Sleeve Gastrectomy: Laparoscopy and Evidence of Benefits

Early sleeve gastrectomies performed in the 1980s were open surgeries. Laparoscopic surgery techniques developed in the 1980s and the first laparoscopic weight loss surgeries were done in the U.S. in the early 1990s. In the early 2000s, the majority of BPD-DS procedures, including the preliminary VSG, were laparoscopic.[10] By now, nearly all vertical sleeve gastrectomies are done laparoscopically, so they require only a few small incisions instead of more invasive cuts into your abdomen. In fact, some laparoscopic sleeve gastrectomy, or LSG, procedures are done with one single cut to really reduce your risk of surgery complications and speed recovery time.[11]

The VSG or LSG has a fairly long history as a preparation surgery for the BPD-DS, but it's relatively new as a stand-alone surgery. Still, the amount of evidence is increasing as more and more patients get the sleeve. It's safer than more extensive techniques and has a low mortality rate. Weight loss is good, at least for the first few years, as long as patients stick to their diets. And, it looks as though high blood pressure, high blood sugar and high cholesterol levels can be drastically improved in the majority of patients.[12]

There's still a lot to learn about the sleeve. Researchers are still investigating how safe it is and how effective it is in the long-term. The Weight Control Information Network at the National Institutes of Health states that some patients who get the VSG may eventually get the BDP-DS to allow their weight loss to continue to meet their goals.[13]

Overview of the VSG Procedure

The vertical sleeve gastrectomy is, quite simply, the removal of most of your stomach. The surgeon removes 80 percent or more of your original stomach from the wider side of the "J." The remainder of your stomach gets made into a long "sleeve," or tube, which goes vertically

Laparoscopic versus Open Surgery: What's the Difference?

Open surgery is probably what you think of when you think of the sleeve or any surgery, for that matter. In open surgery, the surgeon cuts into the abdomen through the skin and tissues to gain direct access to your inner stomach cavity. The surgeon performs the surgery directly and operates the tools with his or her own hands. This is also known as a laparotomy.

Most bariatric surgeries today are laparoscopic. Laparoscopic surgery is minimally invasive because the surgeon only makes a few small cuts into your abdomen. Through these incisions, the surgeon inserts a laparoscope, or tiny camera, and some tiny tools. The surgeon can "view" the surgery site on a screen that displays images from the laparoscope, and can operate the tools using remote controls instead of directly placing his or her hands within the patient's stomach cavity.

These are some of the advantages of laparoscopic procedures compared to open procedures:

- Faster recovery time: Only a few small incisions have to heal; you don't have slow-healing injuries to your muscles as in open surgery.
- Less pain: Deeper incisions into your muscles during open surgery are more painful than surface incisions as they heal.
- Less risk of infection: open surgery requires deeper cuts and a wide open stomach cavity. It's easier to get infections during or after surgery than laparoscopic surgery, where your inner body is not exposed to the air.
- Faster procedure: laparoscopic VSG takes 30 to 60 minutes while an open procedure can take hours.
- Less time in the hospital: Laparoscopic surgery is often an outpatient procedure or may include a single night in the hospital; patients who get open VSG may be in the hospital for two or more nights.

Smaller scars: Smaller, shallower cuts in laparoscopic surgery lead to smaller, less visible scars than deeper cuts in open surgery.

Why wouldn't you go laparoscopic? In most cases you would, but sometimes your surgeon may need to perform open VSG. We'll get to those cases later.

from the esophagus to your intestine. How does that change things? Before the surgery, when you swallow food, it goes down your throat, into your stomach pouch and eventually to your small intestine. After the surgery, when you swallow food, it goes down your throat, through the sleeve and into your intestine. As you can see, the path that food takes is pretty similar before and after surgery. That means that the LSG doesn't have a major effect on nutrient absorption. One benefit of that is that you aren't likely to get dumping syndrome. The other benefit is that you're less likely to develop nutritional deficiencies.

How the VSG Helps You Lose Weight

If the sleeve doesn't change your digestion and absorption process, how does it help you lose weight? As mentioned in Chapter 2, the VSG is a restrictive procedure. That means that it limits, or restricts, the amount of food that you can eat at one time. Let's take a look at how it works.

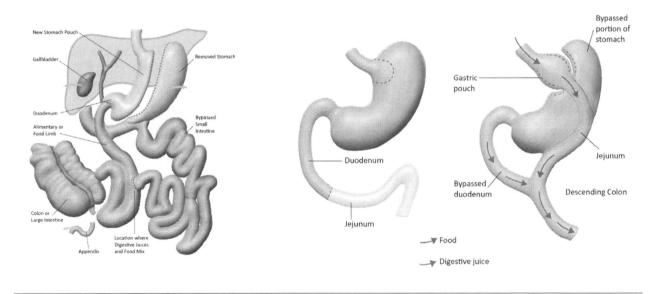

Figure 2: Illustration of the regular stomach (left) versus the sleeve.

You can see the large pouch on the right side of the J-shaped regular stomach. That's where food normally sits after you eat a meal. You don't feel full until the stomach pouch is full. With the sleeve, there's no big pouch for the food to stay. Instead, the theory is that you'll feel full when the sleeve is full – and the sleeve is only 20 percent of the size of the original stomach!

Your Stomach Size May Be Contributing to Your Obesity

This sounds pretty obvious, but it's very true. Think about the regular stomach for a moment. It's big. In fact, its volume is one or two liters—that's four to eight cups, or up to half a gallon! That means that you can eat up to a half gallon of food—*per meal*—before your stomach fills up. That's a lot of food! As an example, a cup of fried rice and a cup of mashed potatoes each have about 230 calories.[14] Eat four to eight cups, and you'll be at 960 to 1,920 calories for the meal! Eat three of those per day, and a few snacks, and you'll understand why it's so easy to gain weight! You could be at 3,000 or more calories per day, when you really only need about 2,000 (or more or less, depending on your body size and activity levels). You could potentially be eating thousands of extra calories if you eat until your stomach is full three times a day—and it only takes 3,500 extra calories to gain a pound of body fat.

Do your stomach size and how much you eat before you feel full really matter that much? Yes! In fact, on average, normal-weight individuals report feeling full when their stomachs contain only 1.1 liters. Obese participants in the same study on average did not report fullness until their stomachs contained 1.9 liters.[15]

Restriction and the VSG: Lasting Weight Loss?

If you never feel full and you think your hunger is causing your obesity, the VSG may be an option to help you lose weight. The VSG limits your stomach capacity to less than 20 percent of its original size by removing the large pouch and creating a narrow sleeve from the remainder of your stomach. The idea behind the sleeve is that the smaller your stomach is, the less you'll want to eat or be physically able to eat. That's the restrictive part of the sleeve; meals will have to be small to avoid feeling sick or having side effects.

You'll lose weight if you eat smaller meals and don't snack much in between them, and that's exactly what the sleeve does for you. It reminds you to eat less.

If you're considering the sleeve gastrectomy after many failed diet attempts, you've probably already lost and regained the same weight multiple times. You're probably wondering how the sleeve can be any different from your previous weight loss efforts. Well, the sleeve is permanent. That means that you can't "go off it" like a diet. That's a benefit if you have a long history of successfully losing weight while dieting but regaining the weight when you stop dieting. With the sleeve, you've lost your stomach and you can never get it back. For the rest of your life, you're limited to the sleeve, so it's much harder for you to overeat and regain the weight.

Hormones and the VSG: Reduction in Hunger

The sleeve may have an additional benefit for losing weight even aside from reducing your stomach capacity. It has to do with an appetite hormone called ghrelin. Ghrelin is known as the hunger hormone because high levels of ghrelin in your bloodstream make you feel hungry.[16] Ghrelin levels increase before a meal so your brain tells you that you're hungry, and ghrelin levels decrease after meals so your brain knows that you're full.

What does this have to do with the VSG? Everything! The key is that certain cells in your stomach make ghrelin and secrete it into the bloodstream. Your pancreas, intestine, and lungs also make ghrelin, but not too much. Your stomach is your body's main source of ghrelin. So what happens when you get the sleeve and 80 percent of your stomach is removed? You guessed it! You'd expect lower levels of ghrelin, and that's exactly what researchers have found

Laparoscopic and open sleeve gastrectomy decrease ghrelin levels.[17] One study found that ghrelin levels dropped by about one-third within a single day of surgery, and the effects lasted through the end of the study at six months after surgery. [18] As expected, the laparoscopic adjustable gastric band (LAGB), which does not change the patient's physiology, does not affect ghrelin levels. The roux-en-Y gastric bypass may reduce ghrelin levels slightly, but not as much as the vertical sleeve.[19]

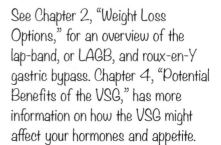

Tip

See Chapter 2, "Weight Loss Options," for an overview of the lap-band, or LAGB, and roux-en-Y gastric bypass. Chapter 4, "Potential Benefits of the VSG," has more information on how the VSG might affect your hormones and appetite.

Your Responsibilities and the VSG: Success Is up to You

Here's another reminder that the sleeve is a just tool for weight loss; it's up to you do decide whether or how to use the tool. It's your responsibility to follow the sleeve diet that you're prescribed. If you cheat on the diet, your weight loss results won't be as good and you'll have a higher risk for complications. Something else to consider is that your sleeve can stretch. It starts out at a very small fraction of your original stomach size, but it can stretch over time if you continuously eat too much. These are some general behaviors to avoid on the sleeve diet. We'll go over your diet in much more detail in Chapters 8 and 9.

- Eating too much food (high volume)
- Choosing high-calorie foods
- Eating too frequently
- Drinking with your meals or immediately before or after
- Drinking high-calorie beverages
- Eating when you're not hungry
- Continuing to eat even when you're full

The Surgery

Now you have a general picture of what the sleeve is and how it may help you lose weight. You know that it's a surgical procedure, but exactly what happens during the operation? In this section, we'll go over the surgical procedure for getting the sleeve. We'll start with the surgeon and other healthcare workers in the operating room so you know who's who.

Key Players in the Operating Room

The surgeon and a few other important figures are responsible for making sure your surgery is safe and the results are as good as possible. You'll meet the surgeon and probably each of the other team members before your surgery as they introduce themselves and explain what their roles during the vertical sleeve gastrectomy procedure.

- The *surgeon* has the lead role in your surgery. The surgeon directs the other members of the team, makes the incisions into your abdomen, controls the laparoscopic medical tools, and makes important decisions such as any changes to plans in the surgical cuts. Compared to the other members of the surgical team, you will probably work more closely with your surgeon both before and after surgery appointments.

- The *anesthesiologist* is responsible for administering the general anesthesia to put you to sleep so that you remain unconscious during VSG. Anesthesiologists are fully licensed physicians with special training. A good anesthesiologist:
  - Provides the right type and amount of anesthesia so that it's enough to help you fall asleep quickly, but not so much that you are groggy for too long after the procedure.[20]
  - Monitors your heart rate and other vital signs during surgery.
  - Monitors and helps to reduce your pain levels after surgery.

- Two *surgeon assistants* are present in the operating room to assist the surgeon.[21] Typically, one stands on each side of you as you are on your back on the operating table. The surgeon assistants help out by handing the surgeon tools as necessary, helping to inflate the abdominal cavity with gas so the surgeon has room to work, watching the screen with the images from the laparoscopic camera and alerting the surgeon if anything doesn't look right.

The Actual Vertical Sleeve Gastrectomy Procedure

You already know the basics of the VSG. Now you can learn a few details about the VSG if you're curious. If you're the queasy type who doesn't want to know the raw details of the VSG, you don't have to read this section. Instead, you can skip to the next section. All you have to know from this section is that with the sleeve gastrectomy, you lose about 80 percent of your stomach and the remainder of your stomach is fashioned into a tube, or sleeve, as described earlier in the chapter.

Laparoscopic Gastrectomy Procedure

Here is the information about the laparoscopic vertical sleeve gastrectomy for our more curious readers. You, the patient, will be lying on your back. Of course you'll be unconscious during the entire surgery, so you'll have no idea what's happening. The surgeon will make one to five incisions through or near the umbilicus (belly button).[22] Then he or she will place six ports, small devices that go under the skin.[23] During surgery, medical ports hold the skin and other tissues in place so the surgeon can easily see and access the surgery site. The six ports go in the following places: [24]

- One at the upper right of your abdomen holds your liver back away from the stomach.

- One port at your lower esophagus, slightly above the top of your stomach, allows access to the hiatus.

- Three ports are used in middle of stomach area, one toward the right, one toward the left, and one at top.

- One port at the upper left holds back the side of stomach so it does not get in the way of any cuts.

The surgeon carefully inserts the laparoscope – that's the tiny camera that'll let the surgeon visualize what's happening– through the slits in your abdomen.

The surgeon or a surgeon's assistant pumps carbon dioxide gas to inflate the peritoneum, the lining around your stomach. That's called creating a pneumoperitoneum, and it gives the surgeon space to work.[25]

What Is a Pneumoperitoneum and Why Do You Get One?

"Pneumo" means "air," and "peritoneum" refers to the lining around your abdominal cavity. "Pneumoperitoneum" happens during laparoscopic surgery when you have carbon dioxide gas pumped into your abdominal cavity. This helps inflate it so the surgeon has room to work – remember, the beauty of the laparoscopic technique is that you only have tiny incisions in your abdomen.

The pneumoperitoneum allows the laparoscopic procedure to occur so that you don't have to have a longer and riskier open surgery. However, there are a few side effects or complications that can happen as a result of having the pneumoperitoneum:

- Nausea, vomiting, and pain after the surgery, especially in your shoulders and neck

- Thromboembolism, or a blood clot that can block blood flow to a leg, arm, your heart, or brain.

- Severe headaches, until all of the extra gas has left your body.

Source[26]

Next, the surgeon cuts from the initial incision near or at the umbilical cord to the esophagus, being careful not to injure the spleen along the way. The cut continues, and the surgeon needs to work slowly to avoid injuring the pancreas. When the surgeon ends the cut, the majority of your stomach tissue can be removed permanently. At this time, you only have a flat area of stomach tissue left, so the surgeon needs to close it up so food can go from the esophagus, or throat, to the intestine.

That's when the sleeve comes in. The surgeon forms a vertical sleeve, or tube, by gently folding the sides of the remaining portion of your stomach over each other. The American Society for Metabolic and Bariatric Surgery suggests guidelines for how wide to make the sleeve.[27] A sleeve that's too narrow will increase your risk for complications, while an overly large sleeve won't be as helpful for weight loss because you'll still be able to eat a higher volume of food.

Surgical staples are used to hold the sides of the sleeve together. Staples are typically 1.5 to 2 millimeters thick because that's the average thickness of the stomach. At the suture line, or line of staples, the surgeon can place a buttress material to reduce the risk of leaks. To finish off the sleeve, the surgeon sews over the staples to protect them. The materials are bio-disposable and do not need to be removed later. The completed sleeve almost has the shape of a banana.[28]

The surgeon then completes the surgical procedure. All of the surgical tools and the laparoscopic camera are removed from your abdomen. You get your initial incisions sewn up, and your surgery is done.

A benefit of the VSG is that a high amount of your regular digestive physiology remains unchanged. For example, the surgeon does not need to cut through the stomach's sphincters, or the ring-shaped valves at the top of the stomach (the esophageal sphincter) and the bottom of the stomach (the pyloric sphincter). The sphincters constrict and relax to allow food to pass through.

Laparoscopic Sleeve Gastrectomy (LSG) versus Open Procedure

The above description is for the laparoscopic vertical sleeve gastrectomy. It takes about 30 to 90 minutes and requires about two nights in the hospital following surgery. The exact time for the surgery and the hospital stay vary by surgeon and patient. One surgeon reported that among 23 patients, LSG surgery time ranged from 80 to 220 minutes, with an average time of 120 minutes. And, these patients spent an average of seven nights in the hospital.[29] Compared to open surgery, the laparoscopic procedure is easier on your body in most ways. The incisions are smaller, and the procedure is faster. Recovery is faster, and you have a lower risk of infections during surgery.

The VSG isn't always that straightforward, though. Some patients aren't able to have the laparoscopic procedure and instead need an open surgery.[30] Your surgeon may know this before starting your surgery, or the surgeon may make the decision to convert your laparoscopic procedure into an open procedure during the surgery. Whether you get the laparoscopic or the open procedure, the basic surgical technique and outcome is the same; in either case, you will have most of your stomach removed.

When might you need an open procedure?

- If you have a weak heart or trouble with your lungs, they may not be able to tolerate the pneumoperitoneum, or carbon dioxide gas in your abdominal cavity, that is necessary for the laparoscopic procedure.[31]

- If you are at a higher BMI than some of the other patients your surgeon sees, your surgeon may have difficulty making the necessary incision(s) through your umbilical cord to properly position the laparoscope, other instruments, or medical ports.

- If your surgeon has trouble placing or manipulating the laparoscope or other laparoscopic instruments in your abdomen, you might be converted to an open procedure during surgery.

Why Is the Pneumoperitoneum a Challenge for Your Circulatory System?

During a laparoscopic procedure, surgeons pump carbon dioxide gas into your abdominal cavity to create a pneumoperitoneum and have more space to work. However, the need for this extra gas is tough on your circulatory (or cardiovascular) system, and so some VSG patients may not be good candidates for the laparoscopic procedure. Instead, they'd need the open procedure. Extra carbon dioxide is a challenge because:

- Your heart needs to beat faster to pump more blood.
- Your lungs need to breathe faster to exchange more air between your body and the outside environment.
- Your blood vessels have added stress because of difficulties with venous return, or getting blood back to your heart from your legs and other body parts.

Cholecystectomy and the Vertical Sleeve Gastrectomy

A cholecystectomy is the removal of your gallbladder. It's a procedure that's relatively common to get at the same time as you get the sleeve.[32] It's not necessarily because anything's wrong with your gallbladder. It's just to reduce your risk of developing gallstones as you lose weight quickly because gallstones are a common side effect of rapid weight loss.

Gallstones occur when bile accumulates in your gallbladder and forms hard balls like pebbles.[33] These gallstones can obstruct, or block, your bile duct, which is part of the system that allows digestive juices to get from your liver and pancreas to your stomach and small intestines. Gallstones can cause abdominal pain, diarrhea, and vomiting after you eat fatty foods.

Rapid weight loss after getting the sleeve increases your risk for developing gallstones. A successful weight loss surgery helps you lose weight much more quickly than you would with diet alone, so you're at high risk for gallstones after you get the sleeve and follow the sleeve diet. Your surgeon may discuss the risk of gallstones with you before your surgery and recommend removing your gallbladder while performing the vertical sleeve procedure.

Gallbladder removal is not a very high-risk operation. Your gallbladder can be removed during a laparoscopic or an open procedure, so it won't complicate your procedure and recovery. Also, even though your gallbladder is normally involved with digestion, you can still digest your food properly without it.

A Few More Vertical Sleeve Facts

Now you're close to being an expert on the sleeve. You know what it is and how the surgery works. It's such an important decision in your life, though, that we're adding a few more tidbits to keep in mind as you continue to think about getting the procedure.

The Sleeve Is Permanent

We've repeated this a few times already, but it's worth repeating because it's such an important point. The vertical sleeve gastrectomy is permanent. You can never get your stomach back after your surgeon cuts it out of your body and throws it away. How does this affect your decision?

- For many sleeve patients, that's fine. They're happy with their decision; they lose weight, and they keep it off for years.
- Some sleeve patients have trouble getting enough nutrients to maintain their weight after hitting their goal weight. Every case is different, but you may find that you're still losing weight because you're having trouble eating enough at your goal weight.
- Pregnancy can be tough after the sleeve because of the additional food you need to eat.

What the Sleeve Does and Doesn't Do

The sleeve isn't magic, but it is a potentially powerful tool against obesity. It is designed to help you lose a lot of weight if you avoid complications and follow your healthcare team's instructions for success. This is what the sleeve should do.

- Provide a constant reminder to limit your food intake because you may vomit if you overeat and fill up your sleeve pouch too full with food.
- Reduce the amount of ghrelin, the hunger hormone, in your body so that you feel less hungry.
- Increase your risk for vomiting, malnutrition, stomach ulcers, and bowel obstruction for the rest of your life.[34]

These are some items that the sleeve doesn't do. It does not:

- Do the work for you; you still need to follow a strict diet plan if you want to hit your weight loss goals.
- Prevent you from making poor choices, because it's up to you to choose healthy foods.
- Dramatically change your regular digestive process, so nutrients from your food still get digested as normal.

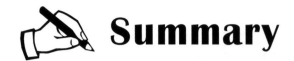 # Summary

☛ After reading this chapter, you should have clearer idea about the sleeve. It's gone from being an abstract idea that sounds promising for fighting obesity to something specific that you can picture in your head. That'll help you think carefully about whether the sleeve still sounds like the answer to your obesity. You're not quite ready to make an informed decision about the sleeve yet, though.

☛ In the next few chapters, we'll get a little more personal. We'll dig deeper into the sleeve to help you decide if it's for you. First, we'll cover the weight loss you can expect, as well as other potential benefits of the sleeve. Then, we'll also go over the sleeve's risks and side effects that can occur with this irreversible surgery.

☛ In the following chapter, we'll guide you through the eligibility criteria and some other considerations for who should get the sleeve.

☛ By the end of the next three chapters, you'll be an expert on the VSG and in an excellent position to make a decision on whether it's for you.

Your Turn: The Sleeve and You

Now that you understand what the gastric sleeve is and how the procedure goes, are you still considering this surgical procedure for weight loss? YES / NO

What did you learn in this chapter that has encouraged you to continue considering the gastric sleeve as a tool for weight loss?

....

....

....

What else do you need to know before you are ready to make your decision?

....

....

....

What are you worried about that makes you hesitant to commit to the gastric sleeve?

....

....

....

Are you ready to make the commitment to get weight loss surgery? YES / NO

Describe what makes you feel that you are mentally prepared to make the necessary lifestyle changes to succeed with bariatric surgery.

....

....

....

A Glimpse into My Life with the Sleeve...Stephanie from Texas

40 years old
Starting Weight: 254 pounds
Current Weight: 132 pounds
Height: 5'7"
Wife and friend
Likes walking and collecting recipes

Stephanie's Story of Getting the Sleeve—Rough but Worthwhile!

Okay, who am I? My name is Stephanie, but my screen name says it all.... 4ALongerLife. That's why I did this surgery.

I weighed 254 lbs in February of 2012, when I first went to see the gastric surgeon that my gynecologist recommended. My gynecologist has been my doctor for over 12 years. He birthed my son, who is now eight years old, and I trust him. So for him to have told me in December, "Girl, you are killing yourself," I knew it was time to be drastic. In the nine months of my pregnancy, my gynecologist never said a word, so I took this seriously.

I had gastric sleeve surgery in March after all the tests indicated that I was an ideal candidate. On my hospital interview form, I indicated that in my last surgery, which was my c-section to give birth my son, I had needed more anesthesia than the norm as my body wouldn't go to sleep. I believe, based on that, the bariatric anesthesiologist gave me too much medication. I don't remember waking up in the recovery room from the surgery, and I hardly woke up the first day.

I was discharged from the hospital two days later. In another two days, I was readmitted with aspiration pneumonia. I stayed in the hospital for five days. I went home and was okay, but a few days later, I was in extreme pain and had very, very shallow breathing. I could no longer sleep in the bed, so I went to a recliner, waiting for the doctor's office to open the next day. They opened at 9:00 a.m., but at 8:45 a.m. I could no longer wait and paged my bariatric doctor. I had shooting pain in my left side and couldn't breathe very deep because it hurt too much. He said go to the ER and that's when I was readmitted with a leak/abscess in my diaphragm – remember that I just got over pneumonia? I was in PAIN!

I was readmitted to the hospital for the leak a few days later and the next day I had revision surgery. The electricity had gone out the day before, and the doctors were concerned that it would happen during my surgery if we didn't wait until first thing the next morning. To say I was scared was an understatement. I made this choice to have the sleeve, but a revision was different. The doctor had to find the location of the tear, and there was a possibility that I'd have to get my tummy rerouted more like a bypass based on where the tear was. Many tears and prayers later, I was revised as a sleeve only. I stayed in the hospital for nine days...I had to have the radiologist drill a hole into my diaphragm, guided by a CAT scan in order to attach what I called an accordion drain into my left side. I had that thing in me for a few weeks, getting rid of what had leaked in my body. I had a PICC (peripherally inserted central catheter) line in the hospital. You name it, I had it. I had TPN (a feeding tube) through my nose. I now say I'm allergic to flagile, which is a strong antibiotic given through your IV that can give some people diarrhea. Imagine sneezing and dirtying yourself. Imagine sneezing every hour! Now remember you have an IV in your arm and a drain in your other side... you cannot clean yourself w/o help ... which means the nurse has to come in as well as the nurse's aid. As a 38 year old woman, I finally lost it. I wanted to be home with my family, stop dirtying myself, and get back to my job that I worried would fire me.

That's not even to mention how much I'd end up paying for my $130,000 hospital bill, since I had a maximum annual limit of $15,000 on my own contractor insurance.

But you know what? My doctor was amazing. He taught me how to fight with the insurance company. He talked to the medical director at the hospital, to the radiology unit, and to any place that I had problems with. He really was an advocate for me. His wife works with him and is a registered nurse. She does his billing, so she too helped me bunches with how to deal with insurance issues. I'm still dealing with them.

The body's a miracle of a device though...it tried to 'fix' my leak by taking the contents and isolating them into my diaphragm. It's odd how that works...but all in all, I'm good now.

Do I regret having surgery? I've had a few moments where I won't lie, I did. But overall, NO. I don't regret the surgery. Surgery is not a 'fast fix', but it's a tool to use. And I'm still learning how to use my tool, hoping for long term success.

Struggles with Weight and Family Personal Issues

Yes, I was a yo-yo dieter. I lost about 50 or 60 lbs on Weight Watchers once at about age 24, and then I think I lost probably 40 pounds the next time I tried Weight Watchers, a few years later. I don't remember how much I had put back on. A few years after that, I ballooned back, since I wasn't watching my diet, and became a workout fiend. I lost 80 lbs the hard way — I literally worked my rear off! That was in 2008. Then my mom, age 56, had a heart attack in her sleep and died. It destroyed me, but not in the way my father's treatment of me thereafter did. He was diagnosed with stage 4 cancer the February after her death, and he passed a few months later, less than a year after my mother's death. There wasn't much, but my siblings made sure they kept everything away from me.

Deciding Moments Leading to the Sleeve

During this time, I succumbed to my food addiction. I became a hermit. I still worked out daily, but ate like a fiend. That lasted until 2011, when my gynecologist gave me a good scare about my health. I was doing five to six miles a day and thought I was watching what I was eating, but I saw all of the commercials for weight loss surgery. I live in the Dallas Fort Worth region, where [former NFL player] Nate Newton is a BIG deal. Newton had the gastric sleeve, so it's a highly publicized thing here.

My gynecologist struggled with his weight for years, but a few years back he did a hormone study and it "fixed" his issues. Based on his own experience, he told me that if he had issues with food still like he's had all of his life, he would consider sleeve and get his neighbor, a bariatric doctor, to do the surgery. I trust my gynecologist and I was miserable. My siblings at least did have the decency to send me a check from my dad's life insurance, so since I hadn't used it after getting laid off from my job, my husband and I decided that we should use it to invest in my health for our long term.

My other "ah-ha" moment was seeing myself in pictures in 2011 at Disney World. We went before the surgery, as I don't have family anymore, and the holidays for me are terrible. In all honesty, I get very lonely and down at that time of the year. In 2011, I said that we were going to change that so since everyone says how wonderful Disney World is at that time of year, we splurged. When I look back at photos, I have a red shirt on and I look like the Michelin girl!

Heart disease runs in my family on the women's side. It took my mom at age 56 and my paternal grandmother at age 50. I am 38. My doctor's conversation the next month just sealed the deal so to speak.

Sources of Support outside the Family

I don't have family, so thankfully I can't tell you how they would have been about the sleeve gastrectomy. I don't talk to my siblings any longer. My husband's family has been rather supportive up until this last leak, which is when my father-in-law told my hubs I should sue my doctor. They don't understand. Heck, I get really frustrated. I get tired of defending my doctor or telling people that some people's bodies react differently to sutures. Unfortunately mine did. Why the leak now? In the good Lord's creation, I have no idea.... I just know I was hurting like crazy in my left flank and my shoulder and thought six months after surgery was too far out to have a leak. So I went to my primary care physician and got it checked out. At first my doctor thought it was osteoarthritis in my shoulder, but a pulmonologist eventually diagnosed me with a leak.

As for how my friends have reacted, well... I haven't told most of them, to be honest. I've been working from home. With all of the worries with my special diet, I just didn't get out like I used to. I told some of my son's PTA moms, and they were all okay. But that's catty PTA moms, and I'm not sure what to say about that. I didn't care what they said, but then again, I really don't care what anyone says anymore. I didn't do this for them or not do this for them. They weren't even considered and aren't going to be should I ever think for an instant that I regret this. Hindsight is always 20/20, but you know what? You can't undo the past. So why regret it? It's just a waste of energy, and I need to focus on losing my remaining weight and getting 100% healthy.

I use the discussion boards [BariatricPal.com] as a resource since I don't have friends or family to discuss this with.

A Few Regrets after Surgery

So, do I regret surgery? Sometimes, yes, I honestly do. But then again...if I get through all of this, and am one of the people in the 80% that never regain their weight, I will always be *thankful for having it. And in a way, I've said it before, it's kind of right that I got all of these complications and not someone else. Who else at my high weight of 254 pounds could do five miles? I was in better shape than most of the population that has this surgery, so...I didn't want these complications, but ...life keeps teaching me what doesn't kill you DOES make you stronger. And that's the journey that we all are on. We have to learn to let go of things that hurt us and believe that we can accomplish whatever our minds allow us to be open to. So am I a success? Hell no...but I'm working on it. And I'll get through this. I'll do my best to be positive through it, but do I worry? Yes, entirely too much. And it's a trigger for me to eat, so I'm struggling in all honesty.*

Plastic Surgery Might be in the Future

I haven't gotten plastic surgery. I don't know that I need it. Don't get me wrong, I've always dreamed of a boob job, but that was even prior to bariatric surgery. I mean hello... do you have kids? Just wait until you breast feed and gain a bunch of weight then lose it. Your body changes a lot as you age... but so far, no ma'am, I don't need it. My skin at the back of my arms and the back of my thighs/inner thighs are starting to droop a little just now. I asked my doctor, and he says that because I don't smoke and don't tan, my elasticity should come back and it'll be fine. Plus who sees these areas? And after all of the issues that I've had, no, I don't foresee undergoing anything for these two areas. Now a boob job, maybe one day, but I don't know... I like me as I am. I wish I didn't have the scars on my belly because my rear is gonna rock that bikini I just got next summer. Of course it'll only be at the beach in Mexico or somewhere that I don't know anyone... I am still very modest too. That hasn't changed.

Plenty of Tips for Other Sleeve Patients

- ***Get active/work out, get active/work out, get active/work out.*** *I don't care if you do 10 minutes three times a day, it's something! It takes 60 to 90 minutes of daily cardio to lose weight. That is what my health behaviorist doctor has taught my support group class. It wasn't until he said that that I truly kicked it up a notch and really had the last 20 lbs or so come off really well. You have to 'mix it up' and keep your body guessing. It's frustrating as all get out, but for me, if I don't do it I believe I won't make it to goal as surgery is NOT a magic wand.*

- *Drink water, drink water, drink water. My goal is four cups a day in this mug from the hospital that holds 28 ounces. That's 14 - 8 oz. cups a day. Until I got sick, I was doing this and I swear it helps with the elasticity of your skin as well as pushing weight loss into the rapid zone.*

- ***Get your protein in.*** *Avoid carbohydrates. Carbs make you want more carbs. I love carbs, but I try to avoid the 'bad' ones. I don't always succeed. I do allow myself to have treats (even daily sometimes, then I can see myself slipping and realize I have to stop doing this, and again, I change).*

- ***Track your food intake!*** *Every time I don't, I slip back into bad habits. But I am a food addict to the core. Tracking helps me to remain cognizant of my daily triggers. Whenever you hit a stall, ask three questions. How much do you work out? Do you track and measure what you are eating? How much water do you have? I bet you money that one or more of those needs tweaking. Lo and behold, whenever the change is made, voila!*

- ***Work on your head issues.*** *This one is very hard and one of my struggles. I am a food addict, and many of my issues are deeply rooted in food.*

- ***Stop pressuring yourself.*** *You didn't gain this overnight and even with surgery, you won't lose ALL of your weight overnight. You might lose a large portion quickly, but you'll never get to goal without doing my tips above. I truly believe that.*

- ***Don't compare your weight loss to anyone else's.*** *Unfortunately we are all different, and we react and respond differently, too. You will drive yourself nuts if you compare!*

- ***Weigh yourself only once a week.*** *Once you get closer to goal or after you reach goal, I suggest keeping the scale in the kitchen and noticing how the day plays with your weight. For example, I am currently [at time of interview] 158 to 159 pounds in the mornings. When I get home at 5:00 p.m., I am 161 pounds. When I go to the gym and return home at 8, I am 159 pounds. Before bed, I'm 161. These changes are from changes in water weight, so don't freak out. As you get close to goal, be cognizant of this fluctuation. Only "count" ["record"] the weight on your one day of the week - so if you previously always checked your weight on Monday, then continue to only count the weight on Mondays because you will fluctuate a lot as you get closer to goal.*

- ***Vary your eating choices.*** *Learn to cook at home more than eating out. If you have to be social, then start cooking for others. You save so many calories by cooking food and preparing it yourself. I just really struggle with sticking to plan whenever I don't eat at home.*

1   Lee J. Vertical sleeve gastrectomy. Healthline Web site. http://www.healthline.com/adamcontent/vertical-sleeve-gastrectomy. Updated November 4, 2009. Accessed August 27, 2012.

2   Gendron JP. The first bariatric surgery: the single procedure jejunoileal bypass (1954-1980). Sci Can, 2010;33(1)29-70.

3   Rosenthal RJ, International Sleeve Gastrectomy Expert Panel. International Sleeve Gastrectomy Expert Panel Consensus Statement: Best practice guidelines based on experience of > 12,000 cases. Surgery for Obesity and Related Diseases, 2012;8(1):8-19.

4   Weight Control Information Network, National Institutes of Health. Bariatric surgery as a treatment for obesity. National Institute of Diabetes and Digestive and Kidney Diseases. 2011, June. Accessed August 30, 2012 from http://win.niddk.nih.gov/publications/gastric.htm

5   Saber AA, Elgamel MH, McLeod, MK. Bariatric surgery: the past, present and future. Obesity Surgery Including Laparoscopy and Allied Care, 2008;18(1):121-8.

6   Rosenthal RJ, International Sleeve Gastrectomy Expert Panel. International Sleeve Gastrectomy Expert Panel Consensus Statement: Best practice guidelines based on experience of > 12,000 cases. Surgery for Obesity and Related Diseases, 2012;8(1):8-19.

7   Johnston D, Dachtler J, Sue-Ling HM, King RF, Martin G. The Magnestrasse and Mill operation for morbid obesity. Obes Surg, 2003;13(1):10:6.

8   Baker MT. The history and evolution of bariatric surgical procedures. Surgical Clinics of North America. 2011;91(6).

9   Carmichael AR, Johnston D, King RF, & Sue-Ling HM. Effects of the Magenstrasse and Mill operation for obesity on plasma leptin and insulin resistance. 2001;3(2):99-103

10 Ren CJ, Patterson E, Gagner M. Early results of laparoscopic biliopancreatic diversion with duodenal switch: a case series of 40 consecutive patients. 2000;10: 514-523.

11 Huang C. Single-incision laparoscopic bariatric surgery. J Minimal Access Surg. 2011;7(1):99-103.

12 Moy J, Pomp A, Dakin G, Parikh M, Gagner M. Laparoscopic sleeve gastrectomy for morbid obesity. American Journal of Surgery. 2008;196(5).

13 Weight Control Information Network, National Institutes of Health. Bariatric surgery as a treatment for obesity. National Institute of Diabetes and Digestive and Kidney Diseases. 2011, June. Accessed August 30, 2012 from http://win.niddk.nih.gov/publications/gastric.htm

14 National nutrient database for standard reference. National Agricultural Library, Agricultural Research Service, USDA. 2012, January 30. Accessed August 30, 2012 from http://ndb.nal.usda.gov/ndb/foods/list

15 Geliebter A. Gastric distension and gastric capacity in relation to food intake in humans. Physiol Behav. 1988;44(4-5):665-8.

16 Inui A, Asakawa A, Bowers CY, Mantovani G, Laviano A, Meguid MM, Fujumiya M. Ghrelin, appetite and gastric motility: the emerging role of the stomach as an endocrine organ. 2004;18(3):439-456.

17 Iannelli A, Dainese R, Piche T, Facchiano E, Gugenheim J. Laparoscopic sleeve gastrectomy for morbid obesity. World J Gastroenterology, 2008;14(6)821-827.

18 Langer FB, Reza Hoda MA, Bohdjalian A, Felberbauer FX, Zacherl J, Wenzl E, Schindler K, Luger A, Ludvik B, Prager G. Sleeve gastrectomy and gastric banding: effects on plasma ghrelin levels.Obesity Surgery, 2005;15(10):1501-2.

19 Lee WJ, Chen CY, Chong K, Lee YC, Chen SC, Lee SD. Changes in postprandial gut hormones after metabolic surgery: a comparison of gastric bypass and sleeve gastrectomy. Surg Obes Relat Dis. 2011;7(6):683-90.

20 Physicians and surgeons. The Bureau of Labor Statistics. Web site. http://www.bls.gov/ooh/healthcare/physicians-and-surgeons.htm. 2012, March 29. Accessed September 1, 2012.

21 Moy J, Pomp A. Laparoscopic sleeve gastrectomy for morbid obesity. American Journal of Surgery. 2008;196(5).

22 Bhimji S, Zieve D. Vertical sleeve gastrectomy. Medline Plus. Web site. http://www.nlm.nih.gov/medlineplus/ency/article/007435.htm. 2011, January 26. Accessed September 1, 2012.

23 Lee J. Vertical sleeve gastrectomy. Healthline. Web site. http://www.healthline.com/adamcontent/vertical-sleeve-gastrectomy#1. 2009, November 4. Accessed September 1, 2012.

24 Moy J, Pomp A. Laparoscopic sleeve gastrectomy for morbid obesity. American Journal of Surgery. 2008;196(5).

25 Neudecker J, Sauerland S, Neuebauer E, Expert Panel. The European Association for Endoscopic Surgery clinical practice guideline on the pneumoperitoneum for laparoscopic surgery. Surg Endosc. 2002;16(7):1121-43.

26 Neudecker J, Sauerland S, Neuebauer E, Expert Panel. The European Association for Endoscopic Surgery clinical practice guideline on the pneumoperitoneum for laparoscopic surgery. Surg Endosc. 2002;16(7):1121-43.

27 Rosenthal RJ, International Sleeve Gastrectomy Expert Panel. International Sleeve Gastrectomy Expert Panel Consensus Statement: Best practice guidelines based on experience of > 12,000 cases. Surgery for Obesity and Related Diseases, 2012;8(1):8-19.

28 Bhimji S, Zieve D. Vertical sleeve gastrectomy. Medline Plus. Web site. http://www.nlm.nih.gov/medlineplus/ency/article/007435.htm. 2011, January 26. Accessed September 1, 2012.

29 Catheline JM, Fysekidis M, Dbouk R, Boschetto A, Bihan H, Reach G, Cohen R. Weight loss after sleeve gastrectomy in super superobesity. J Obes. 2012.

30 Holzheimer RG, Mannick JA, eds. Complications of laparoscopic surgery. Surgical Treatment, Evidence-Based and Problem-Oriented. Munich:Zuckschwerdt; 2001.

31 Neudecker J, Sauerland S, Neuebauer E, Expert Panel. The European Association for Endoscopic Surgery clinical practice guideline on the pneumoperitoneum for laparoscopic surgery. Surg Endosc. 2002;16(7):1121-43.

32 Bhimji S, Zieve D. Vertical sleeve gastrectomy. Medline Plus. Web site. http://www.nlm.nih.gov/medlineplus/ency/article/007435.htm. 2011, January 26. Accessed September 2, 2012.

33 Cholecystectomy – Open and Laparoscopic. Medline Plus. Web site. http://www.nlm.nih.gov/medlineplus/tutorials/cholecystectomyopenandlaparoscopic/htm/_no_50_no_0.htm Accessed September 2, 2012.

34 Lee J. Vertical sleeve gastrectomy. Healthline Web site. http://www.healthline.com/adamcontent/vertical-sleeve-gastrectomy. Updated November 4, 2009 Accessed September 2, 2012.

4

Potential Benefits of the VSG

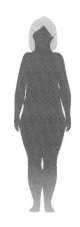

The last chapter talked about the sleeve: what it is, how you get it and what it does. You're thinking that the sleeve that may be your answer to years of struggling with obesity, just like it has been the answer for thousands of patients. But you still need more information before making your final decision about the sleeve. It has pros and cons, and you have to meet certain criteria to be eligible to get the sleeve. It's time to talk about whether the sleeve is right for you. This chapter along with the next two will help you do just that.

We'll start by discussing the potential benefits of the sleeve in this chapter. This is what you'll find information on as you continue to read:

- Weight loss with the sleeve: how much, how fast and how likely?
- A deeper look at how the sleeve may help you lose weight
- Physical health benefits: better health and fewer medications?
- Going beyond the numbers and recognizing that quality of life is just as important.

By the end of the chapter, you'll have a much better idea about whether your expectations for the sleeve are realistic and in line with the amount of weight you hope to lose.

How Much Weight Will You Lose with the sleeve?

Finally, it's time to talk about what you really want to know: *How much weight will I lose with the sleeve*? We can't answer that for every individual patient. Your own weight loss depends on things such as your starting weight and BMI, how well you follow the sleeve diet, your exercise program, your surgeon's skill, your follow-up care and so many more factors! Even though we can't tell you for sure exactly how much weight you'll lose, we can give you some general estimates.

In this section, we'll talk about the amount of weight loss other patients have had with the sleeve. That'll give you some idea of what to expect if you get the sleeve. Always keep in mind that your results with the VSG depend on your own choices. The more closely you follow your VSG instructions and the more consistent you are with your diet, the more likely you are to hit your weight loss goals.

So, How Much Weight Will You Lose?

We can try to answer this question by looking at some of the published research studies on the vertical sleeve gastrectomy. First, let's talk a little bit about the ways to measure weight loss.

Measuring Weight Loss

We're about to go over some of the available information on weight loss after getting the gastric sleeve, but let's get the terminology down first. Each individual has a different amount of weight to lose. Different research studies might use the following measures of weight loss. You can refer back to this list as you read through this chapter and do your own research on the sleeve.

Ideal Body Weight Is Just an Estimate

It's important to remember that your ideal body weight falls within a range. You can be just as healthy with a BMI of 20 or 21 as you can with a BMI of 23 or 24, so you don't have to worry about setting your goal weight at that exact BMI of 22. It's okay if you end up a few pounds below or above the "ideal" of 22 as long as you're eating healthy foods and feeling great.

- **Pounds lost:** This one's pretty simple, and it's probably what you think of when you're thinking about your own weight loss. The problem with pounds lost comes when you're reading about the results of a study with many sleeve patients. An average loss of 75 pounds after, say, two years is very different if the average starting weight was 200 pounds than if the average starting weight was 400 pounds.

- **Excess Weight Loss (EWL):** Let's start with excess weight. Excess weight is the number of pounds that you weigh above a number called your ideal body weight. By definition, the ideal body weight is the weight of someone at your height with a BMI of 22, which is right in the middle of the normal, healthy range of 18.5 to 24.9. So, let's say, for example, that your height is 5 feet, 4 inches. Your ideal body weight, or your weight with a BMI of 22, is 128 pounds (you can check that on the table in chapter one or use an online calculator). If you weigh 228 pounds, you are 100 pounds above your ideal body weight. This means that your excess weight is 100 pounds. Your excess weight loss, or EWL, is the amount of this "excess weight" (100 pounds, in the above example) that you lose after weight loss surgery. It's expressed in percent. Going back to the above example, let's say that you start off with a pre-surgery weight of 228 pounds, or an excess weight of 100 pounds. If you lose 60 pounds within the first year after your sleeve, you will have an excess weight loss of 60 percent. Your excess weight loss will be 100 percent when you hit your goal weight of 128 pounds. Excess weight loss, or EWL, is usually expressed in terms of percent so that you can know how much weight loss to expect and compare your weight loss progress to the progress people with different starting weights and different amounts of excess weight.

- **Excess BMI Loss (EBMIL):** Remember how the BMI is a way to compare your own weight to someone else's, even if you both have different heights? (If not, take a look at Chapter 1 for an explanation of BMI.) Well, the EBMIL has a similar idea. Your excess BMI is defined as the BMI you have over an "ideal BMI" of 22. So, if your pre-surgery BMI is 62, your excess BMI is 40. The excess BMI loss is the percent of excess BMI you lose. Let's say you get down to a BMI of 32 after surgery. That means that you've lost 30 BMI points, or 30 out of your initial 40 excess BMI points. That's an EBMIL of 30 divided by 40, or 75 percent.

- **Sufficient weight loss:** There's no single definition for this. Researcher may define it by:
  - Number of pounds lost, such as 75 within a year

- EWL, such as 40 percent in a year
- BMI, such as BMI under 351
- Certain EBMIL, such as 50 percent

How Much Weight Do People Lose after Getting the Sleeve?

You can estimate the amount of weight you might lose after getting the sleeve by looking at a variety of research studies that follow patients who get the sleeve. Several studies have been done among patients with an average starting BMI between 30 and 47.[2]

> **Too Much Information to Sort Through?**
>
> You don't have to sort through the numbers. Just scroll down to the handy chart at the end of this section. It summarizes the weight loss info you need.

- After 12 months, the average weight loss ranged from 28 percent to 75 percent excess weight loss (EWL) after one year, and was 67 percent after three years.

- Other studies found 40 percent EWL at six months, 47 percent EWL after 12 months and 63 to 72.8 percent EWL after three years. [3,4]

- The average drop in BMI in one study was 12 points.[5]

- Longer-term studies found at least 53 percent EWL after five to nine years.

As you look through these numbers, remember that these are averages from large studies. Each individual patient's results vary and may be as low as 10 percent EWL or as high as 100 percent EWL. [6]

The sleeve appears to be a relatively effective option for treating extreme morbid obesity. That's important because this type of obesity is the most likely to cause health problems for you. Another reason why having the VSG as an option for treating extreme morbid obesity is that other forms of surgery can be especially dangerous if you're in this group.

One study looked at individuals whose pre-surgery BMI was at least 60. The surgery led to an EWL of 34 percent after six months, 50 percent after a year and 53 percent after three years. Out of the 23 patients in the study, 17 had a BMI under 35 at three years after surgery.[7] The average weight loss by that time was 123 pounds, or 51 percent of EWL.[8] Another study in patients with an average starting BMI of 66 found an average excess weight loss (EWL) of 46% after eight years.[9] Other results among individuals with a starting BMI over 60 have found similar results.[10]

Here's a Summary

The above section has a lot of numbers. *Table 12* is a good cheat sheet to summarize what you might expect to lose with the sleeve.

Measure	Likely Value or Range to Expect
At 6 months	
Excess weight loss (EWL)	34% to 40%
At One Year (12 Months)	
Percent excess weight loss (EWL)	47% 53%
Reduction in BMI points	12 (in a study whose average BMI started at 44)
Percent excess BMI loss (EBMIL)	65.6%
At Three Years (36 Months)	
Excess weight loss (EWL)	51% 72.8%
Five to Nine Years (60 to 108 months)	
Excess weight loss (EWL)	46% to 69%
BMI lost	17

Table 12: Summary of weight loss you might expect with the sleeve

What if You Don't Lose as Much as You'd Hoped?

Not all sleeve patients hit their weight loss goals. And some of the patients who do hit their initial weight loss goals find themselves regaining the weight. What happens in that case? Your choices depend on the reason why you're not controlling your weight as well as you'd hoped. These are some of the possible reasons and the actions to take to take charge.

Poor Diet

You can regain weight if you're not being honest with yourself about your diet. You won't hit your weight loss goals if you sneak in foods or beverages that aren't allowed or eat portions that are too large. Another cause of a poor diet for weight control is accidentally making mistakes on your sleeve diet. This often happens after the initial period of time after your surgery or when you've hit your goal weight. You may *think* you've memorized the entire diet or you can estimate ("eyeball") portions without measuring them, but soon the bad habits kick in. Be sure to look over your instructions carefully and to consult your surgeon and/or dietitian. Another great tip is to check in with BariatricPal.com for some advice from other sleeve patients who thought they were following their diets but realized that they were making mistakes that were hurting their weight loss.

Lack of Restriction—Stretching of the Sleeve

Right after surgery, your sleeve is only about 15 percent of the original volume of your full stomach, with a capacity of just two to three ounces.[11] Your sleeve is made from the same stretchable tissue as your stomach. Over time, if you eat meals that are too big, the sleeve can stretch so that you no longer feel full on a small amount of food. The best way to prevent this is to measure your portions and avoid overeating.

Poor Support

A lack of post-surgery support can make you lose motivation and leave you without the information you need to meet your weight loss goals. Choose a surgeon with a comprehensive aftercare program. If you have already had the sleeve surgery and you need more support, don't be afraid to look to another surgeon, clinic or peer support group for help. BariatricPal.com is another source of support, and you can get information and advice from thousands of other sleeve patients.

The Sleeve Simply May Not Work for You

For a variety of other reasons, some patients don't lose the amount of weight they wanted when they have the sleeve. For example, taking another look at the weight loss data we talked about above, you can see that in one study, 17 out of 23 patients hit their three-year goal BMI of under 35; that means that six did not. It may be that the other six patients lost a great deal of weight but started out at a high BMI and had not yet reached a BMI of 35. Or, it could be that for some reason, the sleeve did not work for those patients. Some surgeons will suggest another surgery. You might get revisional surgery to get your sleeve re-done, known as a re-sleeve,[12] or have your procedure converted to a roux-en-Y gastric bypass or duodenal switch.[13]

Losing Weight with Restriction and Hormonal Changes

The vertical sleeve works in a few ways to help you lose weight. The smaller sleeve compared to your original stomach makes the sleeve a restrictive procedure. The idea is that your sleeve fills up sooner after a meal with the sleeve than with an entire stomach, so you feel full sooner, eat less, and lose weight. Another way the sleeve may work is through its effects on your hunger hormones.

Changes in Hormones after the Sleev

Where's your mind at?! Don't be silly – we're not talking about *those* kinds of hormones. We're talking about hormones that affect your hunger and appetite. The VSG can help you lose weight and improve your health because it changes your body's levels of some of these hormones. We already mentioned ghrelin in Chapter 3, and there are some others whose levels may change after surgery. The gut hormones (produced by your gut) that we'll talk about are ghrelin, peptide-YY, or PYY, glucagon-like peptide-1, or GLP-1, and cholecystokinin, or CCK. The VSG also affects insulin and leptin, known as the "peripheral adiposity" hormones—or, to put it in plain language, hormones that circulate in the blood and affect your metabolism.[14]

Have you ever wondered what makes you hungry? A lot of it is related to the effects of these hormones. And the sleeve changes the amount of these hormones in your body.

Ghrelin: Ghrelin is also known as the hunger hormone. It's produced and secreted cells in your stomach, and it makes you feel hungry. You have higher levels of ghrelin circulating in your bloodstream before meals. Levels decrease after meals so you feel full, but obese individuals tend to have higher levels of ghrelin—more potential for hunger—than normal weight individuals. Patients with the VSG have lower levels of ghrelin because so much of your stomach is removed. This can help you feel less hungry, eat less, and lose weight. There's a greater decrease in ghrelin after the VSG than after the roux-en-Y gastric bypass.[15]

Peptide-YY (PYY): PYY increases your feelings of fullness after a meal. Levels are higher in obese individuals than normal-weight people, and they tend to increase after getting the sleeve — which may contribute to your weight loss.[16]

Glucagon-Like Peptide-1 (GLP-1): Glucagon-like peptide-1, or GLP-1, is a gut hormone that helps you feel full. Levels of GLP-1 are lower between meals and higher after meals. A high amount of GLP-1 tends to make you eat less. Obese individuals have lower levels of GLP-1 than normal-weight individuals. The VSG leads to lower GLP-1 levels, which might help you lose weight. Together, GLP-1 and PYY are part of the "ileum brake." It's called that because these hormones work to make you feel full when food gets toward the further end of your small intestine — the ileum. [17]

Cholecystokinin (CCK): Cholecystokinin, or CCK, is a gut hormone that comes from your small intestine. It stimulates your pancreas to secrete digestive enzymes and your gallbladder to secrete bile when you eat.18 CCK may reduce food intake by promoting satiety, or a feeling of fullness. Levels of CCK decrease after getting the sleeve, so that's another way the sleeve may help you lose weight.

Leptin: Leptin is a hormone that comes from your fat cells and is involved in appetite control. Leptin may reduce appetite, but obese individuals have higher leptin levels than normal weight individuals. That may mean that obese individuals respond differently to leptin. The sleeve may improve the effects of leptin on your appetite, but the research results aren't yet clear. If your body really does become more responsive to leptin after getting the sleeve, that would be another reason why the VSG can help you lose weight.

Insulin: We've already talked about insulin in the section on diabetes in Chapter 1, and we'll talk a bit more about it in the following section on the potential benefits of the sleeve. It's the hormone that's responsible for keeping your blood sugar levels from getting too high, but it also makes you hungry. Insulin levels may decrease after getting the sleeve.[19]

Weight Loss Is Largely Up to You!

You can see from the above studies that your possible weight loss falls within a wide range; that is, you might lose only a few pounds or you might hit your goal weight within the first year of getting the sleeve. The amount of weight that you lose is largely up to you. These steps can increase your chances of losing your goal amount of weight:

- Following the sleeve diet that your surgeon, dietitian or clinic recommends
- Exercising regularly
- Choosing an experienced surgeon for your procedure
- Taking your post-surgery aftercare program seriously[20]

Other Factors Affecting Your Weight Loss with the VSG

You play the largest role in your own success with the sleeve, but other factors also affect your weight loss.[21] We'll get deeper into how you can use this information to your advantage in Chapter 5 as you start to plan for your surgery. Factors affecting your weight loss include the following:

- Surgeon differences: technique and experience
- Degree of comprehensiveness: of your post-surgery follow-up care plan
- Biological factors: You're more likely to lose more weight if you have a lower pre-surgery BMI, if you don't have type 2 diabetes before surgery, and if you are normally physically active. You can be aware of these factors and adjust your weight loss expectations in order to avoid disappointment.

Other Potential Benefits of the Sleeve

Weight loss is the first benefit that comes to mind when you think of success with the sleeve. After all, the vertical sleeve gastrectomy is a *weight loss surgery*. Successful sleevers may experience a variety of other benefits, too. You might have better physical health and notice psychological and social benefits. These are some potential benefits of the sleeve:

- Lower risk of chronic diseases—since many of them are related to obesity.
- Having lower doses of medications or being able to stop your medications entirely (of course, never change your medications without your physician's recommendations)
- Better mood
- Ability to move more easily

Possible Health Benefits of the VSG

The gastric sleeve is designed to help you lose weight, and the physical health benefits that you might experience after getting the sleeve surgery are results of losing weight. As discussed in Chapter 1, obesity can cause or increase your risk for chronic conditions, including type 2 diabetes and heart disease-related conditions, such as high blood pressure and high cholesterol levels. You'd expect to have improvements in these and other chronic conditions after losing weight, and in fact, many sleeve patients do.

Type 2 Diabetes and Blood Sugar Levels

Nearly all cases of type 2 diabetes are related to obesity, so you're probably not surprised that successful sleeve patients see improvements in their diabetes. Up to 100 percent of patients in some research studies have seen improvements in their diabetes.[22] Again, though, the numbers vary between studies. One study found that only 19 percent of patients with type two diabetes got their diabetes resolved after getting the surgery, [23] while a third and fourth study found that 50 to 77 percent of patients had improved diabetes control at one year after surgery.[24],[25]

What kind of improvements might you see?

- Reduced need for medications or the ability to get off your medications entirely (but always remember, only change your medication dosage with your doctor's recommendation).
- Lower blood glucose values. Blood sugar levels dropped an average of 88 points in one study! [26]
- Lower insulin levels, which is a sign of better glucose control.[27]
- Decreased levels of glucagon-like peptide-1 (GLP-1) and peptide-YY (PYY), leading to a healthier (smaller) insulin response. [28]

Lower blood sugar and less severe diabetes are expected when you lose weight, but the gastric sleeve may have benefits for diabetes that go beyond what you'd expect from the amount of weight you lose.[29] That is to say that after the sleeve gastrectomy, you might have bigger improvements in your type 2 diabetes and blood sugar levels than someone who didn't get the surgery but lost the same amount of weight. And it happens faster. These benefits are probably because of hormonal changes, as discussed in an earlier section in this chapter. The VSG is more effective at resolving diabetes than the laparoscopic adjustable gastric band (Lap-Band or Realize Band), but less effective than the roux-en-y gastric bypass or BPD-DS.

The Sleeve and Heart Disease

Weight loss and the vertical sleeve can be powerful weapons in fighting heart disease, the top killer of Americans. High blood pressure and dyslipidemia, or high total cholesterol, high LDL cholesterol, high triglycerides, or low HDL cholesterol are major risk factors for heart disease. High blood pressure and dyslipidemia are related to obesity, too. You're likely to see improvements in these measures and have a lower risk for heart disease as you lose weight after getting the sleeve.

- *Weight loss*: Obese individuals are about twice as likely to have coronary heart disease than normal-weight individuals, so losing weight reduces your risk. [30]
- *High blood pressure, or hypertension*: Studies have shown 60 percent[31] to more than 90 percent[32] of sleeve patients with high blood pressure have better numbers after getting the sleeve.
- *Dyslipidemia*: About 30 percent[33] to 75 percent[34] of patients have lower cholesterol within a year of getting the sleeve.

A Word about the Sleeve and Medications

One of the biggest benefits of getting the vertical sleeve and losing weight is that it may allow you to lower your dose of medications, allow you to get off of some medications entirely, or help you prevent health conditions that would require medication. These may include medications to lower cholesterol, blood sugar or blood pressure, prescription steroids or non-steroidal anti-inflammatory drugs (NSAIDs) to reduce joint pain from osteoarthritis and asthma medications. There are many benefits of avoiding or reducing your prescriptions:

- You don't have to remember to order and refill prescriptions.
- You don't have to remember to take your medications at the proper time.
- You don't have to pay for medications. A single medication for controlling blood sugar can be $1 to $5 or more per day!

Another benefit of avoiding medications is that you won't to worry about their side effects:

- Blood pressure medications (anti-hypertensives) can lead to muscle and joint pain, nausea, constipation and diarrhea, fatigue, and dizziness.
- Cholesterol-lowering medications, such as statins, can cause muscle and joint pain and weakness, nausea, diarrhea, liver disease, and memory loss.
- Glucose or type 2 diabetes medications can lead to hypoglycemia, or low blood sugar, diarrhea, gas and, weight gain.
- Steroids, such as those for fighting osteoarthritis and asthma, can lead to bone mineral density loss and osteoporosis, or a high risk for bone fractures.
- Some asthma medications lead to dry mouth and throat.
- Many NSAIDs are rough on your stomach and can lead to ulcers or stomach discomfort.
- The continuous positive airway pressure, or CPAP, isn't a pill, but it's a treatment for an obesity-related disorder: sleep apnea. Getting rid of your CPAP machine will make sleep more comfortable.

You should not ever stop taking your prescription drug without your doctor's recommendation or take a different dose than what your doctor prescribes. That can lead to even more serious side effects.

Sources[35,36,37]

Other Improvements in Your Physical Health after the VSG

The other improvements in your physical health are probably what you'd expect from losing weight. They're the opposite of the problems caused by obesity that we described in Chapter 1.

- **Sleep apnea**: You'll be able to breathe better at night as you lose weight and don't have as much fat blocking your throat and airways. If your sleep apnea is resolved, you'd be able to sleep through the night without waking up and gasping for air. You might be able to stop using an annoying continuous positive airway pressure, or CPAP, machine without worrying that you'll stop breathing in the middle of the night. One study found that 62 percent of patients had improvements in their sleep apnea 12 months after surgery.[38]

- **Gastroesophageal reflux disease (GERD)**: GERD is a chronic condition with frequent heartburn. It occurs when the highly acidic contents of your stomach backtrack up into your lower esophagus and you feeling a burning sensation in your chest. If you have GERD before surgery, the vertical sleeve gastrectomy might reduce or get rid of your symptoms. One study reported that about half of patients had their GERD resolved within six or 12 months after getting their LSG done.[39] In a different study, 89 percent of patients had their symptoms reduced or eliminated by the end of 30 months (two and one-half years).[40] How can the sleeve reduce reflux:

  - The sleeve helps you lose weight, of course. Obesity is a major risk factor for GERD. When you lose weight, you don't have as much fat pushing against your stomach (or gastric sleeve) as you did before surgery. This means that you aren't as likely to have your stomach contents forced back up into your esophagus.

  - You eat more slowly. You'll probably be eating way more slowly than you did before you got the sleeve – and eating too fast can lead to reflux. Before the sleeve, some of your reflux symptoms may have come from eating too fast.

  - Smaller meals. Your sleeve is only fraction the size of your original stomach, so your meals are smaller. Smaller meals can help you prevent heartburn and GERD.

  - Different food choices. Fatty and fried foods, alcohol, and caffeinated beverages are all foods that can trigger heartburn and GERD. These foods are not allowed or are strictly limited on your sleeve diet.[41]

- **Asthma**: There's a chance that the sleeve can help you overcome asthma or other respiratory problems that you had before the surgery.[42] That's because obesity may be the cause of your breathing problems. Extra fat in your abdomen and in the area near your airways can make breathing difficult. Breathing is easier when you don't have excess fat constricting your airways.

- **Osteoarthritis**: Joint pain is often caused by obesity, and losing weight can reduce the amount of pain that you feel each day. Carrying around so much extra weight is hard work for your body. When you lose the weight, you'll probably have less pain and more energy, too, as you'll be carrying around so many fewer pounds.

Additional Benefits from the Sleeve: Better Quality of Life

The sleeve may have additional benefits beyond weight loss and the physical health benefits that we just discussed. Life is more than numbers that your doctor measures at a physical examination and your quality of life score reflects that. Your quality of life, also known as QoL, is an overall indicator of how good your life is. It doesn't just factor in your physical health. It also considers your social life, your psychological health, and how well you can move around and do the things you want to do.

Researchers measure QoL with a variety of tests. They have slight variations, but address the same general questions. One study that found dramatic improvements in quality of life after the sleeve asked these questions as part of its QoL assessment. These questions are known as the Moorehead-Adult Quality of Life Assessment[43] (See *Table 13*).

Question	Answer Scale (on a Continuum)
Usually I feel	Very bad → very good about myself
I enjoy physical activities	Not at all → very much
I have satisfactory social contacts	None → very much
I am able to work	Not at all → very much
The pleasure I get out of sex	Not at all → very much
The way I approach food	I live to eat → I eat to live

Table 13: Moorehead-Adult Quality of Life Assessment

Why does the QoL tend to improve after you get the sleeve? Besides the weight loss and physical benefits, it affects nearly every aspect of your life:

- *You feel better about yourself.* You're proud of how you look. Your confidence in your ability to control your eating may rub off onto other parts of your life.

- *Your social life may improve.* Many other people will notice that you're a happier person, and they'll enjoy being around you more than before. Plus, you'll be better able to keep up with the group during fun activities than when you were morbidly obese.

- *Life's easier.* To put it more formally, you're more functional. You can move around without struggling instead of having your obesity hold you back. Chances are, you'll have better attendance at work and each day will seem easier and more enjoyable.

There are almost an infinite number of possible reasons for an improved QoL when the VSG is a successful tool for weight loss. However, it's important to remember that not all sleeve patients have better qualities of life or are glad they got the procedure done. The most prudent advice is to make sure that you're getting the sleeve for the right reasons. It's a weight loss tool, not a magical cure for obesity. You need to make lifestyle changes—long-term—to be successful with the sleeve.

Why Don't the Numbers Add Up?!

As you continue to research the sleeve, you'll probably start to notice something a little strange. The numbers change. One website might tell you that there's a two percent risk of having a sleeve leak, while another might say one percent. The more research you do, the more you'll notice that the numbers vary between sources. You may have already noticed the apparent discrepancies in this book! Why does this happen? It's not a mistake, and we're not lying to you. It's because there are different sources of data and different ways of calculating the numbers.

Clinical Trials versus Estimated Figures

Sometimes the information comes from clinical trials. These are carefully-planned research studies to investigate patients who get the sleeve. Before surgery, surgeons ask their patients if they are willing to participate in the study. During the entire time of the study, which might be for six months or a year or more after surgery, surgeons and other researchers ask patients about all of their complications. At the end of the study, they try to answer these or similar questions:

- Which side effects or complications occurred? In how many patients?
- Is there a difference between patients who got certain complications and those who didn't?
- How much weight did the average patient lose over the course of the study?
- Is there a difference between patients who lost their target amount of weight and those who didn't?
- Were there any other benefits to the surgery, e.g., health or mood improvements?

Clinical trials are great because they provide trustworthy information, but they have a big problem.

They're too small. Clinical trials focusing on the sleeve might include only 10 or 20 or 50 patients, which just isn't that much compared to the thousands of obese patients who have gotten the sleeve. Some of the figures describing complication rates or weight loss success come from estimates based on reports from thousands of sleeve patients who have told their surgeons that they're having trouble. That's great because there's a lot of data, but not so good because it's not too well controlled. One patient might call to report diarrhea while another patient with the same symptoms might not. This is different from a clinical trial when all patients promise to report all symptoms. So, the numbers coming from clinical trials and patient reports can be different.

Other Reasons for Differences in Numbers

There are other reasons for different numbers from different studies:

- Small number of people in the study: Yes, a difference of one or two cases can make a difference of a few percent when the research study doesn't have that many patients

- Differences between patients: For example, studies whose participants have lower initial BMIs usually find lower complication rates than studies with higher-BMI patients.

- Average age of participants: Older adults tend to have more complications than younger adults.

- Slight differences in surgical procedures: Surgeon experience and whether the surgery was laparoscopic or open can make a difference.

- How good the aftercare program is: A better post-surgery care program leads to more weight loss, patients who are more likely to stick to their diets, and fewer complications.

What This Means for You

You're not an obesity researcher; you're not looking to make comparisons between studies. All you want is to make the best decision for yourself. It's not always easy or even possible to interpret the numbers. Hopefully you've already guessed the next piece of advice, because it's the first thing that should come to mind by now when you have questions. The advice? Talk to your doctor, a surgeon, and anyone else with the background to give you good individual advice. Your surgery decision needs to be based on your own circumstances. You can also gather information from online communities, such as BariatricPal.com, to get a feel for what their experiences have been with the sleeve.

✍ Summary

☛ This chapter provided an overview of some of the likely benefits of the sleeve. Now, you have an idea of how much weight most patients lose and how long it takes. You also know some of the ways that your life can improve with the sleeve, ranging from better health to a better mood and social life.

☛ The next chapter covers the other side of the sleeve – the potential complications and side effects. It's just as critical for you to know the risks as you decide whether the sleeve is for you.

☛ It's important as you read to remember that each person is an individual. Your own weight loss results, health consequences, and rest of your sleeve gastrectomy experiences are likely to be better, worse, or simply different than someone else's. Predicting your own outcomes is impossible, but you can get a much better handle on the likely results when you do more research. So keep on reading – the next chapter's waiting!

Your Turn: How Do You Feel about the Sleeve Now?

This chapter covered some of the potential benefits of the sleeve that you might experience if the surgery goes smoothly and you follow your surgeon's instructions. Let's take a look now at how you're feeling about the sleeve gastrectomy.

Do you recognize the amount of weight that you can reasonably expect to lose if you follow the sleeve diet? YES / NO

Is this an amount of weight that you'd be happy with? YES / NO

Do you understand the additional health benefits that can happen after getting the sleeve? YES /NO

The vertical sleeve is just a tool for losing weight. You are responsible for making the sleeve diet work for you. For each of the following responsibilities, describe what you, the individual patient, must do if you want to write your own VSG success story.

Diet

....

....

....

Exercise

....

....

....

Self-care

....

....

....

Patience/persistence

....

....

....

1   Catheline JM, Fysekidis M, Dbouk R, Boschetto A, Bihan H, Reach G, Cohen R. Weight loss after sleeve gastrectomy in super superobesity. J Obes. 2012.

2   American Society for Metabolic and Bariatric Surgery. Updated position statement on sleeve gastrectomy as a bariatric procedure. Revised 2011, October 28. http://s3.amazonaws.com/publicASMBS/GuidelinesStatements/PositionStatement/ASMBS-SLEEVE-STATEMENT-2011_10_28.pdf Accessed September 6, 2012.

3   Baker MT. The history and evolution of bariatric surgical procedures. Surgical Clinics of North America. 2011;91(6).

4   Himpens J. Long-term results of laparoscopic sleeve gastrectomy for obesity. Ann Surg. 2010; 252(2): 319-24.

5   Peterli R, Steiner RE, Woelnerhanssan B, Peters T, Christoffel-Courtin C, Gass M, Kern B, von Flueee M, Beglinger C. Metabolic and hormonal changes after laparoscopic roux-en-Y gastric bypass and sleeve gastrectomy: a randomized, prospective trial. Obes Surg. 2012;22(5):740-748.

6   van Rutte PWJ, Luyer MDP, de Hingh IHJT, Nienhuijs, SW. To sleeve or not to sleeve in bariatric surgery? ISRN Surgery. 2012.

7   Catheline JM, Fysekidis M, Dbouk R, Boschetto A, Bihan H, Reach G, Cohen R. Weight loss after sleeve gastrectomy in super superobesity. J Obes. 2012.

8   Catheline JM, Fysekidis M, Dbouk R, Boschetto A, Bihan H, Reach G, Cohen R. Weight loss after sleeve gastrectomy in super superobesity. J Obes. 2012.

9   Eid GM, Brethauer S, Mattar SG, Titchner RL, Gourash W, Schauer RR. Laparoscopic sleeve gastrectomy for super obese patients: forty-eight percent excess weight loss after 6 to 8 years with 93 percent followup. Ann Surg;256(2):262-5.

10 American Society for Metabolic and Bariatric Surgery. Updated position statement on sleeve gastrectomy as a bariatric procedure. Revised 2011, October 28. http://s3.amazonaws.com/publicASMBS/GuidelinesStatements/PositionStatement/ASMBS-SLEEVE-STATEMENT-2011_10_28.pdf Accessed September 6, 2012.

11 Bhimji S, Zieve D. Vertical sleeve gastrectomy. Medline Plus. Web site. Updated January 26, 2012. http://www.nlm.nih.gov/medlineplus/ency/article/007435.htm. 2011. Accessed September 8, 2012.

12 Iannelli A, Schneck AS, Noel P, Ben Amor I, Krawczykowski D, Gugenheim J. Re-sleeve gastrectomy for failed laparoscopic sleeve gastrectomy: a feasibility study. 2011;21(7):832-5.

13 American Society for Metabolic and Bariatric Surgery. Updated position statement on sleeve gastrectomy as a bariatric procedure. Revised 2011, October 28. http://s3.amazonaws.com/publicASMBS/GuidelinesStatements/PositionStatement/ASMBS-SLEEVE-STATEMENT-2011_10_28.pdf Accessed September 8, 2012.

14 Suzuki K, Jayasena CN, Bloom, SR. Obesity and appetite control. Experimental Diabetes Research. 2012. http://www.ncbi.nlm.nih.gov/pubmed/22899902. Accessed September 4, 2012.

15 Peterli R, Steiner RE, Woelnerhanssan B, Peters T, Christoffel-Courtin C, Gass M, Kern B, von Flueee M, Beglinger C. Metabolic and hormonal changes after laparoscopic roux-en-Y gastric bypass and sleeve gastrectomy: a randomized, prospective trial. Obes Surg. 2012;22(5):740-748.

16 Peterli R, Steiner RE, Woelnerhanssan B, Peters T, Christoffel-Courtin C, Gass M, Kern B, von Flueee M, Beglinger C. Metabolic and hormonal changes after laparoscopic roux-en-Y gastric bypass and sleeve gastrectomy: a randomized, prospective trial. Obes Surg. 2012;22(5):740-748.

17 Peterli R, Steiner RE, Woelnerhanssan B, Peters T, Christoffel-Courtin C, Gass M, Kern B, von Flueee M, Beglinger C. Metabolic and hormonal changes after laparoscopic roux-en-Y gastric bypass and sleeve gastrectomy: a randomized, prospective trial. Obes Surg. 2012;22(5):740-748.

18 Peterli R, Steiner RE, Woelnerhanssan B, Peters T, Christoffel-Courtin C, Gass M, Kern B, von Flueee M, Beglinger C. Metabolic and hormonal changes after laparoscopic roux-en-Y gastric bypass and sleeve gastrectomy: a randomized, prospective trial. Obes Surg. 2012;22(5):740-748.

19 Peterli R, Steiner RE, Woelnerhanssan B, Peters T, Christoffel-Courtin C, Gass M, Kern B, von Flueee M, Beglinger C. Metabolic and hormonal changes after laparoscopic roux-en-Y gastric bypass and sleeve gastrectomy: a randomized, prospective trial. Obes Surg. 2012;22(5):740-748.

20 Keren D, Matter I, Rainis T & Lavy A. Getting the most from the sleeve: the importance of post-operative follow-up. Obesity Surgery. 2011;21(12):1887-1893.

21 Kaplan LM, Seeley RJ, Harris JL. Myths associated with obesity and bariatric surgery – myth 5: patient behavior is the primary determinant of outcomes after bariatric surgery. 2012;9(8):8-10.

22 Moy J, Pomp A, Dakin G, Parikh M, Gagner M. Laparoscopic sleeve gastrectomy for morbid obesity. American Journal of Surgery. 2008;196(5).

23 Lee WJ, Chen CY, Chong K, Lee YC, Chen SC, Lee SD. Changes in postprandial gut hormones after metabolic surgery: a comparison of gastric bypass and sleeve gastrectomy. Surg Obes Relat Dis. 2011;7(6):683-90.

24 Hutter MM, Schirmer BD, Jones DB, Ko CY, Cohen ME, Merdow RP, Nguyen NT. First report from the American College of Surgeons Bariatric Surgery Center Network: laparoscopic sleeve gastrectomy has morbidity and effectiveness positioned between the band and the bypass. Annals of Surgery. 2011;254:410-420.

25 Eid GM, Brethauer S, Mattar SG, Titchner RL, Gourash W, Schauer RR. Laparoscopic sleeve gastrectomy for super obese patients: forty-eight percent excess weight loss after 6 to 8 years with 93 percent followup. Ann Surg;256(2):262-5

26 American Society for Metabolic and Bariatric Surgery. Updated position statement on sleeve gastrectomy as a bariatric procedure. Revised 2011, October 28. http://s3.amazonaws.com/publicASMBS/GuidelinesStatements/PositionStatement/ASMBS-SLEEVE-STATEMENT-2011_10_28.pdf Accessed September 6, 2012.

27 Peterli R, Steiner RE, Woelnerhanssan B, Peters T, Christoffel-Courtin C, Gass M, Kern B, von Flueee M, Beglinger C. Metabolic and hormonal changes after laparoscopic roux-en-Y gastric bypass and sleeve gastrectomy: a randomized, prospective trial. Obes Surg. 2012;22(5):740-748.

28 van Rutte PWJ, Luyer MDP, de Hingh IHJT, Nienhuijs, SW. To sleeve or not to sleeve in bariatric surgery? ISRN Surgery. 2012.

29 Kaplan LM, Seeley RJ, Harris JL. Myths associated with obesity and bariatric surgery – myth 4: "diabetes improvement after bariatric surgery is dependent on weight loss."Bariatric Times. 2012;9(7):12-14.

30 Gagnon L, Sheff Karwacki EJ. Outcomes and complications after bariatric surgery. AJN. 2012;112(9):26-36.

31 Hutter MM, Schirmer BD, Jones DB, Ko CY, Cohen ME, Merdow RP, Nguyen NT. First report from the American College of Surgeons Bariatric Surgery Center Network: laparoscopic sleeve gastrectomy has morbidity and effectiveness positioned between the band and the bypass. Annals of Surgery. 2011;254:410-420.

32 Gagnon L, Sheff Karwacki EJ. Outcomes and complications after bariatric surgery. AJN. 2012;112(9):26-36.

33 Hutter MM, Schirmer BD, Jones DB, Ko CY, Cohen ME, Merdow RP, Nguyen NT. First report from the American College of Surgeons Bariatric Surgery Center Network: laparoscopic sleeve gastrectomy has morbidity and effectiveness positioned between the band and the bypass. Annals of Surgery. 2011;254:410-420.

34 Gagnon L, Sheff Karwacki EJ. Outcomes and complications after bariatric surgery. AJN. 2012;112(9):26-36.

35 Dugdale DC, Zieve D. High blood pressure medications. Web site. http://www.nlm.nih.gov/medlineplus/ency/article/007484.htm. Updated 2011, June 10. Accessed September 10, 2012.

36 Humphries A, Workman T, Balasubramanyam A, Fordis M. Medicines for type 2 daibetes: a review of the research for adults. Web site. http://effectivehealthcare.ahrq.gov/index.cfm/search-for-guides-reviews-and-reports/?pageaction=displayproduct&product ID=721. 2011, June 30. Accessed September 10, 2012.

37 Mayo Clinic staff. Statins: are these cholesterol-lowering medications right for you? http://www.mayoclinic.com/health/statins/CL00010. 2012, March 13. Accessed September 10, 2012.

38 Hutter MM, Schirmer BD, Jones DB, Ko CY, Cohen ME, Merdow RP, Nguyen NT. First report from the American College of Surgeons Bariatric Surgery Center Network: laparoscopic sleeve gastrectomy has morbidity and effectiveness positioned between the band and the bypass. Annals of Surgery. 2011;254:410-420.

39 Hutter MM, Schirmer BD, Jones DB, Ko CY, Cohen ME, Merdow RP, Nguyen NT. First report from the American College of Surgeons Bariatric Surgery Center Network: laparoscopic sleeve gastrectomy has morbidity and effectiveness positioned between the band and the bypass. Annals of Surgery. 2011;254:410-420.

40 Keren D, Matter I, Rainis T & Lavy A. Getting the most from the sleeve: the importance of post-operative follow-up. Obesity Surgery. 2011;21(12):1887-1893.

41 Snyder-Markow G, Taylor D, Lenhard MJ. Nutrition care for patients undergoing laparoscopic sleeve gastrectomy for weight loss. J Am Diet Ass. 2010;110(4):600-7.

42 Gagnon L, Sheff Karwacki EJ. Outcomes and complications after bariatric surgery. AJN. 2012;112(9):26-36.

43 Keren D, Matter I, Rainis T & Lavy A. Getting the most from the sleeve: the importance of post-operative follow-up. Obesity Surgery. 2011;21(12):1887-1893.

5

VSG: Risks and Considerations

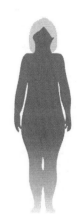

Chapter 4 covered weight loss, health improvements, and other possible advantages of the sleeve. The focus on the sleeve's benefits made the chapter upbeat, and it may have been enough to convince you that you are ready to get the sleeve. The gastric sleeve does have risks, though. This chapter will go over some of the possible problems that the VSG can cause.

- Complications from the open or laparoscopic surgical procedure for the SG.
- Serious and less serious complications that the gastric sleeve can cause.
- A comparison of the sleeve with your other options for treating obesity.

This is another chapter that will be pivotal in your decision on whether to get the sleeve. By the end of it, you'll be better able to weigh the benefits and risks of the sleeve to make a decision that makes you comfortable.

Risks of the Vertical Sleeve Gastrectomy

In this section, we'll take a look at some of the risks from the surgery and complications that can develop later. This information will help you know what to expect and what can happen if you get the sleeve. An important question when deciding about the VSG – or any medical procedure, for that matter – is whether the positives outweigh the negatives. Compared to some other medical procedures, knowing all of the risks is especially important for the sleeve because the sleeve is a permanent, one-way change to your body.

Any Surgical Procedure Has Risks

The first risks of the VSG come during or immediately after surgery. You take a risk any time you have a surgical procedure done, and these are some of the possibilities[1]

- *Allergic reaction to the anesthesia:*[2] Your doctor will ask you about your medical history.
- *Bleeding:* You can lose a great deal of blood during the procedure if you are prone to bleeding or if your body does not respond well.
- *Infections:* Another risk of surgery is infections. Infections can occur during surgery if the surgical environment is not sterile and contaminated air or surgical equipment comes into contact with your lungs, bladder, or kidney. Surgical cuts can also get infected.
- *Blood clots, heart attack, or stroke:* Your risk increases during surgery and within the first couple days after a surgery. This may be related to the need to go off of blood-thinners (to prevent excessive bleeding) before surgery.

There Is a Risk of Death from Surgery

Nobody wants to think about it, but you can die from complications of surgery. The overall rate of death in bariatric surgery is 0.15 to 0.64 percent, with the rate of death from VSG at about 0.5 percent, or about one in 200 patients.[3] The leading causes are a pulmonary embolism (blood clot in your lungs), heart attack, or other heart complications and severe infections. Leakage, excessive bleeding (hemorrhage), and bowel obstruction can also cause death.

Risks of Laparoscopic versus Open SG

Laparoscopic surgeries, or minimally invasive procedures, have lower risks than open procedures. You're less like to have excessive blood loss or get infections. The laparoscopic procedure does, however, cause more pain due to the need for pneumoperiosteum, or carbon dioxide gas pumped into your abdominal cavity. Also, patients with heart or lung conditions may not be able to tolerate the procedure and may need an open surgery instead. Chapter 3 talks about pneumoperiosteum in detail. The chance of having your sleeve gastrectomy converted to an open procedure during surgery is about one percent.[4]

Risks Specific to the VSG

The gastric sleeve can lead to a variety of complications. Some of them are fairly serious and require another surgery; others might just be unpleasant and they'll resolve themselves. You just have to wait them out. This section describes the most common risks of the sleeve.

Keep in mind that most of the following complications are the ones that patients actually tell their surgeons about. As you read through them, remember that some other patients may have experience less serious complications without reporting them. These may include milder cases of nausea, vomiting, diarrhea, and stomach pain. Most gastric sleeve patients experience at least some of these symptoms at some point.

Leak or Anastomotic Leak

As you know, the vertical sleeve is the small portion of your stomach that remains after your surgeon removes the majority, about 85 percent, of your stomach. The surgeon creates the sleeve by forming the remainder of your stomach into a tube shape that goes from your esophagus to your small intestine. The surgeon uses staples and a buttress, or patch, before finally sewing the sleeve closed. When everything is going well, food that you swallow goes down your throat and travels through the tube, or vertical sleeve, to the small intestine. Leaks occur in about one to four percent of gastric sleeve patients.[5,6]

A leak occurs when the stitches that are holding the sleeve closed are no longer tight. This is also known as dehiscence, when the surgical procedure comes undone. It is the most common cause of death after sleeve gastrectomy.[7] Food or beverages can slip through the openings. There are four types of leaks:[8]

1. Acute leaks occur within seven days of your initial surgery.
2. Early leaks occur within one to six weeks after surgery.
3. Late leaks occur within six to 12 weeks after surgery.
4. Chronic leaks occur after 12 weeks post-surgery.

Your surgeon should test the sleeve for leaks during surgery. One way is to place a brightly colored dye in the sleeve. The dye will be visible outside the sleeve if it leaks out. After surgery, you can get tested for a leak using a fluorescent dye that can be seen using x-ray equipment.

Leaks are serious complications and you should tell your surgeon if you think you may have one. You might have stomach pain, bloating, low blood pressure, or frequent urination.[9] A leak can lead to infections and peritonitis, or inflammation of the lining around your abdominal cavity. This occurs when the bacteria from your digestive tract leak into the abdominal cavity. Symptoms of peritonitis include nausea, vomiting, thirst, and fever.[10] You can get gangrene or go into shock if you don't get your leak treated. Another risk is an intraperitoneal adhesion, or the formation of thick scar tissue,[11] which can eventually cause your bowels, or large intestine, to be blocked.

A stent may be enough to treat an acute leak or one that does not have symptoms.[12] A stent is a small tube that can be used in small spaces in your body.[13] It can be placed using an endoscope, so you don't need another surgery. For a leak, the doctor might coat the stent with a medication and hope that your leak gets stopped up within 30 days.[14]

If not, you'll probably need another surgery. If you have symptoms from your leak, you should get another operation. One option is to try to seal up the staple line of your sleeve. Another option is to convert your vertical sleeve gastrectomy into a gastric bypass. The exact procedure that your surgeon will recommend depends on whether your leak is toward the top of the sleeve (known as a "proximal leak") or nearer the bottom (a "distal leak").

Strictures

A stricture is a narrowing of the sleeve that can make it difficult or impossible for food to pass through your digestive tract. It occurs when the stomach sleeve narrows, or con"stricts" (thus the name "strict"ure). Excessive vomiting is a main symptom of strictures. You will probably have trouble keeping your food down because it will get stuck at the place in your gastrointestinal tract where your sleeve is too narrow.

A stricture can be toward the upper end of the sleeve, near the gastroesophageal junction, or lower down, toward the small intestine. Strictures can occur in about one percent of patients, although, like the other complications of VSG, your individual risk varies depending on your surgeon and your own individual characteristics.[15],[16] You're more likely to get a stricture if your surgeon makes your sleeve too small during the initial procedure. You need to get it treated if you are vomiting to avoid dehydration and malnutrition.

The American Society for Metabolic and Bariatric Surgery, known as ASMBS, divides strictures into early strictures, which appear within the first six weeks after surgery, and persistent strictures, which appear after that.[17] The ASMBS provides four treatment options for surgeons to consider depending on the severity of the stricture. These are the steps:

1. *Observation*: This means paying attention to symptoms and being ready to take action if necessary.

2. *Endoscopic dilation*: This helps to open up the stricture by placing a stent, or small tube as described above (in the section on leaks), into the sleeve. It can be done endoscopically, so it doesn't require a full surgery.

3. *Seromytomy*: In this procedure, the surgeon carefully cuts away the scar-like tissue of the stricture to reopen the passageway.

4. *Conversion to roux-en-Y gastric bypass*: If all of the other options fail, you might need your sleeve converted to a gastric bypass.

Nutritional Deficiencies

The sleeve isn't a malabsorptive weight loss surgery, so it doesn't interfere too much with your nutrient absorption. It's less likely to cause nutritional deficiencies than the gastric bypass or biliopancreatic diversion with duodenal switch.[18] You still need to be careful with your nutrient intake, though. You will be eating relatively few calories after you get the sleeve. With such a low food intake, you'll need to focus on getting key nutrients and your dietitian or surgeon may recommend supplements.

> **Tip**
>
> Chapter 15, "The Sleeve Diet, Weight Loss and Your Health," has more information about nutrition. We'll cover the nutrients you need to be especially careful about and also which supplements you are likely to need.

A high-protein diet can support good health and also support you in your weight loss efforts. These are some of the vitamins and minerals that can be of concern after weight loss surgery.[19] Later, we'll go over the food sources and consequences of deficiency for each of these nutrients in more detail:

- *Vitamin B12* deficiency can lead to anemia and permanent neurological damage.
- *Calcium* deficiency can lead to osteoporosis, or low bone mineral density, and a high risk fractures.
- *Vitamin D* deficiency can lead to osteoporosis.
- *Beta-carotene (plant-based sources of vitamin A)* is not likely to have deficiency symptoms, but indicates a poor intake of fruits and vegetables.
- *Iron* deficiency can cause anemia and make you tired and weak.
- *Magnesium* deficiency can cause nausea and vomiting and harm your bones over the long term.
- *Folate*[20] deficiency can cause anemia and increase your risk for heart disease.

Gastroesophageal Reflux Disease (GERD)

Gastroesophageal reflux disease occurs when contents of your stomach come back up into your lower esophagus.[21] Heartburn feels like a burning sensation in your esophagus because of the high acidity of your stomach. Other symptoms are nausea, a feeling of choking and regurgitation, or food coming back up. Untreated GERD can lead to a stricture, Barrett's disease (which is a change in your esophageal lining and a risk factor for cancer), and asthma.

You're more likely to get GERD after getting the VSG if you have a hiatal hernia, so your surgeon should check for a hernia and try to repair it during your sleeve surgery.[22] The risk for developing GERD after the sleeve and requiring a second surgery to fix it is about 0.7 percent.[23] GERD appears more often in LSG patients than gastric bypass patients at the end of one year, but less often in LSG patients than gastric bypass patients at the end of three years.

GERD is an unpleasant condition that can make the sleeve less attractive to you, but you should also remember that obesity can cause GERD. In addition, about 50 percent of patients who get the sleeve have their GERD resolved within six to 12 months.[24]

Other Possible Complications

There are a number of other complications that can happen after the sleeve. These are some of the other conditions that can occur after getting the sleeve:[25]

- General gastrointestinal symptoms (more likely if you go off the sleeve diet)
  - Abdominal pain and cramping
  - Vomiting
  - Nausea
  - Diarrhea
- **Dumping syndrome**: You get symptoms of dumping syndrome when food from your stomach empties too quickly into your small intestine. The food is therefore mostly undigested, and you can become nauseous, have cramps, diarrhea, sweating, and faintness.[26] Dumping syndrome is far less common after getting the sleeve than after getting more extensive bariatric procedures, such as the bypass or biliopancreatic diversion with duodenal switch. That's because the pyloric sphincter, which slows down the passage of food from your stomach to intestine, remains intact and fully functional. However, one study found that 29 percent of VSG patients developed symptoms of dumping syndrome when they ate a high-sugar meal.[27] You're at higher risk for dumping syndrome after you eat high-sugar, high-fat foods and if you had GERD, high cholesterol, or type 2 diabetes before surgery.[28]
- **Excessive bleeding**: Intra-abdominal can happen not only during surgery, but even when your surgery is over. About 2.4 to 8.6 percent of sleeve patients have excessive bleeding, and one-third of those need a another surgery.[29],[30] A subphrenic hematoma is also a type of internal bleeding that occurs below the diaphragm.
- **Gallstones (cholelithiasis)**: Gallstones, also known as cholelithiasis, are painful hard plaques that can block up your gallbladder duct. You're likely to get gallstones when you lose weight quickly, such as after getting the sleeve. Chapter 3 already talks a bit about what gallstones are, their symptoms, and the possibility of getting your gallbladder removed during your initial sleeve surgery. About one-third of sleeve patients develop gallstones within a few months. Most of them resolve themselves, so

you can just wait them out.[31] If they don't go away on their own, your surgeon may need to do another surgery to get them out.

- **Gastric fistula**: This is essentially a hole in your stomach wall that creates an opening between your stomach and your abdominal wall.[32]

- **Conversion to open surgery**: This can happen if your surgeon or anesthesiologist starts to notice that you're having trouble during the laparoscopic procedure. Unexpected conversion to an open sleeve gastrectomy procedure is pretty rare. Some studies report that not a single patient needed a conversion to an open procedure;[33], in other studies, one to two percent of patients had their surgeries converted to an open procedure.[34],[35]

- **Food intolerances**: A food intolerance occurs when you don't digest your food very well. It's similar to dumping syndrome because it can cause unpleasant symptoms including diarrhea, bloating, and stomach pain after you eat. You might develop one or more food intolerances after getting the vertical sleeve because of minor changes to your digestive system. Food intolerances can occur with almost any food, and they have been observed in the following nutritious foods:[36]
  - Red meat, white-meat chicken and fish
  - Salads and cooked vegetables
  - Bread, rice, and pasta

- The VSG tends to cause fewer food intolerances than some other bariatric procedures, such as Roux-en-Y gastric bypass, biliopancreatic diversion with duodenal switch (BPD-DS), or the adjustable gastric band.[37] You're less likely to develop severe symptoms of food intolerance if you have a comprehensive aftercare program and follow your diet very carefully. If you develop intolerances, you may eventually be able to overcome them by taking smaller portions and chewing your food slowly.

You can lower your risk for many of the above complications by being especially careful to follow your sleeve diet: only eat the allowed foods, instead of high-sugar or high-fat foods, and stick to small portions so you don't stretch your sleeve or cause nausea, heartburn, or pain. You're at higher risk for developing complications if before the surgery you already have certain conditions, such as type 2 diabetes, GERD, or sleep apnea. On the other hand, these conditions are likely related to your obesity and can cause their own complications (as discussed in Chapter 1).

The Need for Another Surgical Procedure

As mentioned in the various sections on complications, you may need to have a second surgery after the sleeve. As with the other complications, your risk of needing a second procedure is higher if your surgeon is inexperienced. In one study, as many as 12 percent of patients needed a second procedure, with the majority of these converting their surgery to a roux-en-Y gastric bypass because of poor weight loss or regained weight.[38] However, only 3.2 percent of patients needed a second surgery in another study.[39]

A Summary of Your Risks

Table 14 is a quick summary of the risks that we talked about above so that you can see the different possibilities in one convenient place.

Complication	Estimated Frequency of Occurrence
Overall complication rate (any reported complication requiring medical attention – does not include self-resolving symptoms; excluding nutritional complications and gallstones)	15%
Death	0% to 0.5%
Second surgical procedure	2.2% to 11.6%
Conversion from laparoscopic to open procedure	0% to 2%
Gastric fistula	4.3%
Leak	1 to 3.7%
Pulmonary embolism	4.3%
Gastroesophageal reflux (GERD) requiring re-surgery	0.7%
Nutritional deficiencies	Varies by nutrient; up to 40% or more
Stricture	0.6% to 1%
Gallstones or cholelithiasis (can be self-resolving)	33%
Subphrenic hematoma (intrabdominal bleeding) (may require re-surgery)	2.4% to 8.6%

Table 14: Summary of risks for the second surgery

Reducing Your Risk of Complications

You can reduce your risk of developing complications from the sleeve gastrectomy:

- Choose a surgeon whose patients have low rates of complications.
- Follow instructions from your surgeon and other members of your healthcare team.
- Do not cheat on your diet or recovery program.

> **Tip**
>
> Chapter 6, "Are you a Good Candidate for the Sleeve?" will include tips on choosing a good surgeon to lower your risk of developing complications.

Your risk of developing complications isn't simply about your own post-surgery behavior.[40] It depends partly on things you can't control, such as your pre-surgery BMI. Your risk for complications increases if you have pre-surgery obesity-related diseases, or comorbidities, such as type 2 diabetes, sleep apnea, and high cholesterol.[41]

Comparing the Sleeve to Your Other Weight Loss Options?

As you get closer to making the decision about whether to get the sleeve, it makes sense to compare the sleeve to your other weight loss options. As we talked about in Chapter 1, your other options are:

- To do nothing.
- To diet, exercise, or do both:
- To try weight loss drugs, probably in combination with a diet.
- To opt for another weight loss surgery, such as the gastric band, Roux-en-Y gastric bypass or complete biliopancreatic diversion with duodenal switch, or BPD-DS, starting with the sleeve as a first surgery.

Let's take a quick look at each of these in a table to help you think more clearly about your options.

Alternative Weight Loss Approach	Benefits of the Alternative Approach	Benefits of the Sleeve
Doing Nothing Doing nothing gets you...nothing.	• Don't have to pay for surgery • Easy • No risk of complications • Keep your natural stomach	• Can help you lose weight • Likely savings on obesity-related medical costs • Unlike doing nothing, the VSG has a chance of treating your obesity • Can lead to improved health, social life and self-esteem.
Dieting, Exercising or Both It didn't work before; will it work now?	• Look and feel better • Will see health benefits if you follow a healthy diet and exercise regularly • No risk of surgery-related complications • Don't have to pay for surgery • Some people do lose weight and keep it off by committing to a healthy lifestyle.	• More likely to keep the weight off long-term • Will see health benefits if you follow a healthy diet and exercise regularly • May save money by not needing expensive diet plans • Diets and exercise haven't worked for you in the past.

Alternative Weight Loss Approach	Benefits of the Alternative Approach	Benefits of the Sleeve
Weight Loss Drugs There's no evidence to show that they're a long-term solution.	• Everyone wants to take a pill to solve their problems! • Can help you lose a few pounds, which can be enough weight loss to improve your blood sugar control, blood pressure, and cholesterol levels42 • Need to follow a low-fat diet, which can be healthy • Easy and convenient to take • Can take over-the-counter or prescription weight loss drugs • Don't need extensive planning and preparation	• Less risk of deficiencies of vitamins A, D, and E with a careful diet • Lower risk of fatty diarrhea and other side effects, such as nausea, vomiting, and dizziness with a careful diet • Won't damage your liver • A permanent change to your body and possible long-term obesity solution, while weight loss drugs are only for a few months or a year. • Extensive pre- and post-surgery support from your surgeon and medical team if you choose them well • Can lose about 12 BMI points within a year 43
Alternative Weight Loss Surgeries Each has its pros and cons.	• The adjustable gastric band (lap-band) is fully reversible. • The lap-band can be adjusted for when your needs change, such as during illness or pregnancy. • The Roux-en-Y gastric bypass helps you lose weight through malabsorption, not just restriction. • The lap-band, gastric bypass and biliopancreatic diversion with duodenal switch (BPD-DS) have been more extensively studied for a longer time. • Gastric bypass leads to greater first-year weight loss on average, with 15 BMI points lost compared to 12 with the sleeve. 44, 45	• Developed specifically to make weight loss surgery safer for super obesity for very high BMIs. • Can be converted to gastric bypass or BPD-DS if weight loss is unsatisfactory. • Is a good middle ground between the lap-band and gastric bypass with complications46 • Reduces hunger by removing your stomach, which is a main source of a hunger hormone called ghrelin • More weight loss expected within the first year than the lap-band, which has an average loss of 7 BMI points.47, 48

Table 15: Comparing the sleeve to other weight loss options

From *Table 15*, you can see that you don't have many choices. Doing nothing is not an option if you're not happy with where you are now. If diet and exercise attempts have failed for you in the past, probably numerous times — there's no reason to think they'll work for you in the future unless you or something in your life changes. Weight loss drugs are almost laughable at this point because they only help you lose a few pounds and you can't take them for long. Bariatric surgery has helped thousands of patients lose weight and keep it off, and 200,000 weight loss surgeries were performed in the U.S. in 2007.[49] Although the VSG is a relatively new procedure, it appears about as effective as other surgeries.

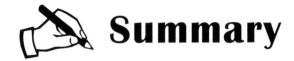 # Summary

- This chapter was another piece in the puzzle of the sleeve. Hopefully you are forming a more complete picture of the sleeve.

- After reading this chapter and the previous one, you now know the potential benefits and risks of the sleeve. This information will help you think logically about whether the vertical sleeve gastrectomy sounds like something you want to treat your obesity.

- The next chapter assumes that you're still interested in the sleeve. The chapter goes over some of the personal considerations of the sleeve, such as whether you're eligible. By the end of that chapter, you will be about ready to make your decision.

Your Turn: Are the Risks Worth Taking?

This chapter described some of the risks of the VSG and side effects that can happen after the surgery. For some people, the risks aren't worth the benefits. For others, the chance of having complications is small compared to the potential benefits for your weight loss and health.

Where do you stand? Do you feel that the benefits outweigh the risks?

....

....

....

What do you intend to accomplish by getting the sleeve gastrectomy? In addition to weight loss, you might, for example, answer that you intend to gain control of your eating and make healthy choices.

....

....

....

What are the biggest problems in your life? For each, what role, if any, do you see the sleeve playing in solving them? Follow the examples and add your own.

Obesity: The sleeve can be a tool to help me lose weight.

Low self-esteem: Now I feel ashamed to go out with my family. The sleeve can help me lose weight so I can go out with my family and keep up with my friends instead of saying no to their invitations.

Anxiety that I won't be there for my family. Losing weight with the sleeve can help me be healthier and not have diabetes

Add your own

....

....

....

....

....

....

....

....

1 Lee J. Vertical sleeve gastrectomy. Healthline Website. http://www.healthline.com/adamcontent/vertical-sleeve-gastrectomy. Updated 2009, November 4. Accessed September 3, 2012.

2 Bhimji S, Zieve D. General anesthesia. Medline Plus Website. http://www.nlm.nih.gov/medlineplus/ency/article/007410.htm. Updated 2011, January 26. Accessed September 3, 2012.

3 Gagnon L, Sheff Karwacki EJ. Outcomes and complications after bariatric surgery. AJN. 2012;112(9):26-36.

4 Hutter, M.M., Schirmer, B.D., Jones, D.B., Ko, C.Y., Cohen, M.E., Merdow, R.P., & Nguyen, N.T. (2011). First report from the American College of Surgeons Bariatric Surgery Center Network: laparoscopic sleeve gastrectomy has morbidity and effectiveness positioned between the band and the bypass. Annals of Surgery, 254:410-420.

5 American Society for Metabolic and Bariatric Surgery. Updated position statement on sleeve gastrectomy as a bariatric procedure. Revised 2011, October 28. http://s3.amazonaws.com/publicASMBS/GuidelinesStatements/PositionStatement/ASMBS-SLEEVE-STATEMENT-2011_10_28.pdf Accessed September 7, 2012.

6 Lacy A, Obarzabal A, Pando E, Adelsorfer C, Delitala A, Corcelles R, Delgado S, Vidal J. Revisional surgery after sleeve gastrectomy. Surg Laparosc Endosc Percutan Tech. 2010;20(5):351-6.

7 Himpens J, Dapri G, Cadiere. Treatment of leaks after sleeve gastrectomy. Bariatric Times. 2009, September.

8 Rosenthal RJ, International Sleeve Gastrectomy Expert Panel. International Sleeve Gastrectomy Expert Panel Consensus Statement: Best practice guidelines based on experience of □ 12,000 cases. Surgery for Obesity and Related Diseases, 2012;8(1):8-19.

9 Gagnon L, Sheff Karwacki EJ. Outcomes and complications after bariatric surgery. AJN. 2012;112(9):26-36.

10 Heller JL, Zieve D. Peritonitis – secondary. Website. http://www.nlm.nih.gov/medlineplus/ency/article/000651.htm. Updated 2010, June 28. Accessed September 7, 2012.

11 Vorvick L, Storck S, Zieve, D. Adhesion. http://www.nlm.nih.gov/medlineplus/ency/article/001493.htm. Updated 2012, February 26. Accessed September 7, 2012.

12 Rosenthal RJ, International Sleeve Gastrectomy Expert Panel. International Sleeve Gastrectomy Expert Panel Consensus Statement: Best practice guidelines based on experience of □ 12,000 cases. Surgery for Obesity and Related Diseases, 2012;8(1):8-19.

13 National Heart Lung and Blood Institute. What is a stent? Website. http://www.nhlbi.nih.gov/health/health-topics/topics/stents/. 2011, November 8. Accessed September 7, 2012.

14 Rosenthal RJ, International Sleeve Gastrectomy Expert Panel. International Sleeve Gastrectomy Expert Panel Consensus Statement: Best practice guidelines based on experience of □ 12,000 cases. Surgery for Obesity and Related Diseases, 2012;8(1):8-19.

15 American Society for Metabolic and Bariatric Surgery. Updated position statement on sleeve gastrectomy as a bariatric procedure. Revised 2011, October 28. http://s3.amazonaws.com/publicASMBS/GuidelinesStatements/PositionStatement/ASMBS-SLEEVE-STATEMENT-2011_10_28.pdf Accessed September 7 2012.

16 Lacy A, Obarzabal A, Pando E, Adelsorfer C, Delitala A, Corcelles R, Delgado S, Vidal J. Revisional surgery after sleeve gastrectomy. Surg Laparosc Endosc Percutan Tech. 2010;20(5):351-6.

17 Rosenthal RJ, International Sleeve Gastrectomy Expert Panel. International Sleeve Gastrectomy Expert Panel Consensus Statement: Best practice guidelines based on experience of □ 12,000 cases. Surgery for Obesity and Related Diseases, 2012;8(1):8-19.

18 American Society for Metabolic and Bariatric Surgery. Updated position statement on sleeve gastrectomy as a bariatric procedure. Revised 2011, October 28. http://s3.amazonaws.com/publicASMBS/GuidelinesStatements/PositionStatement/ASMBS-SLEEVE-STATEMENT-2011_10_28.pdf Accessed September 8, 2012.

19 Gagnon L, Sheff Karwacki EJ. Outcomes and complications after bariatric surgery. AJN. 2012;112(9):26-36.

20 Aarts EO, Janssen, IM, Berends, FJ. The gastric sleeve: losing weight as fast as micronutrients? Obes Surg. 2011;21(2):207-211.

21 Longstreth GF, Zieve, D. Gastresophageal reflux disease. Medline Plus. Website. Updated August 11, 2011. http://www.nlm.nih.gov/medlineplus/ency/article/000265.htm. Accessed September 9, 2012.

22 Rosenthal RJ, International Sleeve Gastrectomy Expert Panel. International Sleeve Gastrectomy Expert Panel Consensus Statement: Best practice guidelines based on experience of □ 12,000 cases. Surgery for Obesity and Related Diseases, 2012;8(1):8-19.

23 Lacy A, Obarzabal A, Pando E, Adelsorfer C, Delitala A, Corcelles R, Delgado S, Vidal J. Revisional surgery after sleeve gastrectomy. Surg Laparosc Endosc Percutan Tech. 2010;20(5):351-6.

24 Hutter, M.M., Schirmer, B.D., Jones, D.B., Ko, C.Y., Cohen, M.E., Merdow, R.P., & Nguyen, N.T. (2011). First report from the American College of Surgeons Bariatric Surgery Center Network: laparoscopic sleeve gastrectomy has morbidity and effectiveness positioned between the band and the bypass. Annals of Surgery, 254:410-420.

25 Gagnon L, Sheff Karwacki EJ. Outcomes and complications after bariatric surgery. AJN. 2012;112(9):26-36.

26 Zieve D, Rogers A. Dumping syndrome. Medline Plus. Website. http://www.nlm.nih.gov/medlineplus/ency/imagepages/19830.htm. Updated 2012, June 4. Accessed September 9, 2012.

27 Tzovaras G, Papamargaritis D, Sioka E, Zachari E, Baloyiannis I, Zacharoulis D, Koukoulis G. Symptoms suggestive of dumping syndrome after provocation in patients after laparoscopic sleeve gastrectomy. Obes Surg. 2012;Jan 22(1):23-8.

28 Gagnon L, Sheff Karwacki EJ. Outcomes and complications after bariatric surgery. AJN. 2012;112(9):26-36.

29 Lacy A, Obarzabal A, Pando E, Adelsorfer C, Delitala A, Corcelles R, Delgado S, Vidal J. Revisional surgery after sleeve gastrectomy. Surg Laparosc Endosc Percutan Tech. 2010;20(5):351-6.

30 Catheline JM, Fysekidis M, Dbouk R, Boschetto A, Bihan H, Reach G, Cohen R. Weight loss after sleeve gastrectomy in super superobesity. J Obes. 2012.

31 Gagnon L, Sheff Karwacki EJ. Outcomes and complications after bariatric surgery. AJN. 2012;112(9):26-36.

32 Catheline JM, Fysekidis M, Dbouk R, Boschetto A, Bihan H, Reach G, Cohen R. Weight loss after sleeve gastrectomy in super superobesity. J Obes. 2012.

33 Catheline JM, Fysekidis M, Dbouk R, Boschetto A, Bihan H, Reach G, Cohen R. Weight loss after sleeve gastrectomy in super superobesity. J Obes. 2012.

34 Moy J, Pomp A, Dakin G, Parikh M, Gagner M. Laparoscopic sleeve gastrectomy for morbid obesity. American Journal of Surgery. 2008;196(5).

35 Lalor PF, Tucker ON, Szomestein S, Rosenthal RJ. Complications after laparoscopic sleeve gastrectomy. Surg Obes Relat Dis. 2007;98(10):1345-55.

36 Keren D, Matter I, Rainis T & Lavy A. Getting the most from the sleeve: the importance of post-operative follow-up. Obesity Surgery. 2011;21(12):1887-1893.

37 Overs SE, Freeman RA, Zarshenas N, Walton KL, Jorgenson JO. Food intolerance and gastrointestinal quality of life following three bariatric procedures: gastric banding, Roux-en-Y gastric bypass and sleeve gastrectomy. Obes Surg. 2012;22(4):536-543.

38 Weiner RA, Theodoridou S, Weiner S. Failure of laparscopic sleeve gastrectomy – further procedure? Obes Facts. 2011;4 Suppl1:42-46.

39 American Society for Metabolic and Bariatric Surgery. Updated position statement on sleeve gastrectomy as a bariatric procedure. Revised 2011, October 28. http://s3.amazonaws.com/publicASMBS/GuidelinesStatements/PositionStatement/ASMBS-SLEEVE-STATEMENT-2011_10_28.pdf Accessed September 8, 2012.

40 Kaplan LM, Seeley RJ, Harris JL. Myths associated with obesity and bariatric surgery – myth 5: patient behavior is the primary determinant of outcomes after bariatric surgery. 2012;9(8):8-10.

41 Gagnon L, Sheff Karwacki EJ. Outcomes and complications after bariatric surgery. AJN. 2012;112(9):26-36.

42 Mayo Clinic Staff. Prescription weight loss drugs: can they help you? Website. http://www.mayoclinic.com/health/weight-loss-drugs/WT00013/METHOD=print Updated 2012, July 27. Accessed September 15, 2012.

43 Hutter MM, Schirmer BD, Jones DB, Ko CY, Cohen ME, Merdow RP, Nguyen NT. First report from the American College of Surgeons Bariatric Surgery Center Network: laparoscopic sleeve gastrectomy has morbidity and effectiveness positioned between the band and the bypass. Annals of Surgery. 2011;254:410-420.

44 Jackson TD, Hutter MM. Morbidity and effectiveness of laporscopic sleeve gastrectomy, adjustable gastric band and gastric bypass for morbid obesity. Advances in Surgery, 2012;46:255-68.

45 Jackson TD, Hutter MM. Morbidity and effectiveness of laporscopic sleeve gastrectomy, adjustable gastric band and gastric bypass for morbid obesity. Advances in Surgery, 2012;46:255-68.

46 Jackson TD, Hutter MM. Morbidity and effectiveness of laporscopic sleeve gastrectomy, adjustable gastric band and gastric bypass for morbid obesity. Advances in Surgery, 2012;46:255-68.

47 Hutter MM, Schirmer BD, Jones DB, Ko CY, Cohen ME, Merdow RP, Nguyen NT. First report from the American College of Surgeons Bariatric Surgery Center Network: laparoscopic sleeve gastrectomy has morbidity and effectiveness positioned between the band and the bypass. Annals of Surgery. 2011;254:410-420.

48 Jackson TD, Hutter MM. Morbidity and effectiveness of laporscopic sleeve gastrectomy, adjustable gastric band and gastric bypass for morbid obesity. Advances in Surgery, 2012;46:255-68.

49 Gagnon L, Sheff Karwacki EJ. Outcomes and complications after bariatric surgery. AJN. 2012;112(9):26-36.

6

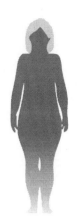

Are you a Good Candidate for the Sleeve?

The last two chapters talked about the pros and cons of the sleeve. Chapter 4 talked about the amount of weight that many patients lose with the VSG and the other likely health benefits of getting the surgery and following the recovery and diet instructions carefully. Chapter 5 introduced some of the risks related to the surgery and sleeve as well as your likelihood of experiencing them.

You're still reading along, so you're probably either leaning toward getting the gastric sleeve or at least interested in finding out more. The sleeve's not a realistic option for everyone who's obese, though. This chapter helps you figure whether the sleeve really is for you. This is what you'll find in the following pages:

- Criteria for getting the sleeve
- Conditions (known as contraindications) that may prevent you from getting the sleeve
- Pregnancy and the sleeve
- Getting the sleeve as a revisional surgery
- The sleeve and adolescents: special considerations
- Review of the sleeve as you approach your decision

By the end of this chapter, you'll have a much better idea about whether the vertical sleeve gastrectomy is for you.

Eligibility Criteria for the Sleeve

So far, this chapter and the one before have discussed the sleeve's potential benefits and risks for causing complications. At this point, the vertical sleeve may seem like a good option for you: you've thought about the benefits and risks, and believe that this weight loss surgery can be the answer to your obesity.

But not everyone is a good candidate to get the sleeve. You have to meet certain requirements, known as eligibility criteria, before you can get the vertical sleeve. This section will cover the eligibility criteria so you can figure out whether you meet them. Also, we'll go over the contraindications, or potential reasons that would prevent you from being a good candidate even if you meet the other criteria.

Eligibility Criteria

The first requirement to get the sleeve is that you have a lot of weight to lose. The sleeve is not just to help you lose a few pounds:

- BMI over 40. That's a weight of 233 pounds for someone who's 5 feet, 4 inches tall, and 278 pounds for someone who's 5 feet, 10 inches tall.
- At least 100 pounds over a recommended BMI of 25. That's 245 pounds for someone who's 5 feet, 4 inches tall, and 275 pounds for someone who's 5 feet, 10 inches tall.

- BMI over 35 with an obesity-related comorbidity, such as type 2 diabetes, high cholesterol or osteoarthritis. That's a weight of 204 pounds for someone who's 5 feet, 4 inches tall, and 244 pounds for someone who's 5 feet, 10 inches tall.

In addition to meeting one of the above weight criteria, you will probably need to meet the requirements below before a surgeon will recommend the sleeve for you. These are some of the standard eligibility criteria for the sleeve:

- You have a history of failed diet attempts. You might have lost and regained the same weight, or failed to lose significant amounts of weight while making serious diet attempts.
- Your obesity isn't caused by a metabolic disorder, such as hypothyroidism.[1]
- You are between 18 and 60 years old.[2]
- You understand that you play a major role in your own weight loss after getting the sleeve.
- You are willing to attend post-surgery care appointments and support group sessions.

Different surgeons may change these criteria slightly.[3] For example, some surgeons may be willing to perform the surgery if your BMI is between 30 and 35 and you have a serious comorbidity related to your obesity. Other surgeons might accept older adults or adolescents under age 18. If you don't quite meet the standard eligibility criteria, you'll have to ask surgeons if they believe you should get the surgery. Your insurance policy may have additional requirements, such as following a pre-surgery diet similar to that of the post-surgery sleeve diet that you'll be on for years. We'll cover some of those possibilities in the next chapter.

Contraindications

Contraindications are conditions or circumstances that can prevent you from being a good candidate for the sleeve. They may be health conditions that are made worse by the VSG procedure or they can be health conditions or other factors that make you less likely to succeed with the sleeve. These are some likely contraindications for getting the sleeve[4]

- *Advanced congestive heart failure*: it puts you at very high risk during surgery.
- Substance abuse: surgeons argue that if you can't get over your alcohol or drug addictions, you might not have the mental strength to stick to the VSG diet.
- *Untreated depression or other psychological disorders*: The sleeve lifestyle is a challenge that requires a lot of mental strength. Struggling with a psychopathology while facing your new sleeve lifestyle can make your condition worse or prevent successful weight loss with the sleeve.
- *A compromised immune system*: if you have an infectious disease or weak immune system, you're more susceptible to infections resulting from surgery. They can become serious and even lead to organ failure if your body isn't able to fight them off.
- *A very low pain tolerance*: you'll be in pain after surgery as your surgical wounds heal. If

you know that you're not as good at dealing with pain as some people, you might want to consider another option beside the VSG.

Not all health conditions are automatically contraindications for the sleeve. Even though they may increase some of your risks with the sleeve, they're not considered to be contraindications because the benefits of losing significant amounts of weight with the sleeve may outweigh their risks. Members of the American Society for Metabolic and Bariatric Surgery (ASMBS) agree that these are some conditions are likely not to be contraindications[5]

- Patients at high risk for obesity-related health complications, such as type 2 diabetes
- Individuals with coronary heart disease that is likely to be improved with significant weight loss
- Individuals with cirrhosis or fatty liver disease[6]
- Lack of understanding about how the sleeve works. There's no rush to make your decision. Take your time continuing your research on the VSG until you feel confident that you know enough about the procedure to make the right decision for yourself.

The Sleeve and Pregnancy

Obesity is one of the most common causes of infertility in the U.S. Losing a significant amount of extra body fat can help you conceive a child. If you're a woman, having a healthy body weight during pregnancy can make your pregnancy easier and less risky for you.[7] There are benefits for your child, too. When you're at a healthy weight during pregnancy, your baby is less likely to be:

- Low birth weight
- Premature
- Prone to diabetes
- Overweight or obese as a child or adult

If you are hoping to become a parent, be sure to discuss pregnancy with your primary care physician and surgeon as you decide whether to get the sleeve. You will need to consider the following factors as you plan your pregnancy:[8]

- You should wait at least 12 to 18 months following your surgery before getting pregnant.[9]
- During this time, your hormones are still changing from the VSG and rapid weight loss. These hormonal changes during pregnancy can affect the growth and development of your child.
- The VSG puts you at some risk for nutrient deficiencies, including folate deficiency. It's best to wait until your nutrients are under control before getting pregnant to reduce the risk of having a baby with a neural tube birth defect due to your low levels of folate.

- The sleeve restricts the amount of food you can eat, but you need to get enough nutrients to support a growing fetus. You may need supplements, such as protein shakes.

We'll talk more about pregnancy later in the book so that you can get more information on supporting a healthy pregnancy after getting the sleeve.

The Gastric Sleeve as a Revisional Surgery

Earlier in the chapter we talked about the vertical sleeve being converted into a different procedure, such as the gastric bypass or BDP-DS. Those are options that can happen if for some reason the sleeve doesn't work out for you. The opposite can also happen – that is, the VSG can be a revisional surgery for another kind of weight loss surgery if that first surgery didn't lead to the results you want. You can get the sleeve as a revisional surgery after having a gastric bypass, getting the adjustable gastric band, having the vertical banded gastroplasty, or VBG, or even after an initial sleeve gastrectomy. The most common reasons for a revisional sleeve gastrectomy as a conversion from an original procedure are for disappointing weight loss or weight regain, consistent vomiting and blockage of your throat, or obstruction.[10]

> **Tip**
>
> Chapter 2, "Weight Loss Options," explains the gastric band and the vertical banded gastroplasty. Reviewing them can help you understand how they can be converted into sleeve gastrectomies.

VSG as a Revisional Procedure from the Gastric Band

You can get the sleeve if you are not happy with your results from the adjustable gastric band, which comes in brand names like the Lap-Band and Realize Band. The band is fully reversible; your surgeon just needs to take it out and make sure your stomach and digestive system are fully healed before proceeding with your sleeve gastrectomy. One-quarter of lap-band patients get the device removed eventually.[11]

Why would you opt to get the sleeve gastrectomy after the band? For some patients, the band didn't turn out to be the right tool to meet their weight loss goals. Some patients report that they never feel any restriction with the gastric band, so it doesn't help them with their weight loss. Another reason why some patients choose to get the sleeve instead of the band is that some foods can cause complications. With the band, you might not be able to eat these foods:[12]

- Stringy foods like broccoli, pineapples and asparagus
- Doughy bread
- Sticky foods, such as dried fruit and peanut butter
- Seeds, nuts and popcorn

Best Practice Guidelines: Opinions from the Forefront of the Field

Sometimes, a group of medical experts come together to discuss a certain medical issue. In this case, experts from hospitals and university medical centers discussed bariatric surgery for adolescents. Their purpose was to come up with recommendations, known as best practice guidelines, based on the latest scientific research. The group of experts provided suggestions for:

- When weight loss surgery should be considered for adolescents
- When it's not a good idea
- The pros and cons of different procedures
- Expected results
- Special considerations for planning for and taking advantage of weight loss surgery at this age

Basically, these experts did the research so you don't have to! This section of the chapter summarizes their recommendations for the VSG and adolescents.

VSG as a Revisional Procedure from the Vertical Banded Gastroplasty

The VBG is rarely performed any more in the U.S., but you might have had the procedure done a while ago. [13]Only one out of five VBG patients keeps the weight off for at least ten years. [14] The sleeve can be an option if you're not happy with your weight loss results with the VBG. Another reason to consider the VSG is if the VBG is causing health problems, such as nausea and vomiting, spleen damage heartburn. Another possible complication with the VBG is that it can leak at the staple line and cause infections. With the VBG, you essentially have the larger part of your stomach stapled shut and folded away. During the conversion process, the surgeon removes the staples and the majority of your stomach.

VSG as a Revisional Procedure from the Roux-en-Y Gastric Bypass

The gastric bypass is reversible, although the process isn't so easy. One reason why some gastric bypass patients choose to convert their Roux-en-Y procedure to a vertical sleeve is to reduce discomfort from dumping syndrome, which can cause nausea, diarrhea and weakness after eating high-sugar or high-fat foods. In addition, the Roux-en-Y is a malabsorptive procedure, so it increases your risk for nutrient deficiencies.

Resleeve Gastrectomy: Another Attempt at the Vertical Sleeve

A re-sleeve gastrectomy can be an option if your weight loss after the first procedure didn't meet your goals or if you begin to gain weight again.[15] This is especially likely if the failed first procedure is due to your surgeon leaving too much of your stomach behind, so your food intake isn't as limited as you'd hoped. You may also need a re-sleeve if you have a persistent leak, which can lead to health complications. During the procedure, the surgeon would locate the leak and be sure to sew it up so that it is sealed.

Considerations with a Revisional Bariatric Surgery

Revisional sleeve gastrectomies can work, whether they are converting from a different procedure or a re-sleeve of your first VSG. Different studies have shown that patients are likely to lose weight as expected, and their obesity-related comorbidities, such as type two diabetes, sleep apnea and osteoarthritis, become much less serious on average. Another piece of good news is that the revisional sleeve gastrectomy can usually be laparoscopic, just like if you were getting it as an original surgery. That's true even if your first surgery was an open procedure.[16]

All revision surgeries have higher rates of complications than the first surgery. This includes your risk for damage to the spleen, excessive bleeding, and leakage at the staple line. The risk of leaking is especially high after conversion from Roux-en-Y gastric bypass because that surgery included cuts at the lower esophageal sphincter, which separates the top of your stomach from your lower esophagus, and the pyloric sphincter, which separates the bottom of your stomach from the top of your small intestine.

A critical factor to consider when you're thinking about the VSG as a revisional surgery is why the first surgery didn't work for you. The VSG may be a good option if it's to solve (or at least mitigate) a medical problem caused by your first procedure. And, it might be good if you're not feeling the proper amount of restriction needed to help you lose weight, as some lap-band patients report.

However, the VSG as a revisional procedure is *not* a substitute for dedication to your sleeve diet. If the reason you did not hit your weight loss goals was that you were not following the prescribed diet, you will not hit your weight loss goals with the sleeve unless you change your actions. If you developed complications with your gastric band, the gastric bypass, or the first sleeve because you didn't follow the proper post-surgery eating patterns, you're likely to face the same troubles after the revisional VSG unless you have a new dedication.

For the sleeve to be successful weight loss tool, you must be committed to the required diet for the long term.

What about the Sleeve and Adolescents?

Adolescent obesity is just as big of a public health concern as obesity among adults. Adolescent obesity rates are increasing at a frightening rate, and more than one-third of children and adolescents are overweight or obese.[17] Four percent of children and adolescents, or one out of 25, has extreme obesity.[18] These children and adolescents are more likely to become obese adults. And, just like adults, many of them are already suffering the consequences of their excess weight. These include the following:

- High cholesterol and other risk factors for heart disease
- Type 2 diabetes or poorly controlled blood sugar
- Osteoarthritis
- Sleep apnea
- Higher risk for some kinds of cancer later in life
- Social stigma
- Low self-esteem
- Poorer performance in school

Eligibility for Weight Loss Surgery in Adolescence: Weight Criteria

As with adults, bariatric surgery can potentially be an effective treatment for adolescent obesity. However, the weight criteria for the surgery are different for adolescents than for adults.[19] That's to help prevent adolescents from getting the surgery when they don't truly need it.

- A BMI over 50.
- A BMI over 40 and a less serious comorbidity, or obesity-related condition such as high blood pressure, depression or high cholesterol.
- A BMI over 35 and a serious comorbidity, such as sleep apnea, type 2 diabetes, increased pressure within the skull or liver disease.

Eligibility for Weight Loss Surgery in Adolescence: Maturity

Maturity is the greatest difference between adults and adolescents when considering medical treatments such as weight loss surgery. Insufficient physical and/or psychological maturity can make the sleeve an ineffective or dangerous procedure. Surgeons are likely to ask these questions before recommending the VSG for teenagers:

- Does the adolescent have enough family support? Most adolescents are still living at home and depending on their parents for food and emotional support. Adolescents are more likely to succeed with the sleeve if their families are willing show their support and commit to the lifestyle required for weight loss with the sleeve.
- How old is the adolescent, and at what point in his or her physical development? Adolescents should not get the surgery if they are still early in their growth spurt.
- How psychologically mature is the adolescent? Adolescence, especially early and mid-adolescence, is a time of emotional turmoil for some. The VSG presents a variety of challenges that can be difficult even for the most stable adult to take in stride. Adolescents become more independent and are more likely to be equipped to success with the sleeve when they're closer to adulthood than earlier on.
- Does the adolescent fully understand the procedure and its risks? Does the adolescent understand and accept his or her role and responsibility for success with the sleeve?

VSG in Adolescence: Further Considerations

The sleeve is pretty new as a stand-alone procedure as an obesity treatment, and there still isn't much long-term information about using the sleeve for obese adolescents. The sleeve appears to have potential as an effective obesity treatment in adolescents, and it's less likely to cause nutritional deficiencies than Roux-en-Y gastric bypass. However, because of the lack of definite information and the irreversibility of the procedure, the a panel of experts recommends that the safest option at this point in time is to only opt for the VSG as part of a carefully controlled clinical trial. That way, you'll be under the constant watch of medical professionals.

These are some of the best practice guidelines, or standard recommendations, for adolescents who choose to get the sleeve. They're not absolute requirements, but considering each of these factors when planning the surgery gives you (or your adolescent, if you're a parent) the best chances of success:[20]

- If you are a parent, do not force your child into having the surgery. Adolescents who are forced into getting weight loss surgery are not likely to succeed.
- When possible, the procedure should be done in a bariatric hospital with healthcare team members who have special training in pediatrics or adolescent health.
- The healthcare team should include: a surgeon, a pediatrician, a dietitian, a mental health professional, and a team coordinator
- Adolescents need to be especially careful to get enough iron, vitamin B12 and calcium to prevent deficiencies. Osteopenia, or poor bone mineral density related to inadequate calcium or vitamin D, and thiamine or vitamin B1 deficiency are also threats.
- Female adolescents should understand that they should not get pregnant within at least 18 months of having the surgery.

Weight loss surgery is a serious decision for anyone, and adolescents have even more things to think about. It's a very individual decision that should not be taken lightly. To succeed with the sleeve, an adolescent who gets the sleeve needs to be close to physical maturity, mentally and emotionally capable, and supported at home. Adolescents need to understand the long-term commitment necessary—not only to lose weight and keep it off, but to prevent complications for life.

Likely Effects of the Sleeve

With so much information over the last few chapters, you might be feeling a little confused. It can be hard to pick out the parts that matter most to *you* when you're learning so much information for the first time. *Table 16* summarizes some of the likely effects of the VSG that can be most important to you.

Measure	Likely Effects of the Sleeve
Weight Loss	The sleeve can provide hope for long-term successful weight loss even if you've not been able to overcome your obesity with serious diet attempts. It can lead to hundreds of pounds of weight loss, far more than with any current weight loss drugs.21 The amount of weight that most sleeve patients lose is between what is achieved with the lap-band and gastric bypass.
Likely Side Effects	The sleeve will almost certainly be very painful for the first week or more after surgery. If you go off of the sleeve diet, you might have diarrhea, vomiting, nausea, and cramping. These are comparable to the side effects from weight loss drugs, which can cause dizziness, sweating, nausea, dry mouth, diarrhea, and constipation. However, these weight loss drug effects are largely unavoidable. Other possibilities of side effects from the sleeve are gallstones, resulting from rapid weight loss, and food intolerances.
Possible complications	As discussed in Chapter 5, there is always the possibility of these when you have surgery: • death • excessive bleeding • an embolism or blood clot Other complications with the sleeve can include : • stricture • leakage • gastroesophageal reflux disease, or GERD.
Nutrition	Your current diet is supporting obesity and may still be making you gain weight. The diet likely has these characteristics:22 • high in calories • high in saturated (unhealthy) fat and sugar • low in nutrient-rich foods, such as fruits, vegetables and whole grains The sleeve diet is more likely to have these characteristics: 23 • calorie-controlled • high in lean protein • low in sugar and saturated fat • contains fruits and vegetables You're at nutritional risk from the sleeve because of the low amount of food you'll be eating, but you can prevent nutritional deficiencies by choosing nutrient-dense foods and taking dietary supplements as recommended by your dietitian. Overdosing on supplements can also be harmful.

Measure	Likely Effects of the Sleeve
Health	Maybe your mother, father, sister, or brother had or has an obesity-related health condition, and maybe you've had your own scare. These are some common conditions that can be improved after getting the sleeve and losing weight: • type 2 diabetes • high cholesterol or blood pressure • osteoarthritis and joint pain • sleep apnea and asthma
Quality of Life	The bottom line is that your quality life is the most important reason to get the sleeve. There's no reason to undergo surgery and put in the effort needed for success if your live doesn't get better. Everyone's different, but these are some ways that your life could be affected: • better self-esteem • lower risk for depression • more social confidence • more mobility and stamina so you can participate in fun activities • better ability to get pregnant and more likely to have a healthy pregnancy and baby

Table 16: Likely Effects of the Sleeve

✐ Summary

☛ This chapter was an opportunity for the sleeve to become more real to you. By now, you have a good idea of whether you're eligible and a good candidate for the surgery. You have the information you need about whether to pursue the gastric sleeve gastrectomy to treat your obesity. The next chapter will help you move forward if you think you're going to go for the sleeve. There is a lot of planning to do, so let's get going!

Your Turn: Getting Ready for Your Surgeon Visits

Are you ready and able to take the first steps toward getting the VSG? Table 17 is a quick checklist of some factors to consider when thinking about the sleeve. For each consideration in the left column, highlight or circle the middle box or the right box depending on the accurate answer. Then take a look and see whether you think you're eligible for the sleeve.

Consideration	Candidate for the Vertical Sleeve Gastrectomy	Possible Contraindication
Age	Over 18 years old	Under 18 years old
BMI		
	Over 40	Under 40 with no comorbidity
	35 to 40 with a comorbidity	Under 35
Other medical conditions	none	Heart or lung conditions; bleeding disorders
Pregnancy	No, and not planning to become pregnant within a year	Yes, or planning to soon
Readiness to commit	Yes, completely ready to commit to drastic, long-term dietary changes	No, not sure about commitment or ability to follow the sleeve diet
Understand the process	Yes, recognize my role in weight loss	No, would prefer to depend on a weight loss treatment that will do everything for me
Average ability to tolerate pain	Yes, at least average pain tolerance	No, cannot imagine recovering from a surgery without high doses of pain medications for a long time
Alcohol or drug addictions	No, none.	Yes, abuse alcohol or drugs
Mental conditions	No, none; or, I am under treatment and they are well-controlled	Yes, and they are severe and not always under control.

Table 17: Checklist of factors to consider when thinking about the sleeve

1   Nall R. The ups and downs of vertical sleeve gastrectomy. Healthline. Website. http://www.healthline.com/health/vertical-sleeve-gastrectomy. Published 2012, May 29. Accessed September 13, 2012.

2   Gagnon L, Sheff Karwacki EJ. Outcomes and complications after bariatric surgery. AJN. 2012;112(9):26-36.

3   Nall R. The ups and downs of vertical sleeve gastrectomy. Healthline. Website. http://www.healthline.com/health/vertical-sleeve-gastrectomy. Published 2012, May 29. Accessed September 13, 2012.

4   Gagnon L, Sheff Karwacki EJ. Outcomes and complications after bariatric surgery. AJN. 2012;112(9):26-36.

5   Rosenthal RJ, International Sleeve Gastrectomy Expert Panel. International Sleeve Gastrectomy Expert Panel Consensus Statement: Best practice guidelines based on experience of 12,000 cases. Surgery for Obesity and Related Diseases, 2012;8(1):8-19.

6   Barreto CJ, Sarr MG, Swain JM. Bariatric surgery in patients with liver cirrhosis and portal hypertension. Bariatric Times. 2009, July 14. http://bariatrictimes.com/2009/07/14/bariatric-surgery-in-patients-with-liver-cirrhosis-and-portal-hypertension/ Accessed September 13, 2012.

7   National Heart, Lung and Blood Institute. High blood pressure in pregnancy. National Institutes of Health. Website. http://www.nhlbi.nih.gov/health/public/heart/hbp/hbp_preg.htm. Accessed September 13, 2012.

8   Delamont K. Clinical considerations and recommendations for pregnancy after bariatric surgery. Bariatric Times. 2011;8(10):12-14.

9   Ziegler O, Sirveaux MA, Brunaud L, Reibel N, Quillot D. Medical follow-up after bariatric surgery: nutritional and drug issues. General recommendations for the prevention and treatment of nutritional deficiencies. Diabetes Metab. 2009;35(6 Pt 2):544-547.

10 Berende CAS, de Zoete JP, Smulders JF, Nienhuijs SW. Laparoscopic sleeve gastrectomy feasible for bariatric revision surgery. Obes Surg. 2012;22(2):330-334.

11 Frey R. Vertical banded gastroplasty. Website. http://www.healthline.com/galecontent/vertical-banded-gastroplasty. 2004. Accessed September 12, 2012.

12 Bioenterics Corporation. (ND). Information for patients, a surgical aid in the treatment for morbid obesity: a decision guide for adults. Inamed. Accessed September 12 2012 from http://www.lapband.com/local/files/Surgical_Aid_Booklet.pdf.

13 Berende CAS, de Zoete JP, Smulders JF, Nienhuijs SW. Laparoscopic sleeve gastrectomy feasible for bariatric revision surgery. Obes Surg. 2012;22(2):330-334.

14 Bioenterics Corporation. (ND). Information for patients, a surgical aid in the treatment for morbid obesity: a decision guide for adults. Inamed. Accessed September 12 2012 from http://www.lapband.com/local/files/Surgical_Aid_Booklet.pdf.

15 Iannelli A, Schneck AS, Noel P, Amor IB, Krawczykowski D, Gugenheim J. Re-sleeve gastrectomy for failed laparoscopic sleeve gastrectomy: a feasibility study. Obes Surg. 2011;21(7):832-835.

16 Berende CAS, de Zoete JP, Smulders JF, Nienhuijs SW. Laparoscopic sleeve gastrectomy feasible for bariatric revision surgery. Obes Surg. 2012;22(2):330-334.

17 Centers for Disease Control and Prevention. Childhood obesity facts. Website. http://www.cdc.gov/HealthyYouth/obesity/facts.htm. 2012, June 7. Accessed September 13, 2012.

18 Xanthakos SA. Bariatric surgery for extreme adolescent obesity: indications, outcomes and physiologic effects on the gut-brain axis. Pathophysiology. 2008;15(2):135-46.

19 Nagle A, Zieve D. Weight-loss surgery and children. Website. http://www.nlm.nih.gov/medlineplus/ency/patientinstructions/000356.htm. Updated 2011, July 1. Accessed September 13, 2012.

20 Pratt JSA, Lenders CM, Dionne EA, Hoppin AG, Hsu GLK., Inge, TH, …, & Sanchez VM. Best practice updates for pediatric/adolescent weight loss surgery. Obesity (Silver Spring). 2009;17(5):901-910.

21 Mayo Clinic Staff. Prescription weight loss drugs: can they help you? Website. http://www.mayoclinic.com/health/weight-loss-drugs/WT00013/METHOD=print Updated 2012, July 27. Accessed September 15, 2012.

22 Martinez-Gomez, MA, Garcia-Arellano A, et al. A 14-item Mediterranean diet assessment tool and obesity indices among high-risk subjects: the PREDIMED trial. PLoS One. 2012;7(8):e431-34.

23 Snyder-Marlow G, Tayle D, Lenhard MJ. Nutrition care for patients undergoing laparoscopic sleeve gastrectomy for weight loss. J Am Diet Ass. 2010;110(4):600-607

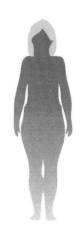

7

Tips When Planning for the Sleeve

So...you've decided to get the sleeve! Congratulations on making your choice – it always feels great to have the decision behind you so you don't have to go back and forth over it any more. This chapter assumes the following basic points:

- You fully understand the VSG and how it works.
- You've looked at the amount of weight that the sleeve is likely to help you lose, and you are happy with that amount.
- You've weighed the pros and cons and decided that the benefits outweigh the drawbacks.
- You understand your role and responsibility in losing weight with the sleeve and are willing to make a long-term commitment to success.

You're excited to take this life-changing step, but where do you even begin? How do you go from being an interested examiner to a sleeve patient? And how do you make sure you get the best possible care? This chapter will explain these topics so you can build a solid foundation for success with the sleeve:

- Learning more about the sleeve
- Finding and choosing a surgeon
- Getting the rest of your healthcare team together
- Paying for surgery: insurance and other options
- Medical tourism: getting the sleeve in another country

This chapter is full of actions for you to take, and you'll be much further in your path toward surgery by the end of this chapter. Ready to get started? Let's go!

Research, Research and More Research

You may have been researching weight loss surgery and the sleeve gastrectomy for years, or it may be a new idea that you just learned about. Maybe the first few chapters of this book are all you know about the sleeve. Regardless of how much or little you already know, more research on the sleeve can always be helpful. Being well-informed lets you take the right steps in your preparation for surgery to improve your chances of successful weight loss with minimal side effects and complications.

What should you be learning about? These are a few questions to start you off:

- How do I choose the best surgeon?
- How can I finance my surgery?
- How do I prepare for surgery?
- What will the recovery be like? How will I feel?
- What dietary changes can I expect?

- Where do most people get the support they need to get through this experience?
- How do I know if I'm emotionally prepared for this change in my life?

Get answers to your new questions, and keep an open mind for additional answers to your old questions. You might get new insights or perspectives when you ask the same question to different people or look in different sources. You're more likely to get better care and have better health when you stay involved in your care. You can't prevent all risks or guarantee a certain amount of weight loss, but you can definitely increase your chances of the results you want by staying informed.

Possible Sources of Information

Where do you go to get information? It can be a little tough to get started, but you'll find that you're able to come up with resources more easily with a little practice. Many of the sources you find will lead you to one or more additional sources, and you'll soon have a wealth of trustworthy possibilities. BariatricPal.com is a great starting point and a source to carry you through surgery and beyond, no matter how much you know!

Reading Material

What can you read beside this book? There aren't too many other books dedicated solely to the sleeve gastrectomy, but that's probably just because it's a pretty new weight loss surgery technique. There will probably be more VSG books soon. In the meantime, there are a ton of weight loss surgery books that cover general points about the surgery. You can learn about things such as:

- Qualifying for surgery
- Paying for surgery with insurance or yourself
- The pre-surgery and post-surgery diets
- How to set goals and work through challenges
- Which side effects and complications can occur
- How other sleeve patients describe their experiences
- How to prepare for the surgery and what to take to the hospital

This book covers these topics and more, but getting the information from additional sources helps you remember it better.

You don't literally have to set foot in the library or a bookstore if that's just not your style. The point is to read everything you can get your hands on. Beside books, magazines can be excellent sources of information. Weight loss-focused or lifestyle-focused magazines may have in-depth articles on specific weight loss patients, procedures, surgeons, or facilities.

> **Tip**
>
> Chapter 6, "Are you a Good Candidate for the Sleeve?" discusses the sleeve gastrectomy as a revisional surgery after a failed lap-band procedure.

Surprisingly, newspapers can be a great starting point for research. Pay close attention each time you see an article about weight loss surgery in general or the sleeve gastrectomy in particular. You can use the article to help you think through your own decisions. For example, you might see a news article, such as one published on Yahoo.com in September of 2012, describing someone who got the sleeve gastrectomy as a revisional surgery after the lap-band didn't work for her.[1] This article might make you think about what allows you to trust a surgeon, what you're looking for with your own surgery, and why the sleeve might work for her when the lap-band didn't.

The News

The news can be a great conversation starter when you're trying to get information about the sleeve. You can ask about an issue that you read about in the newspaper, a magazine or online, see on TV or hear about on the radio. Paying attention to the news gives you a good starting point when you're calling around to find a surgeon or you're talking to sleeve patients whom you don't know that well. Ask their opinions and find out their reasoning to help you get an inside scoop and another perspective—the news media don't always tell the whole story.

The Internet

The Internet is a great resource for research at any point during your sleeve journey. It's an unlimited source of information covering pretty much everything. Start with basic searches, using keywords such as "sleeve gastrectomy" or "vertical sleeve diet." You'll probably soon find that the search engines repeatedly direct you to a few sites, and these are often the most complete and useful. You'll develop your own favorite sources as you get familiar with the options.

Sites for Fact-Finding

Not everything you read on the internet is true. Anyone can post statements and advice online without any verification. You can't always be certain about whether your source is accurate or not, but a few general guidelines can help you make good decisions.[2]

- *Check the website domain, or the three letters at the end of the web address.* Sites ending in ".edu" and ".gov" are typically credible; they're sponsored respectively by educational institutions and the government.

- *Company sites, ending in ".com," and organizations' sites, ending in ".org," can have good information.* Just be aware of their possible causes. Companies are probably going to push a product or service. Organizations may be pushing certain causes, such as pro-weight loss surgery or anti-insurance coverage for the LSG procedure.

- *Think about potential bias.* Does the owner of the website have an obvious interest in trying to persuade you one way or another? A surgeon who specializes in the sleeve, for example, might paint a rosy picture of the VSG while portraying the other weight loss surgeries as particularly negative. Or a company that offers weight loss surgery packages to Mexico might emphasize the high cost of the surgery in the U.S. and the ease of getting the surgery done in Mexico.

- *Check other sites.* Any information that you find on one site is probably going to be findable on other sites if it's true information. This isn't a foolproof method, though; sometimes misinformation is repeated.

- *Use common sense.* Sometimes, you just have to use your best judgment. A good rule of thumb is to avoid making serious decisions based on what you find online if you're not certain about its truth. Instead, pose your questions to a surgeon or another qualified professional, such as a dietitian if you have diet questions.

Online Communities: Others' Personal Experiences and Asking Your Own Questions

Online communities, such as discussion boards and social networks, can be valuable research resources. Members of communities are often willing to share their experiences and advice for each stage of your sleeve gastrectomy process from making the decision to get the sleeve to learning how to live with it. You can ask detailed questions about your particular situation and concerns and get more personalized answers to your questions than when you stick to solely informational sites.

Online communities are abundant, but there are few that are dedicated solely to the sleeve gastrectomy. BariatricPal.com is one of those. It is specifically geared toward sleeve patients and individuals who are considering getting the sleeve or are already scheduled for it. BariatricPal.com has some other advantages, too:

- It has a high standard of courtesy and its moderators are constantly looking out for anyone who violates the zero-tolerance policy.

- It is absolutely free to join and use all the features.

- There are separate discussion boards dedicated to different topics and audiences, so you can find what you need easily whether you're looking for diet information, post-surgery recovery tips or stories from moms who got the sleeve.

- You can use it to help find a surgeon (more about that later in this chapter).

Talking to People to Gather Information

People are among your best resources. In general, people are very willing to share their own experiences, especially if they think they can help you out. It can be tough to get started if you feel shy about considering the sleeve. Also, chances are that you don't know — or don't *think* you know — anyone with the sleeve. Remember, though, that you're not the first person to get the sleeve! Once you start to ask around, you may realize that more people have gotten the VSG than you thought. A great way to find VSG patients is through bariatric surgeons. They might invite you to a weight loss surgery support group meeting so you can meet sleeve patients. Surgeons and clinical staff may also have lists of gastric sleeve patients who have said they're willing to talk to people like you who need information.

Patients whose surgeries were more recent will be able to remember and tell you about many of the changes in their lives. Patients who are further out from surgery have a longer-term perspective, and can offer insights on what works and what doesn't in the long run. These are some of the unique perspectives that you can get from vertical sleeve patients:

- Things they wish they had known before the surgery
- What they would have changed if they could do it over again
- Some of the hardest parts about the surgery and lifestyle changes
- Whether they're glad that they got the surgery

Medical Professionals

Who better to go to for learning about the sleeve gastrectomy than medical professionals who've dedicated their lives to the procedure? These healthcare professionals should be able to answer your questions about the procedure, preparation for and recovery from surgery, the diet, the risks, and what to expect throughout your experience

- Bariatric surgeons
- Dietitians with experience in working with sleeve patients
- Bariatric center staff members, such as nurses and receptionists

You can call their offices, contact them via website contact forms, or even try walking in off the street if you prefer to make face to face contact. They should be well-equipped to answer your questions and offer additional facts that you might not have even thought about since they take care of patients like you every day. Surgeons can show you diagrams of the surgical process and explain the post-surgical care that you'll receive; dietitians can go over sample meal plans, and nurses can describe your in-clinic experience.

Weight Loss Surgery Seminar

Weight loss surgery seminars are excellent opportunities to learn more about the vertical sleeve gastrectomy. Seminars can be the better part of a day or just a few hours. They're typically free, but they may require telephone or online administration days or weeks in advance. Because seminars can get pretty crowded, you might only be allowed to bring one single guest. Usually, the seminar's main speaker is a surgeon; there may be multiple surgeons if the seminar is hosted by a larger facility. There may also be some sleeve and other weight loss surgery patients to share their experiences and answer your questions about personal experiences.

Many bariatric surgery seminars cover the other types of surgeries, too. The seminars may be sponsored by hospital bariatric centers or other clinics specializing in bariatric surgery, and they will probably include a presentation on each type of weight loss surgery that they offer. This is a good chance for you not only to learn more about the sleeve gastrectomy. It also encourages you to reconsider – and possibly reaffirm – your choice of the sleeve over the other weight loss surgeries. Now that you've read the first part of this book and you're a little more familiar with the VSG and the other surgeries, you'll be able to get lot more out of a seminar.

A benefit of attending seminars is that they give you the chance to get to know the presenting surgeon in person. If you like that surgeon, you might end up selecting him or her for your surgery. That's not always practical, since the surgeon may be located too far away from your home to be practical or may not accept your insurance. Still, you can ask the surgeon for his or her recommendations to get a lead on some other possibilities.

While attending the seminar, you'll get tons of questions answered, and probably get answers to questions you didn't even know you had. You might also discover some new questions that you can ask your potential surgeon or a few new aspects to consider as you plan. The seminar may be your first opportunity to ask about your specific situation, so take a list of questions with you and bring pencil and paper to jot down notes.

To summarize, these are some things to think about when you're at a seminar:

- Are you now confident that you understand enough about the VSG process and life after getting the sleeve?
- Are you clear about the risks and benefits of the sleeve, especially as compared to other weight loss surgery options?
- Did the seminar bring up any new concerns about the sleeve?
- Do you like the surgeon who gave the seminar enough to consider choosing him or her for your own procedure?
- Do you now have a list of questions and criteria that can guide you when you're selecting a surgeon?

You can find a seminar by searching online. Another option is to call around to a few local bariatric center clinics and ask them for information about their seminars and other seminars in the region. Don't despair if the seminar schedule doesn't fit with yours or there are no upcoming seminars. Some seminars are offered as live webcasts. That means you can watch them live online from your computer. This type of seminar is often set up to let you participate by typing in your questions and comments. Pre-recorded seminars are options if you just can't make a live or webcast seminar in real-time. Save your questions to ask a surgeon when you get a chance.

Learn Your Terms

Your research isn't helpful if you don't understand what you're reading. Be sure to look up medical terms and other VSG-related words that you don't know. Many of them are located in this book's glossary, but some won't be. That's okay; we've left space for your new terms in the glossary. Just write each new term in the table along with the definition and where you saw it. If you do this, all of your new words and definitions will be in the same easy-to-remember place.

Now we're really getting to the exciting part of your vertical sleeve experience. In the next part of this chapter, we'll go over the process of selecting a surgeon and figuring out where you'll get your surgery done and who the other members of your healthcare team are. It's a challenging job, but we'll give you tips and guidelines to make it easier. You want to make the most you can out of this early stage of your VSG experience.

First, why are choosing a surgeon, locating your clinic and assembling the rest of your team so important? Despite your best intentions, deep commitment, and in-depth research, your own actions aren't the only factor in your success.[3] You are more likely to have better weight loss, fewer complications and a better overall experience if your surgeon is competent, your hospital or clinic has the right amenities, and your healthcare team members are experienced in treating bariatric patients. In addition, a comprehensive post-surgery care program contributes to your success, so it's better to make sure that your surgeon leads one or has provisions for you to be enrolled in one.[4]

If the process is so critical, how can it be fun, too? Here's why. At this point in your life, *you* get to be in charge. *You* are hand-picking the group of experts who will take care of you over the coming months and years. In fact, you might even want to approach the process as though it were a series of interviews. The truth is that each member of your team is applying for the privilege of working with you.

These are some of the basic questions that you need to have answered and should keep in mind when gathering information and making your decision:

- Do you have a formal vertical sleeve gastrectomy or bariatric patient support program that starts before surgery and goes through surgery and for years afterward?
- How much experience do you have with the sleeve gastrectomy? How many sleeve gastrectomies have you done, and how many procedures do you perform in an average month?
- Do you primarily perform sleeve gastrectomies? What other bariatric surgeries do you do, and how many? How do you choose which procedure to perform on a patient?
- Is your facility (clinic or department) dedicated to bariatric patients? Do you treat patients for conditions unrelated to obesity?
- What percent of your patients have their surgeries converted to biliopancreatic diversion with duodenal switch (BPD-DS) or Roux-en-Y gastric bypass? Why does this happen?
- What is the average weight loss of your sleeve gastrectomy patients after a year and after five years?
- What percent of your patients are not hitting their weight loss goals? Why does that happen?

These are just a few questions to keep in mind when you're looking around. We'll go through some more specific tips to consider when choosing each of the members of your team. As you go through this section, you'll understand how to evaluate these questions and what the "right" answers are.

How to Choose a Surgeon

Where do you even start when you want to choose a surgeon? Online searches are a good place to start. You can use a search engine or online directory just as you would when you're trying to find any other kinds of services. Most surgeons are findable online and you can narrow searches by location and ratings.

Personal Recommendations

It's hard to know which ratings and reviews are trustworthy when you're browsing online. They can be posted by paid reviewers who may not have even truly seen the surgeon they are reviewing. A better option than relying strictly on online ratings is to get the opinions from real, live vertical sleeve patients. You can also meet sleeve patients at weight loss surgery seminars.

Ask all the sleeve patients you know how they would rate their surgeon and the overall experience, and whether they have any tips for you as you choose your own surgeon. Be sure to find out why they did or did not like their surgeon. You may not be able to use the same surgeon for reasons such as lack of insurance coverage or bad location for you, but their recommendations are still valuable. They'll help you figure out your own preferences.

BariatricPal.com

You may not personally know anyone with the sleeve. Even after you go to a seminar or two, you still might not be confident that you have all the information that you need to make the right surgeon choice. BariatricPal.com is a resource that can help by offering the following features.

- Thousands of members who are gastric sleeve patients who are willing to offer advice
- A surgeon directory complete with member ratings and reviews—and you can be confident that they're honest, not paid, reviews
- Honest discussions that may bring up important points about choosing a surgeon that you hadn't even considered before

Verifying Surgeon Qualifications

In the U.S., all surgeons are full medical doctors.[5] They completed medical school, went through residency trainings in the area of surgery. Each state has its own requirements for licensure for practicing surgeons, and you can ask your surgeon about his or her current credentials. So far, these requirements are pretty broad and easy to meet, so you might want to ask potential surgeons about a few other criteria.

Specific and Recent Training

A surgeon can become a sleeve gastrectomy surgeon without much formal bariatric, sleeve-specific or laparoscopic education. However, there are a few optional criteria that you can check for to make sure you're choosing a qualified surgeon. Don't be shy about asking because it's *your* body:

- *Being a member, or fellow, in the American College of Surgeons, or ACS.* It's easy to tell if you surgeon is a fellow because surgeons who have fellowship are allowed to place the letters FACS after their name, next to their M.D. for medical doctor. The ACS publishes regular scientific journals and newsletters so that fellows can learn about things such as new techniques and updates on guidelines for better patient care for bariatric surgery patients.[6]

- *Participation in ongoing educational opportunities.* Years or even decades may have passed since surgeons completed medical school and got their licenses to practice surgery. There are a variety of ways that surgeons can choose to enhance their skills and stay updated with the latest developments in bariatric surgery, laparoscopic surgery, and the vertical sleeve gastrectomy. This is especially important for the VSG because of its novelty as a stand-alone surgery for weight loss. There's constantly new information about what will make the sleeve work better in the long-term, and you want your surgeon to be up to date. You can always ask what your potential surgeon is doing to stay current.

- *Surgeons with the PALLS certification have demonstrated their skills in laparoscopic surgery.* That's a good thing because you're less likely to have your vertical sleeve gastrectomy converted to open surgery when you have a surgeon who's better at laparoscopic surgery. The PALLS, or Peer Review of Laparoscopic Surgical Proficiency, certification is from the American Society of General Surgeons[7].

  - This certification from the American Society of General Surgeons requires the surgeon to be at Level I, or advanced laparoscopic surgeon. That's the most difficult level to achieve.

  - To be certified, surgeons have to send in a video of themselves doing a surgery or have an evaluator in the operating room in person to watch the surgeon perform actual surgeries. The surgeon gets evaluated on a variety of specific technical skills and procedures that are important for the sleeve.

- *Membership in the American Society for Metabolic and Bariatric Surgery.*[8] This is another example of a membership that's not required to practice the sleeve gastrectomy, but you may feel more confident in the surgeons you are considering if they are members of the ASMBS.

  - Regular members are certified by the American Board of Surgery or the American Osteopathic Board of Surgery and/or are fellows in the American College of Surgeons, or FACS, or one of the Royal Colleges of Surgeons in the United Kingdom or Ireland. They also have completed at least 25 bariatric surgeries within the past two years.

- Affiliate members are bariatric surgeons who have not met the above requirements but have a letter of recommendation from a current regular member.
- International members have completed at least 25 bariatric surgeries within the past two years and have recommendation letters of support.

Experience and Current Focus

You don't just want a doctor; you don't just want a surgeon and you don't just want a weight loss surgery expert. You want an expert in the sleeve gastrectomy. It doesn't matter how many other skills your surgeon has; you want your surgeon to be the best possible surgeon for your vertical sleeve gastrectomy. Ask whether the sleeve gastrectomy is one of the main procedures that your surgeon does. It's only reasonable to expect that he or she performs other bariatric surgeries, too, but you want to be sure that the VSG is one of the top.

In general, more experience is better. Your procedure is less likely to have complications when your surgeon has had plenty of practice with other patients. Ask potential surgeons when they started doing the sleeve gastrectomy and how many sleeve patients they've had. Also ask how many sleeve gastrectomies they do per week or month. You want to be sure that it's a regular occurrence and not an unusual procedure.

Asking the Tough Questions

Healthcare professionals, especially your own physician, surgeon, and healthcare members, are ethically obligated to provide you the information you need to make the best decisions for your health.[9] Despite this, the majority of patients have unrealistic expectations about the amount of weight they are likely to lose and may not fully understand the risks they take with the procedure.[10] Physicians need to be prepared to tell you about the procedure, the potential benefits and the risks. It's safest to rule out surgeons who won't be open about this information.

Patient Records

It's perfectly legitimate to ask potential surgeons about their patients' records. It can be uncomfortable if you're shy, but you have every right to know what you're getting into. Surgeons who are hesitant to answer your questions or who act offended by them are raising red flags. They should be proud, not embarrassed, to talk about their role in their patients' success and safety. At a minimum, you should ask about the following:

- Average patient weight loss at a few months, a year and several years after surgery
- Percent of laparoscopic procedures that are converted into open surgeries during surgery
- Percent of patients who require a second surgery due to complications
- Rate of complications and which types are most common

Red Flags

The best surgeon for you might not have the "right" answers to every single one of your questions. That's okay as long as you're comfortable with the surgeon and you get the "right" answers to the questions that are most important to you. However, it may be time to rule out surgeons if they show any of these red flags.

- Acting offended when you ask about personal VSG training and experience and patient history of weight loss and complications
- Lack of knowledge about patient weight loss after a few years – a good follow-up program keeps in touch with patients for years
- Unwillingness to discuss what happens if you have complications
- Not treating you as an individual with your own legitimate concerns
- Not well acquainted with each member of the healthcare team
- Inability to answer questions regarding care that's not strictly related to the surgery procedure

Once you get these answers, compare the numbers to the numbers you saw in Chapters 4 and 5 of this book in the discussions on expected weight loss. Of course, you want the weight loss numbers to be among the higher values seen in Chapter 4. Surgeons should be able to tell you their patients' numbers for years after surgery because of long-term participation in post-surgery care programs.

A low rate of complications is a pretty good indicator of a surgeon's ability to perform the VSG. If the surgeon has a relatively high rate of complications, be sure to dig deeper into the possible reasons. Some demographic groups, such as more obese, older men compared to less obese, younger women, can have a rate of complications 20 times higher—and the complications are due to patient characteristics, not to any fault of the surgeon. [11]

Post-Surgery Care or Aftercare Program

Once you're convinced that a surgeon is well-qualified and has good technical expertise, your next step is to really dig into the surgeon's aftercare, or post-surgery care, program. All gastric sleeve surgeons should be able to describe the surgery to you in their sleep. A more revealing feat is to clearly explain the aftercare program. It's a sign that you may not have the aftercare experience you need if your surgeon doesn't know all the details of a comprehensive post-surgery care plan. This can be devastating, since post-surgery follow-up care improves your chances of success. [12]

Basics of an Aftercare Program

The surgery is only an early step in your weight loss journey. A post-operative care plan needs to be comprehensive and mandatory to maximize your chances of good weight loss and minimal complications with the sleeve. A comprehensive plan includes input from your surgeon and provides support for your physical and psychological health, as well as dietary support. Depending on your surgeon's preferences and/or the facility's procedure, the program may be mandatory for just a few months, a year or two, or even life.

Getting the Scoop on Post-Surgery Care

Ask specific questions as you are trying to choose a surgeon. You should be concerned if the surgeon or patient care specialist is unable or unwilling to clarify each component of the post-op care program. It may mean that the program isn't well-structure and that some patients tend to slip through the cracks. You don't want to be one of those patients! Following are some questions that you might want to ask when you're trying to find out about aftercare. Always feel free to ask different people multiple times within one clinic to be sure that you are getting an accurate picture of the program. You might also want to ask patients who you see about their experiences:

- *After the sleeve surgery, how often are patients required to have appointments with the surgeon?* Your surgeon should have you come in at least a few times during the first months to monitor your recovery and the rapid changes in your body, and then less frequently throughout the year after surgery.

- *How often and for how long do you meet with the other members of your medical team?* You should meet weekly or biweekly with your dietitian right after your sleeve procedure, and continue to meet regularly for months after the procedure and as needed for meal plans, recipes, and tips. You should also meet with an exercise physiologist and have ongoing meetings with a mental health professional to make sure that you're doing well.

- *What happens if you miss your appointments?* The clinic might ask you to sign a contract that you will follow through with your aftercare. If you need to miss appointments due to scheduling conflicts and you notify the clinic ahead of time, the clinic should be accommodating and reschedule you as soon as possible.

- *When and how often are support groups meetings held?* What happens if you can't make those meetings because of your schedule? For how long are you required to attend? If you can, choose a surgeon that will connect you with patient peer-to-peer support groups that are convenient for you. Many clinics ask you to attend weekly meetings right after surgery, and monthly meetings for years or for life.

- *How does the clinic help patients who aren't meeting their target weight loss goals?* You want to be sure that if you start to falter, the surgeon will reach out to you and make a special effort to find out what's wrong and what kind of extra help you need. This is your time to be successful, so choose a surgeon who will be there for you when you need it most.

- *Why do some patients not make their target weight loss goals?* You want to be sure that you're not going to become one of them. Some reasons that patients might get off track is if they weren't good candidates in the first place or didn't want to commit to the dietary changes. You need to be cautious if the clinic staff members don't seem to know why some patients don't get the success they want.

- *What happens in the case of an emergency if your surgeon is out of town and you need urgent help with a problem such as slippage or obstruction?* There should always be an available surgeon who is on call to cover for your surgeon if you have an emergency.

- *How experienced are the nurses?* A CBN is a Certified Bariatric Nurse. Nurses with this qualification have at least two years of experience caring for morbidly obese patients.[13] CBNs need to take a recertification exam every four years to maintain their status as a CBN.

Chapter 10 is devoted to recovering from surgery and your post-op care plan. You can find more details in that chapter.

Choosing a Surgeon Based on Insurance Coverage

Often, your choice of surgeons will be partly or completely determined by your insurance plan. If your insurance plan will only reimburse you if you go to a specific surgeon, it's still important to do your background research and find out whether you're comfortable with that surgeon. Chances are that you'll be comfortable with the surgeon that you're offered. If not, continue to explore other options. This is a big step in your life, and you want to be sure that you're going to work well with your surgeon now and in the future.

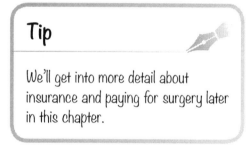

Tip

We'll get into more detail about insurance and paying for surgery later in this chapter.

Choosing a Location for Your Surgery

Choosing a location for your surgery often goes hand in hand with choosing a surgeon. The surgeon you decide on may determine the location of your surgery. Or, you may only be near one or two facilities that offer bariatric surgery, so your location will partially determine your surgeon choice. If you are able to have some say in your facility, there are a few criteria you can look for to improve your chances of a safe and successful experience.

Certified Weight Loss Surgery Centers

In the U.S., the American College of Surgeons Bariatric Surgery Center Network Program, or ACS/BSCNP) and ASMBS have certain criteria for hospitals to become accredited bariatric surgery centers.[14] The Bariatric Surgery Center of Excellence, or BSCOE, program was formerly part of the Surgical Review Corporation. Now, it's a joint program of the ACS and ASMBS.[15] Medicare and many other insurance programs require facilities to be certified to qualify for insurance reimbursement.

Here's a list of some features to look for when you're choosing a facility for your sleeve surgery. Having these amenities will make your surgery safer and your entire experience more pleasant. [16] We'll talk in more detail about some of these next:

- Large and stable wheelchairs, stretchers, and walkers for heavy patients
- Large-sized monitoring devices, such as blood pressure cuffs
- Wide, heavy-duty beds
- Wide commodes and toilets
- Wide doorways, halls, and chairs
- Emergency equipment for large people
- Large scales
- Wide operating table with high weight capacity
- Open MRI and CT scan with high weight capacity
- Specially-trained personnel and appropriate lifting equipment

A Few More Considerations

Other considerations when choosing a clinic are its size, focus and comfort.

Size - The idea of a small clinic with a single bariatric surgeon might be appealing because it seems more personal, but it's not always the best choice. In fact, on average, you're more likely to do better if you get your surgery done at a larger facility that treats a lot of patients like you. Hospitals and large medical centers are examples. These high-volume facilities are typically safer and more effective for a few reasons:[17]

- They have entire departments that are more focused on bariatric surgery. In addition to your bariatric surgeon, these departments may have nurses, mental health professionals and other staff members with special training in bariatric surgery.[18] Bariatric centers should also have special equipment and procedures for lifting patients when necessary.
- They have established protocols. The entire program, from surgery planning through aftercare, is very well-planned and clear. You walk in and there's no hesitation because they know what works and what doesn't. Their experience comes from treating many, many patients just like you, and you'll benefit from this expertise.
- They may have more than one surgeon who is an expert in the sleeve. That means that if your surgeon is away, you can get care immediately and prevent more serious complications if you have a small problem. Even if your own surgeon is the only one at your clinic, a large clinic is more likely to be able to get you an appointment quickly with another, partner clinic.
- The aftercare program is probably more developed. With so many patients, there are probably more opportunities to attend peer-to-peer support groups compared to smaller facilities. There's probably an established schedule of post-surgery follow-up care so that there's no uncertainty about which appointments you'll have with whom.

- There are more support staff, such as dietitians, nurses, exercise physiologists, and psychologists. This makes it easier for you to get appointments and increases the chances of getting all of your appointments scheduled on a single day.

Physical and Emotional Comfort - Between the pre-surgery preparation, the surgery itself, and the post-surgery care, you'll be spending a lot of time at the clinic. You'll do better if you're physically and emotionally comfortable. If you've been obese for years, you already know the huge importance of things such as chairs that are wide enough to sit in, toilets that are easier to sit down on, beds that are big enough for you, scales that can weigh you, hospital gowns that you can fit into and doorways that you can actually get through. Wider wheelchairs and operating tables for obese patients are just a couple examples of amenities that facilities with a lot of experience with obese patients will have for you.

The other part of comfort is your mental comfort. You want to feel comfortable throughout the whole process, from when you walk in the door and the receptionist greets you, to being cared for by nurses, to communicating well with your surgeon to feeling secure talking to your dietitian and other members. You don't ever want to feel embarrassed to bring up your issues or feel like your healthcare team isn't listening. That can lead to problems for your health.

Convenience - When all other things are equal, it's best to choose a facility that's close to your house. It's one thing to get your surgery done in a place that requires a long drive or overnight stay. It's quite another to have to make travel arrangements or take some time off work every time you have to see your surgeon. In most cases, you'll have to see your surgeon several times from your first pre-surgery appointment until you reach your goal weight. It's most convenient to be treated at clinic that is located near you.

It's always nice to get all of your appointments and medical tests done in one trip and in one facility. Choosing a large clinic for your sleeve surgery care can be more convenient. Think about the other services you'll probably be using regularly:

- Dietitian consults
- Blood tests in a lab
- X-rays, or MRI or CT scans in a radiology department
- Group support meetings

In a large facility where everything's located on-site, you can get two or three tasks done in one trip. But if your surgeon is from a small clinic, you might have to go to appointments at different locations. You might not be able to get more than one appointment or service done at once.

Where Should Adolescents Go?

If you're an adolescent or a parent of one who's going to get the sleeve, you may be wondering whether to opt for a pediatric center or a bariatric center in a regular hospital. The ideal scenario would be for adolescents to go to a pediatric bariatric center. That way, they'd get the best of both worlds with age-appropriate treatment and bariatric medical expertise. A children's bariatric center probably isn't available, and experts recommend that adolescents get their procedures done in an adult center to take advantage of the better facilities. [19] The same criteria for adults apply to adolescents: choose a surgeon who is competent and qualified, and who makes you feel comfortable.

It's Too Confusing!

The whole process of choosing a surgeon, building the rest of your healthcare team, and figuring out insurance can be confusing. Often, the information you need to make your decision is in complicated medical or legal jargon. BariatricPal.com is a good resource for translating some of this information into language that you can understand. It's a huge community of gastric sleeve patients and individuals who are considering weight loss surgery. Many of them are willing to help you out by explaining the process and letting you know what's important and what's not when you're choosing your surgeon and trying to fund the surgery.

✎ Summary

☛ This chapter is pivotal. Now you have a surgeon, or know how to go about choosing one. Once you make the decision about a surgeon and where you'll get your surgery done, you have professionals to guide you. From now on, they'll be your main sources of instructions.

☛ In the next chapter, we'll continue with the preparation for surgery. You'll learn about paying for your surgery using insurance or with other options. Let's get going!

Your Turn: Choosing a Surgeon

This chapter covered some of the things you should look for when you're choosing a surgeon and a facility for your weight loss. Every sleeve patient has slightly different wants and needs, though. In this worksheet, you will say how important each of the following characteristics is to you. When you're done, you will have a better idea of how to evaluate your own potential surgeons when you're trying to choose.

On a scale from 1 (not important) to 5 (extremely important), how important to you are the following?

Your surgeon has good user reviews and ratings.

1   2   3   4   5

Your surgeon was recommended to you by someone you know and trust, such as a family member or friend.

1   2   3   4   5

Your surgery is done in a facility (or department of a hospital) that's dedicated to obese patients.

1   2   3   4   5

Your surgeon runs his or her own support group meetings.

1   2   3   4   5

A dietitian is on-site at the clinic or hospital where your surgeon works.

1   2   3   4   5

Knowing that you're going to need to visit your surgeon several times before and after surgery, how far are you willing to travel to see your surgeon?_miles.

A Glimpse into My Life with the Sleeve...Nancy from California

56 years old
Starting Weight: 208 pounds
Current Weight 138 pounds
Height: 5'2"
Loves her dogs and walking

I wasn't a yo-yo dieter. I was always on a diet, but basically all of my efforts were focused on "the last ten pounds" that I had gained during a vacation or birthday or holiday, or just from a binge. I'd lose five to seven pounds and stay there until the next 10-pound gain. My biggest problem was that while I rarely felt hunger, I never felt satisfied unless I ate until I was stuffed. When I tried cutting back my portions, I'd end up eating more throughout the day because I felt like I had eaten nothing when I wasn't stuffed. I eventually evolved to the point where I'd eat one huge meal around lunchtime. I'd have 2,000-3,500 calories. Then maybe I'd have a snack in the evening, while cooking my husband's dinner, and a midnight snack. I had the snacks about 50% of the time. I tried phen/phen and lost 30lbs. I tried different diet pills and lost some weight, but always gained it back. I tried Jenny Craig, but didn't like it. I had spent my whole adult life dieting with no real results, and I knew that unless something changed, I would never get results

Exercise has never been a problem for me. In my twenties I lost weight and kept it off with exercise. At that time I walked four hours a day. After I got married and we moved and there were more time constraints. I cut down to about two hours. In the 30 years I have been walking, I'd say if you added the time where I wasn't walking for whatever reason it won't add up to five years. I think my longest break was six months. Today I walk two and a half hours a day, five days a week and take my dogs for nightly 45 minute walks seven days a week.

Weight Gain Ending in Getting the Sleeve

In my twenties, before I started walking, I weighed close to 150. I got down to 115, stayed there about five years and then started to creep up to my maximum of 220.

I was always interested in weight loss surgery, but wasn't big enough, as most at that time wanted you to be 75 to 100 lbs overweight. That's not to mention the costs, too. A good friend of mine who also is obese found out that our insurance did cover weight loss surgery. At the time, I was interested in the adjustable gastric band, and she was interested in the band as I was. We went to the seminar and both of us liked what we heard about the sleeve and thought that would be the best one for us. My BMI was 38.8 and the co morbidities I had were high blood pressure and high cholesterol. Kaiser, which was my insurance carrier, required a BMI over 40 or a BMI over 35 with comorbidities of sleep apnea or diabetes. So I did not qualify. My friend went through their 12-week session of classes and changed her mind. I read over the paperwork she got in class and read up about it online. I found this site [BariatricPal.com] and others and my mind was made up to get weight loss surgery. I had to go self-pay, but it was worth it. I knew if

I did not do something, I would have some kind of medical weight related crisis. I was borderline diabetic, my latest EKG was borderline abnormal and I was having trouble with my walks on hot days. My heart would pound too fast on the hills.

The reason I choose the sleeve is because it leaves the patient with an intact, normally-functioning stomach. There is little to no chance of dumping syndrome, as with the bypass, or blockage, as with the band. I can still take certain class cardiac drugs in the future should the need arise; with the band and bypass, some are forbidden. Plus I can still take NSAIDs (non-steroidal anti-inflammatory drugs) for my arthritic toe.

I found my surgeon online after doing searches based on pricing and location. I also liked the fact that in my surgeon's package I got one year of follow-up including labs. They had a dietitian who I met with once and could have seen again but did not.

Regular Daily Diet

I typically have a protein shake every morning. I'll have some fruit in the afternoon, and then at dinner I eat what I want. I always eat protein first so that I fill up. If I just eat non-protein foods, I don't feel the restriction. I use to love bread; now it's okay, but not something I usually want. Luckily, it's the same with pasta and rice. I drank tons of diet soda pre-operation; now I may have some on really hot days, but it's a rare thing. I still have my sweet tooth, unfortunately. I try to satisfy it by making my protein shakes super rich and sweet. I use Hood's Calorie Countdown Chocolate Milk to make my shakes and to make sugar-free chocolate pudding. I use protein powder in the pudding. I will add 1/4 cup of the pudding into my morning shakes so that it's a thicker, more shake-like consistency. And I'll either have a glass of skim milk or hard-boiled egg or anything else high in protein before I even think of having anything sweet, which I may do twice a month.

Other Observations

My husband and friends have been all supportive. I did not tell my elderly mother because I didn't want her to worry. The friend who backed out can be negative at times but no overly so. I have never been questioned or treated oddly eating out.

The loose skin does bother me a little, not physically, but cosmetically. The further I am out from surgery, the less it bothers me. I would like to have some plastic surgery but probably won't. That's partly because of the cost but mostly because it feels like a slippery slope. I mean where do you stop? My arms? My thighs? My back? My butt? My stomach? My neck? My breasts? They all have loose saggy skin.

I don't visit the BariatricPal boards that often anymore. But they were great pre-op and post op. I was probably on them daily the first year now maybe once a month.

1   PR Newswire. From "chubby cheerleader to sleeve success with Dr. Michael Feiz." http://finance.yahoo.com/news/chubby-cheerleader-sleeve-success-dr-180700269.html;_ylt=A2KJNTsVp1dQ7kQA_s_QtDMD. 2012, September 12. Accessed September 17, 2012.

2   Evaluating web-based health resources. National Center for Complementary and Alternative Medicine, National Institutes of Health. Website. http://nccam.nih.gov/health/webresources Modified January 2011. Accessed September 18, 2012.

3   Kaplan LM, Seeley RJ, Harris JL. Myths associated with obesity and bariatric surgery – myth 5: patient behavior is the primary determinant of outcomes after bariatric surgery. 2012;9(8):8-10.

4   Keren D, Matter I, Rainis T & Lavy A. Getting the most from the sleeve: the importance of post-operative follow-up. Obesity Surgery. 2011;21(12):1887-1893.

5   Bureau of Labor Statistics. Physicans and surgeons. http://www.bls.gov/ooh/healthcare/physicians-and-surgeons.htm. Published 2012, March 29. Accessed September 20, 2012.

6   American College of Surgeons (n.d.). Retrieved from http://www.facs.org/index.html

7   Education: Peer review of laparoscopic surgical proficiency. (n.d.) American Society of General Surgeons. Retrieved from http://www.theasgs.org/education/education1.html

8   Become a member. American Society for Metabolic and Bariatric Surgery. Website. http://asmbs.org/become-a-member/ Accessed September 21, 2012.

9   Wee CC, Pratt JS, Fanelli R, Samour PQ, Trainer LS, Paasche-Orlow MK. Best practice updates for informed consent and patient education in weight loss surgery. Obesity (Silver Spring). 2009;17(5):885-888.

10 Wee CC, Pratt JS, Fanelli R, Samour PQ, Trainer LS, Paasche-Orlow MK. Best practice updates for informed consent and patient education in weight loss surgery. Obesity (Silver Spring). 2009;17(5):885-888.

11 Wee CC, Pratt JS, Fanelli R, Samour PQ, Trainer LS, Paasche-Orlow MK. Best practice updates for informed consent and patient education in weight loss surgery. Obesity (Silver Spring). 2009;17(5):885-888.

12 Keren D, Matter I, Rainis T & Lavy A. Getting the most from the sleeve: the importance of post-operative follow-up. Obesity Surgery. 2011;21(12):1887-1893.

13 American Society for Metabolic and Bariatric Surgery. CBN Certification FAQ. Website. http://asmbs.org/cbn-certification/. Accessed September 22, 2012.

14 Lautz DB, Jiser ME, Kelly JJ, Shikora SA, Partridge SK, Romanelli JR, Cella RJ, Ryan JP. An update on best practice guidelines for specialized facilities and resources necessary for weight loss surgical programs. Obesity (Silver Spring). 2009;17(5):8911-917.

15 American Society for Metabolic and Bariatric Surgery. Unified national accreditation program for bariatric surgery announced by American College of Surgeons and American Society for Metabolic and Bariatric Surgery. Website. http://asmbs.org/2012/03/unified-national-accreditation-program-for-bariatric-surgery-centers-announced-by-american-college-of-surgeons-and-american-society-for-metabolic-and-bariatric-surgery/. 2012, March 9. Accessed September 20, 2012.

16 Lautz DB, Jiser ME, Kelly JJ, Shikora SA, Partridge SK, Romanelli JR, Cella RJ, Ryan JP. An update on best practice guidelines for specialized facilities and resources necessary for weight loss surgical programs. Obesity (Silver Spring). 2009;17(5):8911-917.

17 Agency for Healthcare Research and Quality. (January 2011). Outcomes/effectiveness research: serious complications from bariatric surgery are fewer when done by high-volume hospitals and surgeons. United States Department of Health and Human Services. Retrieved from http://www.ahrq.gov/research/jan11/0111RA9.htm

18 Lautz DB, Jiser ME, Kelly JJ, Shikora SA, Partridge SK, Romanelli JR, Cella RJ, Ryan JP. An update on best practice guidelines for specialized facilities and resources necessary for weight loss surgical programs. Obesity (Silver Spring). 2009;17(5):8911-917.

19 Pratt JSA, Lenders CM, Dionne EA, Hoppin AG, Hsu GLK., Inge, TH, …, & Sanchez VM. Best practice updates for pediatric/adolescent weight loss surgery. Obesity (Silver Spring). 2009;17(5):901-910.

8

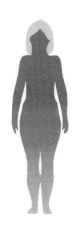

Insurance, Self-Pay and Medical Tourism

The last chapter provided some guidelines on choosing a surgeon and the rest of your medical team. By now you may have some possibilities in mind. Maybe you've already selected a surgeon for your sleeve surgery. This chapter continues with another practical consideration of surgery—payment. Your payment options can be a little confusing, so this chapter will explain the most common scenarios and serve as a guide. We also discuss these topics:

- Investigating whether your health insurance covers the sleeve gastrectomy
- The process of getting your insurance company's pre-approval for reimbursement for the sleeve gastrectomy
- Self-pay and financing options for the sleeve
- Medical tourism: getting the sleeve in another country to lower cost

This chapter takes a giant leap toward making your surgery a reality. By the end of the chapter, you'll know how to pay for it, so the surgery will seem much closer than it was before. Let's start digging!

How much the VSG cost?

Once you've decided to get the sleeve, you're going to have to figure out how to pay for it. Part or all of the cost of the sleeve and related expenses may be covered by your insurance plan. If not, you'll need to pay for it yourself either with cash or a financing plan.

Cost of the Sleeve

How much does the sleeve cost? As with any medical procedure, patients' final charges can vary quite a bit. In addition to asking each facility how much they charge for the procedure, you can get an idea of the cost of the gastric sleeve by searching online. Fair Health Consumer Cost Lookup is a resource that provides estimates based on your zip code and health insurance.[1] These are examples factors that affect the cost of the procedure:

- Different surgeons and clinics charge different prices for their services.
- The state and zip code where you live
- Complications during or after the surgery that require extra medical care
- A health condition that requires special care during, before or after surgery
- Which services are included in this estimate

The vertical sleeve gastrectomy itself may cost about $7,000 to $10,000, but this range can be thousands of dollars higher or lower. Another critical point is that this first figure may not include the other necessary costs of surgery. You need to specifically ask instead of assuming, but it probably includes these services:

- The surgery itself
- Regular post-surgery follow-up appointments with your surgeon

- Anesthesia and pain medications if you use them
- Expected care in the hospital if you have no complications
- Pre-surgery tests to make sure you're a good candidate for surgery

When you're gathering cost estimates, looking up your healthcare coverage and doing your budget, it is absolutely necessary to consider other likely costs, such as:

- Ongoing appointments with a dietitian
- Regular monitoring tests, such as laboratory blood tests for your nutritional status
- Extra care in the hospital if your surgery leads to a longer hospital stay than expected
- Further procedures, such as a re-sleeve, if you have complications
- Diagnostic tests, such as x-rays or MRIs, if you have complications
- Extra appointments with your physician or surgeon to troubleshoot side effects

When you're adding up the costs of the sleeve, don't forget to think about the potential savings, too. The sleeve may end up saving you money if it truly helps you lose weight and get healthier. You won't have to pay for any more fad diets, and you may save money on doctor's visits, medical tests, and prescription drugs if the sleeve works for you. Along with economic concerns, there's also the issue of your health and quality of life. Do you expect your weight loss, health, and general quality of life to improve enough to be worth the investment in the sleeve?

Will Insurance Cover the VSG?

Health coverage is becoming more common for bariatric surgery in general and the sleeve gastrectomy in particular.[2] The government's largest plans, Medicare and Medicaid, removed the SG from Non-Covered status on October 1, 2012.[3] The gastric sleeve now recognized as a potentially reimbursable obesity treatment in Medicare.[4] ASMBS cites Aetna Inc. and United Health as examples of large private medical insurance providers that now cover the gastric sleeve, and there are many more examples.[5]

If you've been considering weight loss surgery for a few years and your healthcare coverage didn't cover it before, it's probably worth checking again. There's a chance that now your plan covers the sleeve. It seems increasingly clear that covering the sleeve makes good business sense for insurance companies.

Figuring out your insurance coverage can be tough, and we'll try to guide you through it over the next few pages. Some of the main sources of information on whether the procedure is covered or whether a specific surgeon takes your insurances include:

- The specific surgeon or his or her office
- Your healthcare coverage insurance customer service representative
- The human resources department at your workplace
- The insurance coverage map from ASMBS, which is a work in progress and should be a valuable resource when it is complete[6]

Identifying Which Type of Insurance Plan You Have, and Getting Information about VSG Coverage

The first step is to figure out what kind of insurance plan you have. Then, you need to figure out how to get information about your specific benefits. You might already be familiar with all of these aspects, especially if you have medical problems that you have to deal with on a regular basis. Your experience will help you now!

But, if you're lucky enough to have good insurance and you've never had to worry about your medical costs because you've never asked for anything extra, you might not have ever really thought about health insurance. For many of us, health insurance is a blurry concept that doesn't really come into focus until we need something specific—right now, it's the sleeve and the other costs that come along with it. This section will walk you through getting any reimbursement that you're entitled to. This section will include this information:

- Types of private insurance plans, and how they work
- National health insurance coverage: Medicare and Medicaid, and how they work
- Getting information about what's covered by your insurance plan
- Asking for pre-approval for reimbursement and appealing a denied claim

Private Insurance: HMOs and PPOs

Private health insurance is insurance that you or your employer pays for. You need to know what kind of insurance plan you have so that you know how to get the benefits you are entitled to and where to find information.

HMOs and PPOs: The most common systems of private health insurance are health management organizations, or HMOs, and preferred provider organizations, or PPOs.

- *HMO.* In an HMO, you typically get all of your medical care done by healthcare providers within the network. You need a referral from your primary care physician in order to get reimbursed for care by specialists, such as the sleeve surgeon. An HMO will most likely only reimburse you for the sleeve gastrectomy if you go to a surgeon within the network. If the entire network only has a few LSG surgeons, you may need to travel out of town to get your surgery done by an approved surgeon. This can make aftercare difficult and inconvenient, as you will need to see your surgeon multiple times in the weeks and months after surgery. However, you may be allowed to see a more local doctor within the HMO for your post-surgery follow-up.
- *PPO.* If you are part of a PPO, you are usually covered for care when you see any provider in the network. You might need a referral for seeing a specialist, depending on what the rules are with your PPO. Relatively expensive or major procedures, such as the VSG, are more likely to require referrals before you can get reimbursed.

Coverage with Fully-Insured and Self-Insured Insurance Plans: A *fully-insured* insurance plan is one that you pay for directly to the insurance company or your employer pays part or all of it for you. A *self-insured* insurance plan is one that your employer has negotiated with the insurance company; the exact list of services that are covered may be different than what the insurance company offers to other companies and individuals. Either plan can be an HMO or PPO.

Why does it matter whether you have a fully-insured or self-insured plan? This information is a clue to where you can find information about the coverage. On a fully-insured plan, the information you need is in the *Summary of Benefits* (SOB) or *Certificate of Coverage*. With a self-insured insurance plan, you'll need the *Summary Plan Description (SPD)*. There isn't a big difference between these two items, but knowing the proper terms will help you track down the documents you need.

Once you have those documents, look through them carefully for information about weight loss surgery coverage. This can take a while because the documents aren't usually very easy to read. They're full of jargon that is tough to wade through. These are a few key words to look for as you skim through your policy:

- *Exclusion clauses*: These sections list services that *are not* covered by the policy. An exclusion clause might list all obesity treatments, including weight loss surgery, as excluded services — they are not covered at all by your policy.

- *Inclusion clauses*: These sections list services that *are* covered by the policy. Your policy might state that the open or laparoscopic sleeve gastrectomy is covered, or it might state that some types of bariatric surgery are covered. It might be as general as stating that many types of obesity treatment are covered. If the policy does not specifically state the LSG as an included procedure, you'll need to call your representative.

- *Expenses Covered* or *Expenses Not Covered*: These might come in the middle of an exclusion clause or an inclusion clause, or they might come in their own separate lists elsewhere in the policy. Again, if you don't see the sleeve gastrectomy mentioned anywhere, it's time to call an insurance representative.

Do your best with the dense, legal-style language and medical terminology. Whether you think you understand it or not, it's a good idea to check with a representative from the insurance company (if you have a fully-insured plan) or with an insurance expert in your human resources department (if you have self-insured insurance coverage). Ask them to explain anything that you don't understand. Also, ask them to mail you a copy of everything related to obesity treatment so you can read it at your leisure.

As you investigate reimbursement for the sleeve, don't forget about the other treatment that you'll need — and that cost money. You'll need to have multiple pre-surgery and post-surgery appointments with your surgeon, as well as the dietitian, psychiatrist, and other members of the medical team:

- Each service may require a pre-approval separate from the sleeve pre-approval.

- Some services may not be covered even if the sleeve is.

- These other services may be covered even if your sleeve gastrectomy isn't. This can make the entire procedure affordable for you.

A Few Tips to Make the Insurance Process Easier

Dealing with health insurance companies is challenging. Getting information from them can take hours. You can feel as though you're going around in circles because of so many phone calls with so many different representatives. These are a few tips that can help prepare you for possibly frustrating encounters with the company:

- *Take notes:* That includes having a pen and paper in hand so you can take notes whenever you make a phone call or look something up online. Keep records of all your phone calls, noting the time and date.

- *Be patient and persistent:* You might be on hold, you might get a rude representative, and you might get an answer that you're sure is wrong. Take a deep breath and try again. Keep your eye on the prize, which could be as much as several thousand dollars for a life-changing medical procedure.

- *Be prepared with the following information:* insurance provider's contact information (name, fax number, phone number, email address, website).

- *Make sure everything is verifiable:* Get all promises in writing and ask for your customer service rep's name each time you make a call. Don't depend on your memory or on a spoken promise.

- *Do not give up:* Keep trying until you're satisfied with the answer and you have any promises for reimbursement in writing.

Be especially careful to read the fine print if you're looking into the sleeve as a revisional surgery to convert the lap-band into a sleeve or if you're getting a re-sleeve. Many plans have an exclusion policy for all bariatric surgeries that aren't your first. That means that insurance companies will only reimburse you for your first weight loss surgery, even if your previous surgery was with another insurance company or you paid for it yourself.

In some cases, your insurance coverage might be comprehensive. Often, however, it has limits on the total cost or type of services that you can receive in a year. If this is the case, you can find out your out-of-pocket fees, or the amount you'll be paying yourself.

- Add up the total cost of the sleeve surgery and related costs of pre-surgery and post-surgery care.
- Find out the maximum amount of reimbursement.
- Then subtract the amount of reimbursement from the total cost to find out your out-of-pocket fees.

Getting Pre-Approval from Your Insurance Provider

Getting pre-approval in writing is critical! The last thing you want is to pay for and get the gastric sleeve, thinking you'll get reimbursed because someone on the phone said you would, and find out later that you aren't getting a dime from insurance.

The pre-approval process usually isn't too complicated. Usually, someone at your surgeon's office will fill out the paperwork for you requesting coverage for the surgery. They'll send it to your insurance carrier, who should approve it if it's part of your plan.

If your surgeon doesn't take care of the paperwork for you, you can do it yourself. Write a letter explaining the procedure, the amount you are asking for and the surgeon and other health professionals that you will be purchasing services from. Identify the sleeve procedure and the reasons why you qualify for it using official codes.

- **Current Procedural Terminology, or CPT, Code**: The CPT Code is an official designation published by the American Medical Association.[7] There is a different CPT for each medical procedure. The CPTs get updated often, so check the AMA's website for the sleeve gastrectomy's code when you're ready to write your letter. After years of being lumped in with general bariatric procedures, the open and laparoscopic sleeve gastrectomy just got their own CPT codes.[8] This should reduce confusion over which procedure you're asking for.

- **International Classification of Diseases, 9th Edition, or ICD-9**: Each ICD-9 describes a health condition or disease that is a justification for asking for medical treatment. Most insurance companies use the ICD-9 to decide whether to provide reimbursement.

Explain that you need pre-approval in writing. Mail your letter using certified mail so that someone at the insurance company has to sign for delivery and you have proof that your letter got there safely.

Appealing a Denied Claim

Your insurance company might refuse to grant pre-approval, or prior approval, for your sleeve surgery the first time you or your surgeon's office submits the request. This happens pretty often, and you shouldn't panic or lose hope if you get denied after your first try. What you can do is appeal the denial. Your surgeon's office might automatically resubmit the claim for you and try to get the denial overturned. Or, you might need to submit the appeal yourself. In that case, call your insurance representative and request an explanation in writing so that you can address each point. You are legally entitled to an explanation in writing.

Look carefully at the reason for the denial to increase your chances of getting the denial overturned:

- If your insurance company denied your request claiming that you did not give a sufficient reason for the sleeve gastrectomy, make sure that you filled in the ICD-9 number correctly and that you submitted a letter from your physician recommending that you get the sleeve.

- If the company claims that the procedure is experimental and therefore not covered, you can use existing research on the sleeve's safety and effectiveness. Your surgeon should be able to provide a letter backing you up.

- If the insurance company says that the procedure is excluded but you are certain that your policy covers the gastric sleeve, double-check to make sure that the CPT Code you entered was correct.

- If you're under a self-insured plan from your employer, you can ask your employer to add the sleeve to the list of covered procedures. Remember, a self-insured plan includes only those services that your employer chooses, and your employer has the ability to change the service plans.

These are a few tips for composing a letter to your insurance company or insurance representative in your employer's human resources department.

- If you filled out the initial pre-approval form wrong or you believe you were denied because of an error, specifically point out which parts were mistakes. It may be that you filled in the wrong ICD-9 or CPT Code or that the insurance company wrongly interpreted your entitlement or request.

- Include specific information about the health consequences and economic costs of obesity. Chapter 1 of this book is a good place to start when you're gathering your data. You don't have to make it too long, but you can point out that obesity can cause a high risk of diabetes and cardiovascular disease, a shorter life expectancy and more than $1,000 per year in extra medical costs. Your surgeon can help with this part.

- Describe the data showing that weight loss surgery can be more effective than diet and exercise, and that the sleeve has been successful for many patients who haven't been able to lose weight through dieting.[9] Again, your surgeon can help here.

- Briefly describe your personal situation. State how long you have struggled with obesity and describe your obesity-related health conditions. Explain that you feel that the sleeve because you have already tried diets and have not been able to find a successful long-term solution for your weight. You don't need to tell a sob story or your entire life history. It just needs to demonstrate that you've exhausted other options and the sleeve looks like the most promising option that's left.

- Keep your letter as short as possible. You're sending it to someone who doesn't you personally and who may receive hundreds of similar letters each day. The person reading your letter may take only seconds to decide whether to pursue your appeal. You don't want your letter tossed in the garbage (or placed in the pile of rejected appeals) just because it's too long. Do your best to balance the necessary information with keeping the letter short.

The Obesity Action Coalition, or OAC: *A good resource.* The OAC is a non-profit organization whose purpose is to advocate for people with obesity. The OAC publishes a variety of educational materials that you can get for free from the OAC's website. One resource is an excellent brochure for when you are trying to figure out whether your insurance will reimburse the gastric sleeve.[10] The brochure is called, "Working with Your Insurance Provider: A Guide to Seeking Weight Loss Surgery."

Medicare and Medicaid

In the U.S., the two main public health insurance systems are Medicare and Medicaid. They're run by the Centers for Medicare and Medicaid Services, or CMS, which is part of the Department of Health and Human Services. Both programs have covered bariatric surgery for years.[11] Medicare recently removed the gastric sleeve from the list of excluded services for patients who meet at least the minimum criteria of a BMI over 35, at least one obesity-related health condition and a history of unsuccessful medical treatment for obesity.[12]

Medicare is the national insurance coverage plan for individuals age 65 and older. It's designed to help with your medical bills after you retire if you've been paying into your Medicare plan during the years that you were working. Medicare also covers younger individuals with disabilities. Your Medicare eligibility and benefits are pretty standard throughout the U.S. because the federal government has a lot of control over funding and administration.

Medicaid is a health insurance program for low-income individuals. It's a health insurance premium payment program, or HIPP, which is a type of managed care program. That means that the state government pays for you to enroll in a private insurance plan. Each state is responsible for paying for a high proportion of Medicaid to supplement the federal government's funds. Compared to Medicare, there's a lot of flexibility in each state's eligibility criteria and benefits with Medicaid. Each state has its own name for its Medicaid program. For example, California's Medicaid program is called Medi-Cal, Oregon's program is the Oregon Health Plan, Oklahoma has Soonercare and Tennessee has TennCare. You can find the Medicaid program for your state from Medicaid's website at www.Medicaid.gov.[13]

You need to go to a qualified surgeon if you want Medicaid or Medicare to cover your gastric sleeve surgery. Only some surgeons meet CMS requirements for the procedure. To qualify, surgeon facilities need to have certification either as a Level 1 Bariatric Surgery Center as defined by the American College of Surgeons, or as a Bariatric Surgery Center of Excellence, as defined by the American Society for Bariatric Surgery. You can search for surgeons that are under your coverage and within your region at the CMS site.[14]

Extra Requirements for Surgery Reimbursement

You already saw the eligibility criteria for the sleeve listed in Chapter 6. To qualify for reimbursement through your healthcare coverage, you may need to meet one or more of these additional requirements:

- Provide your insurance company with a Letter of Medical Necessity from your doctor.
- Lose a certain amount of weight before your surgery.
- Follow a pre-surgery diet under the supervision of your surgeon and dietitian.
- Have a psychological evaluation.
- Choose a facility with ASMBS BSCOE certification for covering sleeve gastrectomy.[15]

Many of these requirements are the same as the ones that most surgeons would require you to do anyway before getting the SG.

What Does "Cost-Effective" Mean, and How Does It Translate into Better Coverage for the Sleeve?

Something that is cost-effective means that it is at least as valuable as its price. Insurance companies are interested only in making profits, so they conduct cost-benefit analyses pretty much all the time to decide:

- Whether they should cover certain procedures
- Which of their customers should receive which procedures
- How much their patients' contributions should be

For example, most insurance companies cover regular physical exams. The cost-benefit analysis is likely to show that the cost to the insurance company for you to get regular blood cholesterol and blood pressure tests is way less than the cost of paying for your treatment for advanced heart disease or a stroke that might happen if you don't get the early screening tests. Therefore, screening for high cholesterol and high blood pressure is considered cost-effective.

The sleeve gastrectomy and other weight loss surgery procedures are generally considered to be cost-effective, especially as they become more common and we learn more about their effects. Researchers in one published study found that the cost of a successful weight loss surgery, including the surgery and aftercare, pays for itself within a few years. That's due to better overall health when you lose weight. You and your insurance company save money on so many doctor's appointments to monitor your health conditions, a bunch of medications to lower your blood pressure, cholesterol, and glucose, glucose testing kits if you had diabetes, and hospital stays if you had a serious obesity-related health condition like heart disease.

Sources[16,17,18]

Financing Options

Personal financing, paying out-of-pocket and self-pay all mean the same thing: you need to pay for it yourself. You're going to have to pay a good chunk of money if:

- You don't have health insurance.
- Your insurance doesn't cover the gastric sleeve.
- Your insurance only covers a portion of the sleeve, leaving you responsible for the rest.
- Your insurance doesn't cover the related expenses, such as follow-up care or regular post-surgery medical tests.

Is It Really That Expensive?

Now that you know how much money is going to be coming out of your own pocket, are you sure that it's worth it? It's worth it if the benefits and cost-savings are more than the cost. If you successfully lose weight with the sleeve, how will the sleeve save you money?

Obesity is an expensive condition, and the cost will only increase as you remain obese. It's impossible to know the exact cost of obesity for each individual, but there are some estimates. On average, an obese person has medical costs of $1,723 per year.[19] Those are just the direct medical costs, but obesity is expensive in other ways, too. Have you considered these costs:

- How much do you spend on food? If you get a lot of restaurant or prepared snacks and meals, it might be a lot more than you'd like to admit.

- How much have you spent on diets? Be honest here. How much have you spent on diet plans, prepackaged diet food, special types of food and diet supplements? How many times have you paid to lose the same 50 or 100 pounds? The sleeve is designed to be a permanent solution if you use it well.

- How much have you spent on gym memberships and exercise equipment that you don't use?

- How much do you spend on clothing? How many times have you thrown away the larger clothes when you're dieting, and thrown away the smaller clothes when you gain the weight back? How much have you spent on sets of clothing in various sizes?

- How many days of work do you have to take as vacation days because you're home sick and you've already used up all of your sick days? You may be sick so often because of your obesity.

- How much do you spend on medical bills, including trips to the doctor, medical tests, prescription medications, and other obesity-related health costs?

Life's not just about money. Even if you weren't going to save money on healthcare and food costs, there's another reason to shell out a few thousand dollars for the VSG. It's your *quality of life*. We've talked about it before. Being obese is unpleasant. It makes you uncomfortable. It makes people think they have the right to look down on you. It makes you tired during the day and restless at night. You may be at the point where all you can think of is food and your body. You deserve better than that!

How much is being at a healthy weight worth to you? If you're willing to pay for the sleeve and commit to following the healthy lifestyle changes that you'll need in order to succeed, self-pay might not seem so bad after all.

Financing Plans and Options

One self-pay option is to pay in cash or put the sleeve on your credit card if you have a high enough credit limit. There few other options are available in case you don't have the cash on hand right now to pay for your sleeve surgery. You can get a loan from a bank or another lending institution.

Another option is to do medical financing. This is similar to any other financing plan for a major purchase. You may have a down payment and monthly payments due for a few years until you've paid off the amount you agree on. These are a few examples of companies that offer financing plans for bariatric surgery:

- CareCredit
- Credit Medical
- Med Loan Finance
- My Medical Loan
- SurgeryLoans.com
- Surgical Services International/APF USA[20] (Advanced Patient Financing)

Some banks and credit card companies also have special programs for financing medical expenses. You can find more financing options by searching online. If you can't tell whether they cover the vertical sleeve or if you have other questions, just call them. If a company isn't easy to get a hold of, just go on to the next company on your list. You don't want to get started with a company that's not helpful!

Most medical facilities clinics accept one or more types of financing plans. Your surgeon's clinic may recommend a specific plan, or it may accept a variety of payment plans.

As you would whenever you sign up for financing, take personal responsibility for your money:

- Find out the upfront cost, the interest rate and the total cost.
- Make each payment on time.
- Check how much each payment will be, and compare those amounts to your income. Do you have enough money to pay for it?
- Read the terms and conditions. Find out the interest rates and penalties for late payments.
- Consider what might happen if you have an unexpected complication with the sleeve. Will you be able to finance the medical care you may need *while still making* your original sleeve payments?

If you are understand the terms of your loan plan and feel able to commit to them, the plan can be your ticket to getting the sleeve if you weren't able to afford it otherwise.

Medical Tourism: Is it A Viable Option?

Medical tourism is what it's called when you go to another country to get a medical procedure done. Some bariatric patients from wealthier countries, such as the US, Canada and European nations, choose to go to foreign nations where they can get the VSG cheaper. Mexico, Venezuela, and India are examples of destinations for medical tourism. Don't count on a lot of sightseeing when you go abroad for medical tourism. The whole time you're there, you'll be prepping for surgery, at the hospital and recovering from surgery.

Medical Tourism to Reduce Costs

The main reason to opt for medical tourism is to save money. You might consider it if you're not getting insurance coverage for the sleeve and you don't want to or can't pay the price in the U.S. Places including Mexico and Venezuela offer cheaper medical services because their lower per capita gross domestic products, or per capita GDPs, are less than one-third that of the US. That means that average person makes far less money than the average American, and products and services tend to be cheaper. The sleeve can be about one-third the cost in Mexico than in the US.[21]

All about Getting a Current Passport

If you're going abroad for to get your sleeve surgery, you'll need a passport that's good for at least six months from the time you leave the US and enter the other country. This is a requirement for Venezuela, and a recommendation for American visitors to Mexico. The US Department of State provides information and instructions for renewing your old passport or getting your first one at travel.state.gov.

You need to apply in person if:

- Your previous passport was lost, stolen or damaged.
- Your previous passport was issued more than 15 years ago.
- You have never had an American passport before.
- You are under age 16 (unlikely, but possible, for VSG patients)

You can do the entire process by mail if all of these are true for you:

- Your previous passport is intact and you still have it.
- Your previous passport is less than 15 years old.
- You are more than 16 years old.
- You have not legally changed your name since your last passport was issued.

Getting your passport takes approximately 4 to 6 weeks for regular service. You can pay for expedited service, including overnight shipping both ways, and shorten the time to two or three weeks. In either case, you can see that planning ahead is necessary to keep your sleeve surgery on schedule!

Sources:[22,23,24]

Package Deals to Make Planning Easier

Getting the vertical sleeve is already a pretty big deal because it is such a life-changing event. Plus, it requires a lot of research and planning. As you've seen in this and previous chapters, for example, you need to select a surgeon and facility, get the rest of your medical team together and figure out your financing situation. Medical tourism may be your best option, but it can be a challenge to make all of the necessary plans. Some companies offer package deals so that everything's covered and you don't have to make each individual plan yourself.

Why Would You Get a Package Deal?

You might be interested in a package deal if one or more of these describe you:

- You don't know how to get started. Do you know what paperwork is necessary, whether your passport is current, which airport you'll land at, where to stay, how you'll get there and how to get to and from the hospital—especially after surgery when you'll be in no condition to start calling around for a taxi? Some people actually do know how accomplish these things, but if you don't even know where to get started, a package deal might be your best bet.

- You're not an experienced traveler. Traveling on your own comfortably takes some practice. If you don't often travel, you may experience anxiety or stress at being in a foreign country with nobody to take care of things for you. This anxiety will not help your surgery go better!

- You are pretty sure you want to get your surgery done in another country, but you're not sure about how to choose a hospital that has an English-speaking staff and surgeon and performs up to American standards of care and cleanliness. A medical tourism company can act as a go-between between you and the hospital.

- You like the idea of having everything taken care of for you, from your pre-surgery and post-surgery food to having an assistant available so you are not alone.

- Your family is coming with you and you are interested in having them entertained as part of the package deal.

Examples of Medical Tourism Bundles

You can get medical tourism bundles from a variety of private companies. Some of the more established clinics may have their own bundles that you can find out about by contacting them directly. Surgical Services International/APF USA ("Advanced Patient Financing) is an example of a typical medical tourism company that provides package deals for the sleeve gastrectomy in Mexico or on the Caribbean island of Isla Margarita in Venezuela. [25,26] A typical bundle starts at $4,000 and includes the following:

- All pre-surgery consultations and follow-up appointments

- The surgery and related normal fees, including surgeon fees, cost of anesthesia, hospital care, hospital meals, and pain medications
- Ground transportation to and from the airport, hospital, and patient recovery house
- Accommodations at an affiliated patient recovery house
- All meals at the patient recovery house

You will need to pay for any non-included expenses, such as the cost of medical care from unexpected complications. You'll also need to pay extra if you stay in the patient recovery house longer than the originally expected length of time.

Investigating International Locations for Your Surgery

If you're getting the sleeve done outside the U.S., your facility won't be accredited by the ACS and ASMBS. Instead, you can check whether it's an International Center of Excellence, or ICE, as designated by the Surgical Review Corporation[27]. International Centers of Excellence must meet 10 requirements:

1. *Institutional commitment to excellence.* Hospitals show their commitment to excellence and dedication to improvement by defining surgery guidelines for their programs.
2. *Surgical experience and volumes.* Surgeons who lead bariatric surgeries at the center must have completed at least 25 bariatric surgeries in their lifetimes.
3. *Designated medical director.* This ensures that there's always a specific person overseeing the bariatric program and maintaining standards.
4. *Responsive critical care support.* Hospitals need to be ready to respond to any medical emergency.
5. *Appropriate equipment and instruments.* This may mean purchasing new, larger-sized equipment and instruments to safely and accommodate extremely obese patients.
6. *Surgeon dedication and qualified call coverage.* Surgeons show their dedication by becoming certified by a respected organization.
7. *Clinical pathways and standardized operation procedures.* Hospitals should include programs such as pain management, patient instruction and evaluation, research or pre-surgery workups.
8. *Bariatric nurses, physician extenders, and program coordinator.* These staff members ensure that the bariatric program remains focused on weight loss surgery and meets patient needs.
9. *Patient support groups.* These are almost indispensible for success. Support groups keep you motivated, provide information and demonstrate the surgeon and facility's commitment to you.
10. *Long-term patient follow-up, including participation in BOLD (Bariatric Outcomes Longitudinal Database).* Long-term follow-up helps improve your weight loss by keeping you accountable for longer after the surgery. The Bariatric Outcomes Longitudinal

Database is the world's largest database of bariatric surgery patients.[28] Publicly reporting patient results to BOLD gives hospitals and surgeons an extra incentive to work hard for your weight loss success.

Getting your VSG in another country can be stressful because it's hard to evaluate the facility's quality. The ICE designation can help you increase your confidence in your choice because you know that the facility is experienced, well-equipped, and well-staffed.

Similarly, you can check to see whether the surgeon you're considering has a Bariatric Surgeon of Excellence, or BSOE designation.[29] Surgeons who have this have completed 125 weight loss surgeries in their lifetime, and at least 100 of these surgeries per year. They comply with the requirements of ICE hospitals, too.

Additional Advice for Choosing a Surgeon and Clinic

You probably won't be able to meet your surgeon in person before getting your sleeve procedure done abroad. Instead of being able to use your own instinct when choosing a surgeon, you'll have to depend more heavily on the surgeon's qualifications and other people's recommendations. In addition to the guidelines listed above, here are a few more tips for choosing a surgeon without meeting him or her first:

- Ask all of your questions. This might take a lot of emailing back and forth, but your surgeon should be willing and able to clearly answer your questions without evading any of them.

- Ask about travel arrangements and what happens in case of unforeseen complications that force you to stay in the hospital a little longer than planned.

- Get recommendations from people who have had the bariatric surgery done during a medical tourism experience. They can provide names of medical tourism companies and surgeons.

- Once you've narrowed down your search to a few surgeons, ask them if you can contact some of their patients. They should be willing to do this for you.

Considerations with Medical Tourism

Medical tourism can be a great solution to high costs in the US, but there are some additional things to think about before you make your choice and as you plan your trip. Consider an English-speaking facility, your personal safety, what to pack, and how to choose a surgeon in another nation.

Potential for Language Barriers: If your Spanish isn't fluent, you'll be depending on your caregivers to speak English so that you can communicate. So many Americans go south for the sleeve that this may not be a problem; many surgeons and their clinics promise that you will not encounter any language barriers during your entire experience because of their fluency in English. Furthermore, many surgeons who participate in medical tourism were originally Americans, so they and some of their staff may be native English speakers.

BariatricPal.com: An Unbiased Source for Surgeon Information

Unbiased opinions are valuable when you're considering medical tourism and you're looking for a surgeon in another country. BariatricPal.com is a community dedicated to the sleeve community, and many of its members have chosen to get the sleeve done in a foreign nation. Their experiences, surgeon reviews and recommendations can help you make your own decisions with more confidence.

When you visit the site and look at the main page of discussion topics, you'll notice an area that is dedicated to discussions among special groups. These discussions are open to the public, but they're more focused than the general discussions on the board. Among the special groups is an entire forum dedicated to self-pay and medical tourism sleeve patients. Everyone's welcome to join the conversations and ask your own questions.

A simple step make sure you'll be able to communicate when you're at the clinic is to call the facility on the phone or using an online services, such as Skype, which is usually cheaper. The person answering the phone should have no trouble understanding you or speaking in English; if he or she does, you should be able to be connected within seconds to someone who is fluent. If not, it's probably not worth your while to consider that hospital or clinic for your surgery.

Even if the front desk sounds convincingly fluent, it can be a challenge to figure out exactly how great the language barrier will be. It's possible that everyone from the nurses to your surgeon to the driver of your shuttle to your hotel will speak perfect English. On the other hand, it's possible that only the surgeon and the receptionist, who might be your only contacts before you go to the clinic, are fluent in English. The other staff, such as the nurses and anesthesiologist, might not speak English. That can be a problem if you have urgent needs while you're under their care. To protect yourself, ask your contacts at the clinic whether everyone at the clinic speaks English. If not, ask whether there is always someone available to translate.

Safety in Foreign Countries: Mexico and Venezuela have high rates of crime, including violent crime and theft. Venezuela has one of the highest murder and crime rates in world; visitors to Isla Margarita are fingerprinted before entering.[30] In Mexico, drugs, street crime are not as bad as reported in the news in drug-ridden rural areas, but the US Department of State warns travelers to be aware of their surroundings and the potential for crime.[31] A travel warning, inspired by increases in kidnappings and disappearances, was issued in February of 2012.[32]

Some medical tourism companies make special efforts to prevent these facts from scaring away gastric sleeve patients. Surgical Services International, Inc., promises a personal assistant to accompany you so that you'll never be alone during your stay. You also get a cell phone to use.[33]

Complication Rates and Medical Tourism: You always have a risk for complications when you get the sleeve. Your risk of complications may be higher when you go abroad for

Don't Depend on Your High School Spanish!

You may have been a star Spanish student in high school, but don't depend on those skills unless you've continually practiced speaking since then. Even if you do remember as much as you think, you may have trouble being clear and understanding well when you're under a stressful situation, such as being in the hospital for the sleeve surgery.

your procedure in a nation that's not as wealthy as the U.S. Facilities might not be as up-to-date or hygienic as in the U.S., and that can increase your risk for complications during or after your procedure. Some research shows that there are more complications among patients who choose medical tourism for bariatric surgery, although there are certainly a high number of perfectly safe clinics abroad.[34]

Physical Challenges of Travel: Regardless of how easy the trip is or how nice the accommodations are, the truth is that traveling is tough on your body. Almost everyone sleeps better in their own beds compared to even the nicest of luxury hotels. You might have jet lag or extra anxiety making you tired and putting you at risk for getting infected. A minor infection, such as the common cold, makes your immune system work harder and can make your recovery from surgery more challenging.

Traveler's diarrhea is another challenge to your body when you're doing medical tourism. Between 30 and 70 percent of all tourists to foreign nations some form of traveler's diarrhea.[35] Along with diarrhea, you might also have symptoms of vomiting, bloating and stomach pain. These are especially unpleasant when your body's already fighting hard to recover from the sleeve gastrectomy.

Post-Surgery Care and Medical Tourism

You're not likely to be able to see your surgeon during your aftercare program if your surgeon lives in another country. Be sure that your post-surgery care is arranged before you get the sleeve. You might end up participating in a local surgeon's care program that includes appointments and support group meetings. Your surgeon overseas should be able to help you find a surgeon who will accept you as a patient and treat you as well as if you got your gastric sleeve in the U.S. It is absolutely necessary that you have someone near your home to go to for emergencis.

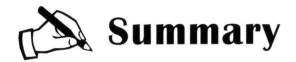 **Summary**

☛ This chapter covered the cost of the sleeve. You may get reimbursed by your health insurance or you may be stuck paying for the entire VSG yourself.

☛ You may need a finance plan to be able to afford the sleeve right now, and many are available to choose from.

☛ Also, you can opt for medical tourism as a cheaper option to self-pay in the US.

☛ Now, as you are thinking about money and payment, is another good time to re-examine whether the sleeve is worth it to you. If it is, full speed ahead!

☛ The next chapter covers your preparations for the actual surgery as the time get closer.

Your Turn: Paying for the Sleeve

This chapter talked about paying for the sleeve with or without the help of insurance coverage. This worksheet can guide you as you figure out your own payment options.

Will your insurance cover the sleeve? YES / NO

If yes, what other expenses remain? These might include things such as dietitian appointments and additional lab work. ....

If no, will your insurance cover any part related? YES / NO

How much will you need to pay out of pocket? ....

Is the surgery worth it to you? YES / NO

Can you afford cash or do you need financing? ....

How much can you afford to pay each month? ....

1   FAIR Health, Inc. Fair Health Consumer Cost Lookup. Website. http://fairhealthconsumer.org/. Copyright 2012. Accessed September 24, 2012.

2   Picot, J., Jones, J., Colquitt, J.L., Gospodarevskaya, E., Loveman, E., Baxter, L., Clegg, A.J. (2009). The clinical effectiveness and cost-effectiveness of bariatric (weight loss) surgery for obesity: a systematic review and economic evaluation. Health Technology Assessment, 13:1-90.

3   American Society for Metabolic and Bariatric Surgery. Access update: sleeve gastrectomy. Website. http://asmbs.org/2012/09/asmbs-access-update-news-from-washington-dc/. August 31, 2012. Accessed September 17, 2012.

4   Rosenthal RJ. The Centers for Medicare and Medicaid Services endorse sleeve gastrectomy as a valid treatment modality for patients with morbid obesity; United States FDA approves prescription weight loss drug Lorcaserin. Website. http://bariatrictimes.com/2012/07/18/the-centers-for-medicare-and-medicaid-services-endorse-sleeve-gastrectomy-as-a-valid-treatment-modality-for-patients-with-morbid-obesity-united-states-fda-approves-prescription-weight-loss-drug-lorca/. Bariatric Times. 2012, July. Accessed September 25, 2012.

5   Aetna Inc., United Healthcare to cover sleeve gastrectomy – ASMBS announces support of policy changes. Bariatric Times. 2010, April. News item. http://bariatrictimes.com/2010/05/19/aetna-inc-unitedhealthcare-to-cover-sleeve-gastrectomy%e2%80%94asmbs-announces-support-of-policy-changes/. Accessed September 26, 2012.

6   American Society for Metabolic and Bariatric Surgery. National insurance coverage map. Web site. http://asmbs.org/2011/12/national-insurance-coverage-map/. 2011, December. Accessed September 26, 2012.

7   American Medical Association. CPT – current procedural terminology. Website. http://www.ama-assn.org/ama/pub/physician-resources/solutions-managing-your-practice/coding-billing-insurance/cpt.page. 2012. Accessed September 27, 2012.

8   Blackstone RL. ASMBS news and update. Bariatric Times. http://bariatrictimes.com/2011/09/22/asmbs-news-and-update%e2%80%94september-2011/. 2011, August. Accessed September 27, 2012.

9   Kaplan LM, Seeley RJ. Myths associated with obesity and bariatric surgery: myth 1: "weight can be reliably controlled by voluntarily adjusting energy balance through diet and exercise. Bariatric Times. Mars Initiative Series. http://bariatrictimes.com/2012/04/18/myths-associated-with-obesity-and-bariatric-surgery/. 2012. 9(4):12-13. Accessed September 27, 2012.

10   Obesity Action Coalition. Working with your insurance provider: a guide to seeking weight loss surgery. Website. http://www.obesityaction.org/educational-resources/brochures-and-guides/oac-insurance-guide/reviewing-your-insurance-policy-or-employer-sponsored-medical-benefits-plan. 2009. Accessed September 27, 2012.

11   Centers for Medicare and Medicaid Services. (2009). National coverage determination (NCD) for bariatric surgery for treatment of morbid obesity. Retrieved from http://www.cms.gov/medicare-coverage-database/details/ncd-details.aspx?NCDId=57&ncdver=3&bc=BAABAAAAAAAA&

12   Jacques L, Jensen TS, Schafer J, Chin J, Ciccanti M. Decision memo for bariatric surgery for the treatment of morbid obesity (CAG-00250R2). Centers for Medicare and Medicaid Services. Memorandum. http://www.cms.gov/medicare-coverage-database/details/nca-decision-memo.aspx?NCAId=258&NcaName=Bariatric+Surgery+for+the+Treatment+of+Morbid+Obesity&CoverageSelection=National&KeyWord=obesity&KeyWordLookUp=Title&KeyWordSearchType=And&where=index&nca_id=219&basket=nca*3a$00397N*3a$219*3a$Surgery+for+Diabetes*3a$Open*3a$New*3a$5&bc=gAAAABAAIAAA&. 2012, June 27. Accessed September 27, 2012.

13   Medicaid. Medical enrollment by state. Centers for Medicare and Medicaid Services, Department of Health and Human Services. http://www.medicaid.gov/Medicaid-CHIP-Program-Information/By-State/By-State.html. Accessed September 27, 2012.

14   Centers for Medicare and Medicaid Services. Bariatric surgery. Department of Health and Human Services. http://www.cms.gov/Medicare/Medicare-General-Information/MedicareApprovedFacilitie/Bariatric-Surgery.html. 2012. Accessed September 27, 2012.

15   American Society for Metabolic and Bariatric Surgery. ASMBS BSCOE Benefits. Website. http://asmbs.org/wp-content/uploads/asmbs_bscoe_benefits1.pdf. September 20, 2012.

16   Picot J, Jones J, Colquitt JL, Gospodarevskaya E, Loveman E, Baxter L., Clegg AJ. The clinical effectiveness and cost-effectiveness of bariatric (weight loss) surgery for obesity: a systematic review and economic evaluation. Health Technology Assessment, 2009;13:1-90.

17   Maklin S, Malmivaara A, Linna M, Victorzon M, Koivukangas V, Sintonen H. Cost-utility of bariatric surgery for morbid obesity in Finland. Br J Surg. 2011;98(1):1422-9.

18   Salem L, Devlin A, Sullivan S, Flum DR. A cost-effectiveness analysis of laparoscopic gastric bypass, adjustable gastric banding and non-surgical weight loss interventions. Surgery for Obesity and Related Disease. 2008;4:24-32.

19   Tsai AG, Williamson DF, Glick HA. Direct medical cost of overweight and obesity in the USA: a quantitative systematic review. 2011;12(1):50-61.

20   Frequently asked questions. Surgical Services International, Inc. Website. http://www.surgicalservicesinternational.com/faq.htm. 2005. Accessed September 17, 2012.

21   Gastric sleeve surgery. Surgical Services International, Inc. Web site. http://www.surgicalservicesinternational.com/gastric_sleeve.htm. 2005. Accessed September 17, 2012.

22   Renew passport. U.S. Department of State. Website. http://www.travel.state.gov/passport/renew/renew_833.html. Accessed October 2, 2012.

23 First-time applicants. U.S. Department of State. Website. http://www.travel.state.gov/passport/get/first/first_830.html. Accessed October 2, 2012.

24 Processing times. U.S. Department of State. Website. http://www.travel.state.gov/passport/processing/processing_1740.html. Accessed October 2, 2012.

25 Gastric sleeve surgery. Surgical Services International, Inc. Website. http://www.surgicalservicesinternational.com/gastric_sleeve.htm. 2005. Accessed September 17, 2012.

26 Gastric sleeve surgery in Mexico. Surgical Services International, Inc. Website. 2005. Accessed September 17, 2012.http://www.surgicalservicesinternational.com/gastric_sleeve_mexico.htm

27 Surgical Review Corporation. ICE designation requirements. Website. http://www.surgicalreview.org/ice/requirements/. Accessed September 20, 2012.

28 Surgical Review Corporation. BOLD overview. Website. http://www.surgicalreview.org/bold/overview/. Accessed September 22, 2012.

29 Surgical Review Corporation. Bariatric Surgeon of Excellence Program. Website. http://www.surgicalreview.org/international/bsoe/. Accessed September 20, 2012.

30 Venezuela: Country Specific Information. U.S. Department of State. Website. http://travel.state.gov/travel/cis_pa_tw/cis/cis_1059.html. Accessed September 17, 2012.

31 Mexico: Country Specific Information. U.S. Department of State. Website. http://travel.state.gov/travel/cis_pa_tw/cis/cis_970.html. Accessed September 17, 2012.

32 Travel Warning. Bureau of Consular Affairs, US Department of State. Website. http://www.travel.state.gov/travel/cis_pa_tw/tw/tw_5665.html. 2012, February 8. Accessed September 17, 2012.

33 Surgical Services International, Inc. Website. http://www.surgicalservicesinternational.com/gastric_sleeve.htm. 2005. Accessed September 17, 2012.

34 Birch, D.W., Vu, L., Karmali, S., Stoklassa, C.J., & Sharma, A.M. (2010). Medical tourism in bariatric surgery. American Journal of Surgery, 5: 604-8.

35 Connor, B.A. Chapter 2: The pre-travel consultation: self-treatable conditions: traveler's diarrhea. Yellow Book, Centers for Disease Control and Prevention: Atlanta, GA. Retrieved from http://wwwnc.cdc.gov/travel/yellowbook/2012/chapter-2-the-pre-travel-consultation/travelers-diarrhea.htm. Updated 2012, February 9. Accessed September 28, 2012.

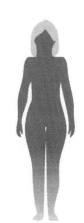

9

Pre-Surgery Preparations

The last couple of chapters have taken you from knowing that you want the sleeve to knowing how you're going to get it. You have your surgeon and medical team all picked out, and you know how you're going to pay for the surgery. You can really start to feel as though your life is changing as your surgery approaches.

This chapter will take you through the weeks or month of pre-surgery preparation that you'll need. This is some of the information that's in the chapter:

Medical appointments before your surgery: surgeon, dietitian and psychologist

- Medical tests to determine that surgery is as safe as possible for you
- Getting your psychological evaluation
- Meeting with the dietitian and following the pre-surgery diet
- Scheduling your surgery within your busy schedule

By the end of the chapter, you'll know what to expect in the weeks and months before the sleeve. This information will keep you right on track with these early stages of your weight loss journey. It's time to get going!

Meeting With Your Surgeon

Your surgery date is likely to be a few weeks or months from when you make the final decision about getting the gastric sleeve. During this time, you'll probably have one lengthy pre-surgery appointment with your surgeon. It's a chance for you to ask all of your additional questions and clarify anything you don't understand. Your surgeon will be able to verify that you're a good candidate for the procedure before setting a date for surgery. From now on, you'll be working closely with your surgeon. It's critical to establish mutual trust and have good two-way communication.

Questions that Your Surgeon Might Ask

Most of your time during your pre-surgery appointment might be spent talking. The most likely questions that your surgeon will ask are about your medical history. This includes past doctor's visits, test results, and medical treatment, plus current health conditions and treatments, including prescription medications.

If you're in a managed care plan, such as an HMO, a PPO, or Medicare, your medical information should be available on electronic health records, also known as EHR or e-records.[1] That means your surgeon and any of your other caregivers who need to know your medical history can access it on the computer from a single, secure database.

Even if your medical information is on an EHR, you may be asked to fill out a medical history form before coming to the clinic or while waiting in the waiting room before your appointment. The form may ask questions that are designed specifically for gastric sleeve candidates. These are some examples:

- Do you tend to throw up easily?
- Do many tastes and smells make you feel nauseous?
- How high is your pain tolerance? Are you more or less sensitive to pain than other people?

These questions help predict your recovery from the VSG and ongoing weight loss success. Your surgeon might ask follow-up questions on any unexpected or unusual answers or information from your medical history. Answers that stand out from the rest don't automatically disqualify you from getting the sleeve. Instead, they're more likely to give your surgeon and the rest of your medical team some guidance in helping you prepare for surgery by addressing your individual characteristics.

Tips for Preparing for Your Pre-Op Appointment

You don't want to run out of time or forget to ask your surgeon something important, so prepare for your appointment! Gather all that you can about your personal medical history and write it down so you can take it to your surgeon. A personal health record, or PHR, is a great way to store your medical information. It's like an EHR, but it's for your own personal use. Your healthcare provider likely offers one and can help you set it up.

Also look into your family's medical history. You can't learn everything detail about your parents and grandparents, but any information that you are able to find can be helpful for you and your surgeon.

Don't rely on your memory! Instead, write down everything you want to ask cover during your pre-op surgeon's appointment, even if you're not usually a list person. You don't want to accidentally forget to ask your surgeon something just because you're feeling nervous, excited, pressured, or distracted at your appointment. These are some of the topics that you might want to ask your surgeon about

- *A review of the vertical sleeve gastrectomy.* You may know the procedure pretty well by now from your research. You may have even seen a surgeon explain it using a lifelike model. However, having your own surgeon explain the procedure can solidify the details in your mind. This explanation also lets you ask questions during the explanation, which may not have been possible at a seminar.
- *"What if…"* You can ask about the "what-ifs" for during and after surgery. What if something goes wrong during surgery? What if you have complications? What if you need care in the middle of the night? What if you have trouble while you're on vacation? Get all of your worries addressed so that you can be confident going into surgery. Your surgeon should be able to answer all of your worries!
- *Your medical conditions.* Even if you've talked about them before, you want to be absolutely certain that you cover everything and give your surgeon time to consider each condition carefully.
- *Your over-the-counter and prescription medications.* Your medications can interfere with nutritional status and your surgeon should know about them. Another important

point is that you won't be eating solid foods right after your surgery, so you won't be able to take your regular pills or capsules. Ask your doctor whether your medications are available in liquid, gel, or powder form. Another option is to grind up medications that are in hard pill forms and dissolve them in water so that you can absorb them. Your surgeon should be able to figure out how you'll take your medications after surgery.

- **Dietary supplements, such as vitamins and minerals.** You're not going to be eating much during the first days, weeks, and even months after getting the sleeve. Dietary supplements help you meet your nutrient needs, but you won't be able to take whole pills or capsules right after surgery. As with medications, multivitamins in gel, powder or liquid form are viable options.

- **Birth control.** If you're currently taking oral contraceptives now is a good time to discuss alternative methods. You might not be allowed to take oral contraceptives for the first few weeks or months after getting the sleeve. Your focus after getting the sleeve should be on weight loss, and most surgeons will recommend waiting for at least 12 to 18 months before trying to get pregnant.[2]

Setting the Date of Your Sleeve Gastrectomy

You and your surgeon might set the date of your sleeve gastrectomy at your pre-surgery appointment. The surgery needs to be at least a few weeks away to give you time to prepare, and it may be a few months away. These are some factors that can affect when your surgery will be:

- **Pre-surgery diet.** At a minimum, you'll need to follow a liquid diet for a few days before surgery. Many patients follow a weight loss diet for a few weeks before surgery. The weight loss and liquid diet make your liver a little smaller to make it easier for your surgeon to see your stomach and esophagus during surgery; this reduces the risk of complications.[3]

- **Your work schedule.** You may be able to return to work seven to 10 days after getting the sleeve; it'll be longer if you have complications or if your job is physically demanding. If possible, choose a time when your work schedule is expected to be a little less hectic than normal. Avoid getting your sleeve during or before conferences or important work events. You want to be able to take an afternoon or day off of work without getting too far behind, and the sleeve can make you miss a few days because you feel nauseous or have surgeon appointments.

- **Your personal schedule.** Minimize the interference with your personal life. If you're a parent, you might want to get sleeved during the school year so that your children away for most of the day. If you're a schoolteacher or an adolescent, it's probably best to set your date at the end of the school year, right before your summer vacation. That will give you time to adjust to your new eating plan and get over the worst of the side effects before going back to school. Take a look at your calendar and make sure your surgery won't interfere with any big events, such as a friend's wedding or a major anniversary party. Of course, these considerations with your personal schedule aren't always practical, and that's okay. The sleeve is a medical procedure that you can fit into your life no matter what if you choose to do so.

- *Facility availability*. Often, hospitals and clinics fill up their bariatric surgery schedules months ahead of time. There's not much you can do about that, and you'll just have to work with the appointment scheduling center to get the soonest possible appointment that works for you. As with other appointments and medical procedures, you might be able to get on a waiting list to be called in case there's a cancellation ahead of you and an appointment slot opens up.

- *Medical tourism*. There is a lot of planning to do if you're going to get the sleeve in another country. Americans don't need a special visa to visit Mexico for the short time that you'll need to stay to get the sleeve and to recover.[4] You need a visa to enter Venezuela, but it doesn't delay your surgery because you can get it on the plane to Venezuela.[5] You also need a current passport for both countries, and your passport needs to be valid for at least another six months from the time you get to Venezuela. Getting your passport renewed can take several weeks, so this can be a factor in pushing back your surgery day. You'll also have to plan for time off of work, and schedule your transportation and hotel accommodations if you're responsible for making your own arrangements rather than having them included as part of a package deal with your surgeon. Travel can be a lot cheaper during the off-season and when you make arrangements far in advance.

You might have to wait a few months to meet all of the requirements and get your sleeve surgery done. That can seem like a long time, but the long waiting period has its benefits:

- You have more time to try out the sleeve diet and lifestyle.
- You have more time to do research on the sleeve so you know what to expect.
- You can lose a little extra weight before surgery to reduce your risk for complications during and after surgery.

Reminder: It's Not too Late to Change Your Surgeon

We want to remind you that it's not too late to change your surgeon. You can change your surgeon at any point up until you go in for surgery. Even after surgery, you can change your surgeon if you feel you're not getting the right aftercare and you can find another surgeon who will give you the post-surgery guidance you need.

Of course it's easier if you choose the right surgeon for you on your first try, but these are some reasons why you might want to change your surgeon.

- Your surgeon makes you feel uncomfortable when you're asking questions.
- Your surgeon doesn't give satisfactory answers to your questions.
- You simply don't have a good feeling about your surgeon.

- Your surgeon does not seem concerned about your personal success and individual concerns.

Don't worry about losing the time and effort that you've already put in toward the surgery. All of your research on the sleeve is still useful. If you already got medical tests done under your old surgeon, your new surgeon will probably accept most or all of the medical tests, dietary assessments, and psychological evaluations that you've gone through.

We're not encouraging you to actively *look* for reasons to change your surgeon, but we do want to remind you that you're still in control of your own health, and always should be. Some patients mistakenly think that they're stuck with a surgeon who doesn't turn out to be as good as hoped for based on their first impressions. That is absolutely not the case!

Medical Tests & Psychological Evaluation

It's a long list…but the tests aren't as bad as they sound! They're necessary for making sure that you're a good candidate for surgery. A lot of them are routine tests that you've had before; they're just checks to make sure your body is working normally and can handle the surgery.

These are some of the tests that you might have done:

- *Ultrasound of your gallbladder*. Rapid weight loss from the sleeve increases your risk of developing gallstones and makes existing gallstones worse. If the ultrasound detects that you already have gallstones, your surgeon might decide to remove your gallbladder during surgery to prevent the need for a second surgery to remove your gallbladder, or cholecystectomy.

- *Gastrointestinal x-rays*. This series of x-rays can verify that your gastrointestinal system has normal physiology; that is, that everything's in the right place. It's helpful for your surgeon to know whether everything's in the usual place before starting the surgery. If you have minor abnormalities, your surgeon can prepare better for the surgery and figure out whether to make different cuts on you compared to on other patients.

> **Tip**
>
> **Why a Chest X-Ray?**
>
> It's very important to make sure that your heart and lungs are healthy enough to undergo the laparosopic or open sleeve gastrectomy. Chapter 3, "Vertical Sleeve Gastrectomy 101," describes the pneumoperitonuem, or air pumped into your abdominal cavity. Chest and heart conditions, or cardiopulmonary diseases, can make a laparoscopic procedure dangerous, so you may need the open procedure instead. Certain conditions can make any surgery too high of a risk to be recommended.

- *Electrocardiogram, or EKG, or ECG*. This test gives you a line graph of alternating peaks and valleys that may look familiar. Each cycle on an ECG graph represents a heartbeat, and it gives a cardiologist a lot of information about your heart function. You get an ECG when a technician sticks some stickers onto the front and maybe back of your torso. Some wires are clipped to the stickers and placed in the ECG reader. The graph displays within minutes.

- *Chest x-ray*. An abnormal chest x-ray or sleep apnea, asthma, or shortness of breath can indicate trouble with your lungs. If you have these symptoms, you might be given additional lung tests, such as a chest CAT scan to give a more detailed image of your lungs, an oximetry or arterial blood oxygenation test to measure the amount of oxygen getting from your lungs to your blood or a spirometry test, which assesses how much and how strongly you can breathe. You may need to see a pulmonologist, or lung specialist, for further testing. Lung function is important because of the extra demands during the laparoscopic procedure.

Likely Blood Tests

You'll have an extensive panel of blood tests, known as a metabolic panel. Almost everyone is used to getting these done – you just need to go to the lab and have your blood drawn. The doctor who orders the tests or a nurse will tell you whether you need to get the tests done in the morning after an overnight fast. If you forget what the instructions are, just call the lab the day before you're planning to get your blood drawn and ask whether you need to fast. The metabolic panel is a basic set of tests that you've probably had a million times before, and probably never looked twice at the results. Chances are, you won't need to look twice at the results now, either. Your tests will probably include some or all of the following:[6]

- *Blood sugar, or blood glucose, test*: The results are pretty predictable if you get your blood sugar or glucose tested regularly. You might already know that you're normal, that you have pre-diabetes or that you have diabetes; or, you might be surprised for your numbers to come back higher than you expected. It's good to know the true value, especially if you have diabetes. That way, you can start treatment for it with a better diet and possibly medications.

- *Carbon dioxide[7] and/or calcium test*: These tests measure acid-base balance in your body. An abnormal acid-base balance can mean that you are having trouble with your kidneys, that you have uncontrolled diabetes, or that your lungs are not functioning well.

- *Serum electrolytes:* Electrolytes maintain fluid balance in your body and include sodium, chloride, and potassium.[8] If your electrolytes are out of whack, you could be dehydrated, have high blood pressure or have trouble with your liver, kidneys, lungs, or heart.

> **Tip**
>
> ### What about Calcium?
>
> A blood calcium test doesn't reflect the amount of calcium you get from the diet. No simple blood test can measure that. The best way to make sure that your calcium intake is adequate is to count up the amount of calcium you're getting from your diet and supplements. We'll go over your daily calcium requirements and good sources of calcium in Chapter 15, "The Sleeve Diet, Weight Loss and Your Health."

- *Kidney tests*: A blood urea nitrogen, or BUN, test and a creatinine test are common ways to check how well your kidneys are working.[9,10] Your kidneys act as filters for your blood, and one of their jobs is to make sure that you don't have too much protein (estimated by measuring creatinine or nitrogen) staying in your blood. BUN doesn't tell you how much protein you get in your diet.

- *Liver function tests*: The standard tests for liver function check your blood levels of aspartate aminotranferase, or AST, and alanine transaminase, or ALT.[11,12] Liver enzymes show you how hard and effectively your liver is working.

- *Nutrient status*: Your surgeon might order a few tests to see whether you're eating enough of key nutrients. These may include thiamin, or vitamin B-1, iron, folic acid, vitamin B-12, and vitamin D. These tests will probably become part of your regular routine after you get the sleeve because you're at higher risk for deficiencies of those nutrients.[13]

You'll have the tests done before your pre-op appointment so that you can go over the results with your surgeon. Don't be alarmed if one or more of your values comes back abnormal. It probably doesn't indicate a serious health problem, and it doesn't necessarily mean you can't get the sleeve. More than likely, it just means that your surgeon or primary care physician should figure out the cause of the out-of-range values and decide whether they will affect your care plan.

Psychological Evaluation

Most surgeons require a psychological evaluation before doing bariatric surgeries. If your healthcare coverage covers the sleeve, your insurance company will probably require the evaluation as a condition for reimbursement. The psychologist and your health team want to be sure that you're mentally and emotionally ready for the sleeve gastrectomy and beyond, because you're going to have to make drastic, long-term changes if you want to achieve your weight loss goals.

A lot of us naturally fear psychological evaluations because it conjures up thoughts of a mysterious person reading your mind and uncovering deep, dark secrets that you didn't even know you had. That's not even close to the truth! In fact, psych evaluations aren't that scary, and getting them done doesn't mean you're weird. The tests are nothing to worry about, and you might even find them kind of fun.

What Are Mental Health Professionals Looking for During Your Evaluation?

These are some of the things that the psych evaluation checks:

- *Your mental preparedness*. The sleeve is just a tool. For you to lose weight and minimize complications, you need to understand what kinds of lifestyle changes are necessary. You also have to realize that it's a lifelong commitment. Getting the sleeve is an irreversible procedure.

- *Your support system*. They may ask you about the role that your friends and family members play in your life, and where else you go for support. If you've gotten involved on BariatricPal.com, you'll have plenty to talk about when the psychologist asks about your support system!

- *Your mental stability*. Untreated mood disorders and other uncontrolled psychological disorders can make it more difficult to cope with changes in your life, such as getting the sleeve and making dramatic lifestyle changes. Losing weight brings its own set of changes, such as how you feel and how others treat you. You also need mental stability to overcome the challenges that you will almost certainly encounter.

- *Your maturity*. Adolescents are still gaining emotional maturity. Only adolescents who are considered relatively mature for their ages should plan to get the sleeve. You need to understand that it's a lifelong, irreversible procedure. You'll always have to be careful about what you eat. You won't be able to eat the same things as your friends, there'll be days when you don't feel well and may need to skip school and you will probably have to face forbidden foods at home on a daily basis.

- *Binge eating disorder and emotional eating*.[14] Binge eating is when you eat abnormally large amounts of food in short periods of time. You may feel out of control. Emotional eating, or compulsive eating, is when you eat to comfort yourself or cope, not to reduce hunger. Emotional eating may lead to binge eating, but it doesn't always. Binge eating and emotional eating can interfere with your weight loss because they show that you're not in control of your food intake. Your food intake needs to be very controlled for you to lose weight and avoid complications with the sleeve. Overeating during binge episodes can lead to sleeve leakage and the need for a second surgery.

- *Night eating syndrome*.[15] You may have night eating syndrome if you eat more than one-quarter of your daily calories late at night, you skip breakfast and are starving by the end of the day, and/or you wake up at night and eat so you can get back to sleep. Night eating is associated with weight gain, and bariatric surgery candidates have higher rates of night eating than normal-weight individuals. Night eating is associated with depression and anxiety, too.[16] Behavioral counseling and/or medications may be treatment options if you and your psychologist determine that you have night eating syndrome. You'll be more likely to succeed with the sleeve if you take care of night eating syndrome before surgery.

- *Drug or alcohol abuse*.[17] An inability to stop abusing drugs or alcohol shows that you may not have the self-discipline that you'll need to stick to the sleeve diet. Surgeons may require you to get over your addiction before agreeing to do the operation.

- *Untreated depression*. Getting the sleeve can improve your life and mood, but it will not cure depression. The large amount of weight loss and sudden changes in your life can even make depression worse. If you have major depressive disorder, it's best to get it under control and understand the reasons for it before going ahead with the VSG. You may need medications to correct a chemical imbalance in your brain, or you may need counseling to resolve underlying emotional issues. Once your depression is under control, you're a much better candidate for surgery.

What to Expect in the Psychologist's Office

There's no standard protocol to determine your psychological eligibility for the bariatric surgery.[18] The experience varies depending on the specific psychologist or psychiatrist that you see. You might even see a social worker to give you all or part of the psychological evaluation.

Face-to-Face Interview - You'll probably start by talking with your mental health professional. The conversation may be free-flowing, or it might involve a list of questions that your psychologist asks one by one. Most likely, there'll be a bit of both in what's called a Structured Clinical Interview. You'll have a lot of open-ended questions to answer, and the doctor will take some notes. The face-to-face interview can be very brief or it can take more than an hour.

Written Evaluation - The other part of your mental testing, or psychological evaluation, is the written part. You might just have a few short questionnaires to fill out, or you might have a bunch of surveys to answer. The questions usually have multiple choice answers, so they're not too tiring for you to answer even though they may seem to be unlimited.

Answer Truthfully! What is the right answer on the tests? The truth. Seriously. Answer honestly without trying to cheat the test and give the psychologist the answer you think he or she is looking for. There are two main reasons for this:

- *Cheating the test is really only cheating yourself.* Yes, it's cliché, and yes, it's true – way truer than it was in grade school when you were "borrowing" your buddy's homework answers. There is no point in getting the VSG if it's not going to work for you. You do not want to spend the rest of your life with only 15 percent of your stomach and still be obese if simply being truthful can prevent it. Don't lie to try to get the sleeve. If it's not right for you, there are other treatments for obesity.

- *You might not even know what the "right" answers are.* There are so many scoring systems and different ways of looking at the results that you might accidentally give some answers that make your evaluations come out unfavorable. If your psychologist tells you that you're ineligible for the sleeve based on your test results, it would be pretty embarrassing to have to explain that you lied on some answers because you were trying to cheat the system but couldn't figure it out!

What Kind of Tests Might You See?

It seems like anything's fair game! Each clinic has its own set of favorite assessments designed to test different aspects of your psychological readiness for surgery. These are a few of the more widely used tests:

- Minnesota Multiphasic Personality Inventory (MMPI) for depression
- Beck Depression Inventory (BDI)
- The Moorehead-Ardelt Quality of Life Questionnaire is a short test for the evaluation of possible mood disorders
- Beck Anxiety Inventory (BAI)
- Mini International Neuropsychiatric Interview (MINI)
- Internalized Shame Scale (ISS)
- University Rhode Island Change Assessment to estimate your readiness to change, or how prepared you are to change your lifestyle.
- Revised Master Questionnaire (RMQ) for the "psychological evaluation of cognitive and behavioral difficulties related to weight management." It aims to uncover reasons why you've had trouble managing your weight and evaluate whether surgery will be helpful for you or whether you'll likely fall into the same patterns.

Psychological testing is a bit tricky because every individual patient is, of course, an individual. Plus, there are so many aspects of mental health that can affect success with the sleeve. That makes it hard to develop a single test or set of tests to evaluate how well you'll probably do with the sleeve.

- For example, the University Rhode Island Change Assessment test sounds pretty useful, but research has found that it might not do a good job predicting your total weight loss or whether you'll have complications.
- A single test doesn't tell the whole story, which is why psychologists need to use a bunch of different tests before they're confident that you're ready for surgery.

It's not as simple as throwing a few tests at you and scoring them on a standard scale. That's where the education and experience of your psychologist comes in. Your psychologist chooses the set of tests that you'll get and looks carefully at the results. You should be asked specifically about anything that looks unusual so that you and your psychologist can make the best decision.

Sources:[19, 20, 21, 22, 23]

Working with a Dietitian is Crucial

You'll start working on your dietary changes before you get the sleeve. You can lose a few pounds during your pre-surgery preparation period. You may meet with a dietitian one or more times to:

- Assess your current diet
- Go over the sleeve diet more specifically to clear up the details
- Point out changes that you'll need to make to follow the sleeve diet
- Develop your pre-surgery weight loss diet meal plan if your surgeon or insurance company requires you to lose weight before surgery
- Get the instructions for the liquid diet that you'll follow before surgery

Working with a dietitian can seem intimidating at first. You may feel embarrassed about your diet because it's clearly not the healthiest for you. However, just like when you see the psychologist, it's important for you to remember that the dietitian is on your side. The dietitian wants to you succeed in losing weight and living a healthy lifestyle. It's no secret that you're getting the sleeve, so be honest about your diet and be open to advice.

Purpose of a Dietary Assessment

Your first appointment with a dietitian will probably include an assessment of your current diet. It's not to make you feel bad about your current choices. Instead, these are these some of the ways in which a dietary assessment can be helpful at this point in your sleeve journey:

- *It gets you out of denial so you can think about your true diet.* You may have been fixating on food and diets, but many of us tend to "forget" the parts that we're not proud of, such as the extra bowl of ice cream or a trip to the local McDonald's just for fun. It's hard to improve your habits when you don't realize or can't admit what you've been eating.

- *It's a starting point.* A diet assessment gets everything down on paper so you can see where you are now, and where you need to be to get to the sleeve diet. You will have to change your food choices, serving sizes, and meal and snack patterns.

- *It makes you think.* When you are forced to do a dietary assessment with a nutrition professional such as a dietitian, you have to think about each little bite that goes into your mouth. That's also what you'll have to do when you have the sleeve. It's best to start now, when you have the dietitian guiding you through the process of remembering the "extra" foods, such as snacks, condiments, beverages with calories, and fat used in cooking.

- It *brings up the question of portion sizes.* As the dietitian asks about how much you eat, you might start to realize that you're not always sure. Once you actually measure your foods, you might be surprised at how many "servings" you actually eat at one time just because you didn't realize how small a serving was. Just cutting back on your serving sizes will really help you lower your calorie intake and help you achieve better weight loss.

Dietary Assessment Using a 24-Hour Recall

How does a diet assessment work? The most common choice for clinical dietitians is a 24-hour recall. Why:

- You don't have to prepare for it.
- It's pretty accurate at estimating your nutrient intake.
- It lets you practice being precise about your diet under the guidance of a dietitian.

It works just like it sounds. In the recall, you identify each food and beverage that you've consumed in the past 24 hours. The dietitian will write each item down and ask you for details, such as serving size, how you prepared it and what else you ate with it. He or she will also ask you if you've eaten normally over the past day, or if whether some reason your meal patterns and food choices were different from your normal diet over the past day.

You'll also tell the dietitian about any nutritional dietary supplements that you take so that your dietitian will have a better idea of your average nutrient intake. These might include the following:

- Individual or combined vitamins and/or minerals, such as iron, calcium and vitamin D, or vitamin B-12.
- Multivitamin and mineral supplements such as a daily tablet or capsule with a variety of vitamins and minerals.
- Omega-three fatty acid supplements, such as fish oil supplements, DHA and EPA or linolenic acid supplements.

Why Does My Dietitian Repeat So Many Questions?

The 24-hour recall can feel repetitive. The dietitian asks you to go over your food and beverage intake a few times, not just once. It's not because your dietitian isn't listening or thinks you're lying. In reality, the dietitian is following a standard method of doing a 24-hour recall. A common choice is the USDA's Multiple-Pass Method, which has you go over your intake five times. Each of the following steps, or "passes," of the Multiple Pass Method is slightly different from the others:

1. Quick list: The dietitian listens without interrupting to each food and beverage you list starting exactly 24 hours ago. This is to get your memory working.
2. Forgotten foods: In this pass, or go-through, your dietitian prompts you to remember items that you might have forgotten. These might include snacks, side dishes, and condiments. The dietitian might ask, for example, whether you had jam on the toast that you listed for breakfast; another question might be whether you had an evening snack after dinner last night.

3. Time and occasion: You go over when, what time, and with whom you ate each meal or snack. This step helps you remember any snacks that you might have forgotten; for example, you might realize that you ate such an early lunch yesterday that you had an extra afternoon snack. Remembering the occasion might help you remember more foods; for example, you might suddenly remember that you had a glass of wine last night to celebrate your wife's birthday. Recording the time and occasion can also help you identify your meal and snack patterns so that you know how you'll need to change your patterns to follow the sleeve diet.

4. Detail cycle: This is when you try to get the details set. The goal for each food is to know what you had with it and how much you had. The dietitian might ask how you prepared each item to see whether you added anything. For example, if you listed fried fish, you probably also had oil or salt, and might have had some sort of batter on it. This is the time to provide details about brand names, if you remember them from food packages. This is also when you estimate your portion sizes. It can be surprisingly tough to remember and try to figure exactly how big your portions were! Now is a good time to start practicing because you'll definitely be using and developing these skills over the next months and years in your gastric sleeve diet! The dietitian might provide various tools to help you with portions as you do your 24-hour recall.

   - Food models are usually made of plastic, and they are very realistic, three-dimensional models of different kinds of foods and beverages in standard serving sizes and realistic shapes. For example, you might see one cup of plastic cereal sitting in one half-cup of plastic milk in a plastic bowl.

   - Pictures of food, plates and utensils. These are usually life-sized photographs of different foods. They often have rulers and other familiar objects, such as pennies, golf balls and decks of cards, in the photos to give you some perspective. Photos are only two-dimensional, but they can help you visualize and figure the amount of each food that you ate.

   - Measuring cups and tablespoons. These are a little more abstract than actual models, but they are, of course, very accurate for quantities. You'll definitely be practicing using measuring cups and tablespoons, so you might as well get their sizes in your head now.

5. Final probe: This is like the proofreading part of the process. You and the dietitian take one last look at the list of foods and beverages to make sure it's as accurate and complete as you can make it. If you haven't already talked about them, this is also when your dietitian will ask about any dietary supplements that you are taking.

You can see that the 24-hour recall has a lot of repetition because you cover the same 24 hours over and over and over again. But, each step has its purpose, and research studies show that this type of approach is relatively accurate.

Source[24]

Other Diet Assessment Methods

The dietitian might choose one of these common methods in addition to or instead of a 24-hour recall:

- *Food frequency questionnaire.* The purpose of a food frequency questionnaire, or FFQ, is to get your diet history—or get a general picture of what you've typically eaten over the past year or so. There are bunch of different types of FFQs; some of the most common are the Block FFQ, the Health Habits and History Questionnaire, and the Harvard University Food Frequency Questionnaires.[25] You do a FFQ by filling out multiple-choice forms that ask you to choose how often you eat different types of foods. The difference between the different kinds of questionnaires is the specific foods and quantities that are listed on them, and how many different foods there are. For example, one FFQ might ask how often you eat fruit, while another might offer distinct choices for apples, oranges, bananas, and other types of fruits. More food choices make an FFQ more accurate, but also make it take longer for you to fill out. FFQs are good because they give a nice general picture of your regular diet and you don't have to remember every detail. They're really good at pointing out general patterns, such as eating a lot of sweets or rarely eating whole grain foods.

- *Food record.* Before your first appointment, at your first appointment or sometime later on your weight loss journey, your dietitian might ask you to fill out a food record, food journal, or food log. That's when you write down everything you eat or drink right as you're eating it or just after the meal. You'll try to write down the same information that your dietitian collects during a 24-hour recall: what you ate, when you ate it, how much you ate, who you were with, and how you prepared it. Usually, food records last for three days, and your dietitian might ask you to complete your record during two weekdays and one day on the weekend. A benefit of a food record is that you're less likely to forget foods compared to doing a 24-hour recall. That's because you can write them down as soon as you eat them. Also, you won't have to be trying to remember your diet while you're on the spot, as you are during an appointment with the dietitian doing a recall. They're kind of annoying at first because you have to remember to write things down and it can feel like a waste of time, but keeping a food journal will probably become a part of your life for at least a few months following surgery. People who keep food journals tend to have better success with weight control, so it's a great idea to get used to keeping a food diary now. It'll get easier pretty soon and won't feel like such a chore.

Figuring Out Your Nutrient Intake

After gathering information about your food intake from a 24-hour recall, an FFQ and/or a food record, your dietitian needs to analyze your diet. That just means changing the foods you listed into values for calories and nutrients. The dietitian can use an online database, such as one provided by the USDA, to calculate your nutrient intake and compare it to your recommendations. Many dietitians use specialized nutritional software to make their jobs easier.

The dietitian will discuss the results will you, and may suggest a few foods or supplements to add to your diet to improve your nutrient intake if you're low in certain nutrients. Up to 80 percent of VSG patients are low in vitamin D, and 13 to 44 percent have low iron and/or vitamin B-12 status before surgery.[26] These deficiencies can cause fatigue, infections, and complications from surgery, so it's best to address them now.

Talking about the Gastric Sleeve Diet with Your Dietitian

Success with the sleeve will depend largely on your motivation to follow the sleeve diet and how closely you follow it. What better time to talk about the diet than before the surgery when you meet with the dietitian? These are some topics you might want to discuss:

- A sample menu showing a few days of sleeve-appropriate eating
- How you will plan your meal and snack timing
- Which foods you won't be able to eat with the sleeve
- Concerns about real-life situations, such as holiday parties, late nights at work, or having company for dinner

Pre-Op Weight Loss, Liquid Diets and Exercise Programs

Many sleeve patients go on a weight loss diet for several weeks or a few months before their surgery. Your surgeon might require this for safety and to demonstrate your ability to follow the sleeve diet. Your insurance company might require you to follow a pre-surgery weight loss diet to show your commitment to the sleeve so that the insurance company feels that the cost is worth it.

Benefits of the Pre-Surgery Weight Loss Diet

This diet will be similar to the diet that you will follow for the months and years following the sleeve gastrectomy as you lose weight and maintain your goal weight loss. The diet will probably include about 800 to 1,200 calories per day, and will emphasize healthy choices and controlled portion sizes. These are some of the reasons why you may be asked follow this diet:[27],[28]

- **It helps you lose weight.** Losing at least five percent of your total body weight before bariatric surgery shortens recovery time and reduces your risk of complications.[29] That's 12 to 25 pounds if your starting weight is 250 pounds, or 15 to 30 pounds if your initial weight is 300 pounds.
- **It's proof that you *can* follow this diet**. Following the sleeve diet before surgery tests your commitment to the sleeve lifestyle and shows that you have the discipline and motivation to change your dietary habits. This gives you confidence in yourself, convinces your surgeon that you're a good candidate for the sleeve, and satisfies your insurance company's requirements for reimbursement.

- **It makes your post-surgery transition easier**. The pre-op diet lets you practice for the post-surgery diet. It's much better to get make your mistakes now, when you're in a low-pressure situation before getting the sleeve, than later, when you have plenty of other things to worry about.

This low-calorie diet can provide enough nutrients for you to stay on it safely for months until your surgery as long as you stay under the care of your surgeon. Make sure to follow your surgeon's and dietitian's recommendations for healthy food choices, getting enough protein, and taking vitamin and mineral supplements as needed.

The diet may be a challenge, especially early on. You might feel hungry and cranky, but you'll get through it. Within a few days, the diet will become much easier. You'll figure out some mental coping techniques, and you might start to realize that you're not really as hungry as you thought you were; at least, you will learn that being hungry is not the worst thing in the world. Keep your eye on the prize – a hard-earned sleeve surgery and the chance to achieve your goal weight for life.

The Pre-Surgery Liquid Diet

The diet that you follow for the final few days or couple weeks before surgery will be even stricter than the longer-term weight loss diet that may have lasted for months. The pre-surgery diet is very low-calorie and unlikely to provide all of the nutrients you need each day. You can only stay on it for a short period before risking health problems, and only under physician supervision. The diet makes your liver smaller by about eight to 14 percent so it's easier for your surgeon to perform surgery.[30]

The preoperative diet is usually a liquid diet, but there may be some flexibility in the guidelines, depending on your surgeon. Many hospitals and dietitians have a prepared flier or brochure that describes the diet, lists what you can and cannot have and suggests a sample meal plan. You might see your dietitian specifically to discuss the liquid diet, or you might just rely on the handout and telephone calls with your surgeon or dietitian to guide you through the diet. You can call your surgeon or dietitian if you have questions. You can also go onto BariatricPal.com to ask post-surgery members about their experiences with their pre-surgery diet.

Foods on a Liquid Diet[31]

Allowed - Liquids	Depends on Surgeon – Pureed Foods	Not Allowed – Solid Foods
• Milk	• Cream of wheat	• Bread, pasta, rice
• Tea, water, coffee	• Applesauce	• Nuts, beans, seeds
• Protein shakes	• Pureed potatoes	• Meats, poultry, fish
• Gelatin	• Oatmeal	• Cheese
• Popsicles	• Other cooked cereals	• Raw fruit
• Ice cream and sherbet	• Strained meats	• Raw vegetables

Table 18: Foods on a Liquid Diet

High-Nutrient, Low-Sugar Choices on Your Liquid Diet

You will probably exchange each of your regular meals for a diet or high-protein meal-replacement beverage, such as a can of regular or high-protein Slim-Fast, a Medifast shake, or a protein shake that is fortified with vitamins and minerals.[32] You can reduce your hunger while following the very low-calorie liquid diet by choosing high-protein and high-fiber options. Also, choose ones that are lower in added sugars so you avoid sugar spikes and crashes.

Be sure to read the nutrition facts label to find out how many calories it contains. Some brands have 100 to 200 calories in a serving, while others have 300 or more calories. You don't want to be eating way more calories than you think and prevent weight loss while on a liquid diet. Avoiding full-sized shakes between meals will also help you limit your calorie intake. Instead, choose calorie-free beverages, such as water, tea and coffee, and low-calorie beverages, such as diet juice drinks and low-calorie flavored waters, such as Crystal Light and sugar-free Kool-Aid.[33] You can also have sugar-free gelatin and popsicles between meals.

Your liquid diet will not allow sugary liquids, such as fruit punch, sports drinks, energy drinks, soft drinks, or sweetened ice coffee or tea. These don't provide important nutrients; they give you a lot of calories, and they can make you feel shaky when you're not eating solid foods with them. You'll also need to avoid carbonated beverages to prevent an upset stomach.

> **Tip**
>
> Chapter 15, "The Sleeve Diet, Weight Loss and Your Health," will cover nutrition labels and ingredients lists on foods and beverages. We'll go over what information you can find on them, how to read them and what to look for when you're choosing your food. You can find out about more about added sugars in Chapter 13, "Recovery and Your Post-Surgery Diet." That chapter also has much more detail on a standard liquid diet, which you'll be following for a few weeks after you get the sleeve, too.

The Liquid Diet and Diabetes

Any special diet is an extra challenge if you have prediabetes or diabetes because your body has trouble keeping your blood sugar levels constant. Your blood glucose levels can skyrocket, which is hyperglycemica, when you get too many calories or too much sugar, such as from a high-carbohydrate meal replacement beverage.

The other consideration is hypoglycemia. This can occur between meals when you haven't eaten any carbohydrates for a while. Before starting your liquid diet, it's especially important to discuss your diabetes and strategies for controlling your blood sugar with your dietitian. You will need to monitor the amount of carbohydrates that you have, and be sure to spread out your intake throughout the day to avoid high and low blood sugar levels.

Pre-Surgery Exercise Program

Some patients can start exercising before surgery. Activity burns extra calories so you lose weight faster; it helps stabilize your blood sugar levels, and it gets you stronger before surgery. Up until now, your obesity may be preventing you from exercising because of embarrassment, pain, asthma, or discomfort while moving.

After you lose weight on the pre-operative diet, you may be able to do light exercise more easily than before. If your physician gives you the go-ahead, you might try gentle stretching, water aerobics, water jogging, or slow walking, either on your own or hanging onto the rails of a treadmill for support.

An exercise program might not be possible if your obesity is still causing too many problems. That's okay. For now, just focus on your eating and on your other preparations for surgery. There'll be plenty of time later for getting into an exercise program and using physical activity as another tool in your weight loss journey with the sleeve.

Tip

Chapter 2, "Weight Loss Options," has a discussion of the health benefits of exercise. Chapter 16, "Staying in Shape with Exercise," lets you know what to expect and how to stay safe when you're starting an exercise program and some ways to stay motivated to exercise regularly.

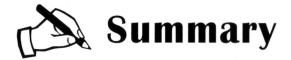 # Summary

- ☛ Surgery's no longer a vague idea in your mind – it's a real event that's about to take place in your life!

- ☛ After this chapter, you know what the typical patient goes through before getting the sleeve. Your role is to follow your medical team's directions and to ask all of your questions so that you have the best chances for success.

- ☛ This chapter covers the months and weeks before surgery; the next chapter goes through the final crucial days and hours before you go in for the sleeve.

- ☛ The goal of this chapter is to prevent you from worrying about overlooking things so you can have peace of mind. Let's get to it!

Your Turn: Getting Ready for Your Surgeon Visits

The chapter talks a lot about visits to your surgeon or other members of your healthcare team. You'll get the most out of each one if you do your homework beforehand. This worksheet should help.

Write down the name, address, telephone number, and email address of your surgeon.

....

....

....

Do the same for each member of your medical team.

....

....

....

Dietitian

....

....

....

Psychologist

....

....

....

Reception desk of clinic or front desk of hospital

....

....

....

Look up everything you can find about your family medical history. Write down any important information here. Try to get at least your parents' information, as well as that of your siblings and any grandparents whose information you can track down.

Name ....

Relationship to you ....

Medical conditions

....

....

....

Name

Relationship to you

Medical conditions

Name

Relationship to you

Medical conditions

Name

Relationship to you

Medical conditions

Write down your own medical information.

Prescription medications

Name brand and generic name

Purpose (why are you taking it: what health condition is it treating?)

Dosage and frequency

....
....
....

———◆———

Name brand and generic name

....
....
....

Purpose (why are you taking it: what health condition is it treating?)

....
....
....

Dosage and frequency

....
....
....

———◆———

Name brand and generic name

....
....
....

Purpose (why are you taking it: what health condition is it treating?)

....
....
....

Dosage and frequency

....
....
....

Write down any other relevant medical history. What conditions do you have? Have you had any medical conditions or major medical procedures in the past?

....
....
....
....

Do you take dietary supplements? This includes vitamins, minerals, herbals, and natural supplements. YES/NO

Write them down here. Include the dosage and how often you take it.

Supplement 1

....

....

....

Supplement 2

....

....

....

Supplement 3

....

....

....

Supplement 4

....

....

....

1   Medicare. Managing your personal health information online. Centers for Medicare and Medicaid Services. U.S. Department of Health and Human Services. Website. http://www.medicare.gov/navigation/manage-your-health/personal-health-records/personal-health-records-overview.aspx. Accessed October 6, 2012.

2   Apovian CM, Cummings S, Anderson W, Borud L, Boyer K, Day K, Hatchigian E, Hodges B, Patti ME, Pettus M, Perna F, Rooks D, Saltzman E, Skoropowski J, Tantillo MB, Thomason P. Best practice updates for multidisciplinary care in weight loss surgery. Obesity (Silver Spring). 2009;17(5):871-879.

3   Apovian CM, Cummings S, Anderson W, Borud L, Boyer K, Day K, Hatchigian E, Hodges B, Patti ME, Pettus M, Perna F, Rooks D, Saltzman E, Skoropowski J, Tantillo MB, Thomason P. Best practice updates for multidisciplinary care in weight loss surgery. Obesity (Silver Spring). 2009;17(5):871-879.

4   Mexico country specific information. Bureau of Consular Affairs, U.S. Department of State. Website. http://travel.state.gov/travel/cis_pa_tw/cis/cis_970.html. Accessed October 2, 2012.

5   Venezuela country specific information. Bureau of Consular Affairs, U.S. Department of State. Website. http://travel.state.gov/travel/cis_pa_tw/cis/cis_1059.html. Accessed October 2, 2012.

6   Basic metabolic panel. Pubmed Health, U.S. National Library of Medicine. Website. http://www.ncbi.nlm.nih.gov/pubmedhealth/PMH0003934/. Reviewed 2011, May 30. Accessed October 2, 2012.

7   CO2 blood test. Pubmed Health, U.S. National Library of Medicine. Website. http://www.ncbi.nlm.nih.gov/pubmedhealth/PMH0003940/. Reviewed 2011, May 30. Accessed October 2, 2012.

8   Chloride test - blood. Pubmed Health, U.S. National Library of Medicine. Website. http://www.ncbi.nlm.nih.gov/pubmedhealth/PMH0003956/. Reviewed 2011, June 1. Accessed October 2, 2012.

9   Creatinine - blood. Pubmed Health, U.S. National Library of Medicine. Website. http://www.ncbi.nlm.nih.gov/pubmedhealth/PMH0003946/. Reviewed 2011, June 1. Accessed October 2, 2012.

10   Blood urea nitrogen – BUN test. Pubmed Health, U.S. National Library of Medicine. Website. http://www.ncbi.nlm.nih.gov/pubmedhealth/PMH0003945/. Reviewed 2011, May 30. Accessed October 2, 2012.

11   .Dugdale DC. Zieve D. AST. MedlinePlus, U.S. National Library of Medicine. Website. http://www.nlm.nih.gov/medlineplus/ency/article/003472.htm. Reviewed 2011, February 20. Accessed October 2, 2012.

12   Dugdale DC, Zieve D. ALT. MedlinePlus, U.S. National Library of Medicine. Website. http://www.nlm.nih.gov/medlineplus/ency/article/003473.htm. Updated 2011, February 20. Accessed October 2, 2012.

13   Apovian CM, Cummings S, Anderson W, Borud L, Boyer K, Day K, Hatchigian E, Hodges B, Patti ME, Pettus M, Perna F, Rooks D, Saltzman E, Skoropowski J, Tantillo MB, Thomason P. Best practice updates for multidisciplinary care in weight loss surgery. Obesity (Silver Spring). 2009;17(5):871-879.

14   Apovian CM, Cummings S, Anderson W, Borud L, Boyer K, Day K, Hatchigian E, Hodges B, Patti ME, Pettus M, Perna F, Rooks D, Saltzman E, Skoropowski J, Tantillo MB, Thomason P. Best practice updates for multidisciplinary care in weight loss surgery. Obesity (Silver Spring). 2009;17(5):871-879.

15   Apovian CM, Cummings S, Anderson W, Borud L, Boyer K, Day K, Hatchigian E, Hodges B, Patti ME, Pettus M, Perna F, Rooks D, Saltzman E, Skoropowski J, Tantillo MB, Thomason P. Best practice updates for multidisciplinary care in weight loss surgery. Obesity (Silver Spring). 2009;17(5):871-879.

16   Striegel-Moore RH, Rosselli F, Wilson GT, Perrin N, Harvey K, DeBar L. Nocturnal eating: association with binge eating, obesity and psychological distress. Int J Eat Disord. 2010;43(6):520-526.

17   Apovian CM, Cummings S, Anderson W, Borud L, Boyer K, Day K, Hatchigian E, Hodges B, Patti ME, Pettus M, Perna F, Rooks D, Saltzman E, Skoropowski J, Tantillo MB, Thomason P. Best practice updates for multidisciplinary care in weight loss surgery. Obesity (Silver Spring). 2009;17(5):871-879.

18   Sogg S, Mori DL. The Boston Interview for gastric bypass: determining the psychological suitability of surgical candidates. Obesity Surgery.14(3):2004.

19   Moorehead AK, Ardelt-Gattinger E, Lechner H, Oria HE. The validation of the Moorehead-Ardelt Quality of Life Questionnaire II. Obesity Surgery. 2003;13:684-92.

20   Nicolai A, Ippoliti C, Petrelli MD. Laparoscopic adjustable banding: essential role of psychological support. Obesity Surgery. 2002;12:857-63.

21   Hayden MJ, Brown WA, Brennan L, O'Brien PE. Validation of the Beck Depression Inventory as a screening tool for a clinical mood disorder in bariatric surgery candidates. Obesity Surgery. 2012. epub ahead of print.

22   Lier HQ, Biringer E, Stubhaug B, Tangen T. Prevalence of psychiatric disorders before and one year after bariatric surgery: the role of shame in maintenance of psychiatric disorders   in patients undergoing bariatric surgery. Nordic Journal of Psychiatry. 2012. epub ahead of print.

23   Corsica JA, Hood MM, Azarbad L, Ivan I. Revisiting the Revised Master Questionnaire for the psychological evaluation of bariatric surgery candidates. Obesity Surgery. 2012;22: 381-8.

24 USDA Automated Multiple-Pass Method. Agricultural Research Services, United States Department of Agriculture. Web site. http://www.ars.usda.gov/Services/docs.htm?docid=7710. Modified 2010, September 29. Accessed October 3, 2012.

25 Thompson FE, Subar AF. Chapter 1: Dietary Assessment Methodology. Nutrition in the Prevention and Treatment of Chronic Disease, 2nd ed. National Cancer Institute: Bethesda, Maryland.

26 Snyder-Marlow G, Tayle D, Lenhard MJ. Nutrition care for patients undergoing laparoscopic sleeve gastrectomy for weight loss. J Am Diet Ass. 2010;110(4):600-607

27 Pre-surgery bariatric diet. Bariatric Choice: The Leading Source of Bariatric Nutrition. Retrieved from http://www.bariatricchoice.com/pre-op-bariatric-diet-for-bariatric-gastric-bypass-surgery-patients.aspx. 2011. Accessed October 4, 2012.

28 Snyder-Marlow G, Tayle D, Lenhard MJ. Nutrition care for patients undergoing laparoscopic sleeve gastrectomy for weight loss. J Am Diet Ass. 2010;110(4):600-607

29 Apovian CM, Cummings S, Anderson W, Borud L, Boyer K, Day K, Hatchigian E, Hodges B, Patti ME, Pettus M, Perna F, Rooks D, Saltzman E, Skoropowski J, Tantillo MB, Thomason P. Best practice updates for multidisciplinary care in weight loss surgery. Obesity (Silver Spring). 2009;17(5):871-879.

30 Goldenberg L. Weight loss before weight loss surgery: what do we know about dropping those preoperative pounds? Bariatric Times. 2010;7(7):18-20.

31 Dugdale DC, Zieve D. Liquid diet – full. Medline Plus, National Institutes of Health. Website. http://www.nlm.nih.gov/medlineplus/ency/patientinstructions/000206.htm. Updated 2010, November 21. Accessed October 4, 2012.

32 Slim-Fast and Medifast are trademarked names, and this book is not affiliated with Slim-Fast or Medifast.

33 Crystal Light and Kool-Aid are trademarked and are not affiliated with this book.

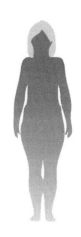

10

Final Preparation for the Sleeve Surgery

Surgery's quickly approaching, and this chapter will get you up to speed so you know exactly what to do to get ready as well as what to expect at the hospital when you go in for surgery. This is some of the information that's in the chapter:

- Planning your home for your post-surgery recovery time
- Packing for the hospital
- Following an overnight fast and adjusting your medications the night before surgery
- Checking into the hospital and going into surgery

This chapter will take you up until you lose consciousness and go into the operating room for surgery. It's a time for excitement and probably a few nerves, but knowing what to expect can calm your nerves and make everything go better than you'd hoped.

Prepare and Make Post-Op Recovery Easier

The suspense is building! Your big day is approaching. You're medically cleared, you've met the surgeon and other members of your medical team, and you know what to expect during and after surgery. It's time to take care of a few logistics to make sure everything goes as smoothly as possible on your surgery day and during your recovery. Some of these tasks are pretty obvious, but it's best to list them out so that you don't forget anything in the excitement of finally getting the vertical sleeve gastrectomy.

Time off from Work

Make sure that you arrange for time off work if you haven't already done so. You'll need to take at least one to two weeks off from work or more if you have an active job or you have complications during or after surgery. If you feel comfortable doing so, let your supervisor know about the possibility of taking off extra time so that it doesn't come as a surprise. Of course, it's up to you whether to tell your supervisor that you may need extra time and whether to give the truthful reason why. A lot of patients choose not to tell their employers about bariatric surgery.

> **Tip**
>
> Chapter 17, 'What to Expect in the First Year after VSG,' talks about whether to tell people about your surgery and how to decide. It's entirely up to you whom to tell or not to tell as well as how much detail you choose to give.

Getting Your Home Ready

You'll be feeling sick and tired when you get home from the hospital after surgery. You won't be in any mood for household chores or grocery shopping, so it's best to prepare ahead of time. Preparing your home before surgery will make recovery easier after surgery.

Pain Medications

You're going to have pain after surgery. Your abdominal area will be hurting from the skin to the places that the surgeon had to make cuts during surgery. You may also have shoulder pain from gas that remains in your body from the pneumoperitoneum portion of the laparoscopic procedure. Talk with your surgeon before surgery to make sure you stock up on the pain medications that you're likely to need. Many are available over the counter, but your surgeon may recommend some stronger prescription medications too.

Non-Steroidal Anti-Inflammatory Drugs (NSAIDs)

Non-steroidal anti-inflammatory drugs, or NSAIDs, are familiar pain medications to most of us. You probably have some in your medicine cabinet already. Some of the many common over-the-counter and prescription pain medications that are NSAIDs are aspirin, ibuprofen, tolfenamic acid, and celecoxib. Using certain prescription NSAIDs after surgery can reduce your need to use opioid painkillers. This is of particular benefit if you have obstructive sleep apnea.[1]

Acetaminophen (Tylenol)

Acetaminophen, whose most common name brand is Tylenol, is an over-the-counter pain medication that is not an NSAID. It can be a good option for post-operative pain management, although you never want to overdose on any pain medication.[2]

Narcotics (Opioids)

Prescription narcotics, or opioids, include codeine, morphine, and oxycodone.[3] Follow your doctor's instructions carefully for use; in most cases, you'll be told to take them only when you need them and not necessarily on a set schedule. Narcotics are strong painkillers that are available by prescription only. Your surgeon will probably write you a prescription in advance so that you can pick up your medications before going into surgery.

It may be a little scary when you start thinking about the pain that you might have after your surgery, but in reality, you'll be fine. It's not a big deal—it's just something to expect and plan for so that it doesn't take you by surprise. If you don't want to think about it, don't. Just know that you may have pain and that you'll deal with it. Following your surgeon's instructions should be enough to manage the pain safely.

You probably won't be taking steroid medications to control pain, even though they're pretty strong. Common names include cortisone, prednisolone, hydrocortisone, and betamethasone. Steroids slow down healing so recovery from surgery can actually take longer.[4]

Getting Your Kitchen Ready for Post-Surgery Recovery

You will be on a clear liquid diet for a couple days following your sleeve gastrectomy. In the beginning, you'll want to have ice chips or crushed ice to suck on, since it's easier than gulping water and aggravating your newly formed sleeve. You can buy ice chips at a convenience store or supermarket if your fridge doesn't make them.

Why Can NSAIDs Be Dangerous after the Sleeve Surgery

You'll probably need some kind of pain relief after the sleeve, but it's best to limit your painkillers to the minimum amounts possible to prevent side effects. Let's take a closer look at NSAIDs and talk about another class of painkillers—steroids—that aren't recommended after surgery.

The U.S. consumes billions of doses of NSAIDs each year. They're available over the counter and by prescription. NSAIDs relieve pain with few serious side effects compared to other drugs. NSAIDs are considered safe enough for many physicians to recommend them to their patients to manage pain from long-term conditions, such as arthritis. So why should you limit their use after the sleeve gastrectomy?

Many NSAIDs are cox-2 inhibitors, which means that they prevent your body from producing cyclooxygenase 2, or cox-2. That's good because cox-2 is a compound that increases your pain and inflammation. However, cox-2 inhibitors also inhibit cox-1, which is necessary for keeping your gastrointestinal tract and stomach lining strong and healthy. When you take NSAIDs that block cox-2 and cox-1, you will have less pain—but will be at a higher risk for developing stomach ulcers. You don't want to mess with your stomach any more than necessary when you've just had 85 percent of it removed and all you want is for it to heal!

Aspirin is a type of NSAID with an additional potential danger. In addition to being an anti-inflammatory cox-2-inhibitor and a pain killer, aspirin is a blood thinner. It reduces blood clotting and helps prevent strokes and heart attacks. Normally, that's a good thing, and you might even take aspirin regularly to prevent heart attacks. However, the ability to thin your blood is exactly why you shouldn't take aspirin right after getting the sleeve. It can increase your risk for bleeding.

These are examples of common NSAIDS:

Aspirin: Ecotrin, Bayer Aspirin, Aspir-trin, and Acutrin

- Ibuprofen: Advil, Motrin, Nuprin, Samson, IB Pro, and Midol
- Dayquil, Ibudone, Dimetapp, and Vicoprofen are each names of mixtures of medications that contain ibuprofen.
- Naproxen: Aleve, Naprosyn, Anaprox, Treximet, and Vimovo also have naproxen in them.
- Salsalate: disalicylic acid and salicylisalic acid

It's easy to tell whether your pain medication is an NSAID or contains one. It probably says on the label. If you're not sure, just ask your doctor or call a pharmacist to find out. These are some of the familiar NSAIDs and some of their brand names.

Sources[5, 6, 7, 8]

These are standard guidelines for a clear liquid diet:[9]

Allowed	Not Allowed
✓ Water	✗ Any solid or semi-solid food
✓ Broth	✗ Nectar
✓ Popsicles	✗ Canned fruit
✓ Gelatin	✗ Milk
✓ Tea	✗ Protein shakes
✓ Coffee	✗ Meal replacement beverages
✓ Sports drinks	✗ Juice with pulp
✓ Pulp-free fruit juices	✗ Cream (e.g., in coffee)

Table 19: Standard guidelines for a clear liquid diet

Other Ways to Make Post-Op Recovery Easier

You'll feel tired, sore, and possibly sick when you get home from the hospital. Your first priority is to recover from the sleeve gastrectomy. These are a few things you might want to take care of before surgery to make your life easier after surgery.

- Do the laundry.
- Clean the house.
- Go grocery shopping for your own liquid diet and for your family's food.

Getting to and from the Hospital

Whether your procedure is inpatient, outpatient, or in another country, you'll probably need to arrange for a ride home from the hospital.

Transportation for Outpatient VSG Patients

A few sleeve patients receive the sleeve gastrectomy as an outpatient procedure. If you're among them, don't try to drive yourself home. You'll be groggy from anesthesia and pain medications, exhausted from the surgery, and in pain. It's safer and easier to get a ride. When you schedule your surgery, your surgeon will be able to estimate what time you'll be ready to go home, assuming that you don't have complications. Keep in mind that the following unpredictable factors can delay your hospital discharge time:

- Changing from a laparoscopic to open procedure
- Complications from surgery that require more care in the hospital
- Taking longer than average for the anesthesia to wear off

Transportation for Inpatient Gastric Sleeve Patients

Most gastric sleeve patients spend two to five nights in the hospital.[10] If you're in the super, super-obese category, with a pre-surgery BMI over 60, you can expect to spend seven or more days.[11] You can leave your car in a long-term patient hospital parking lot. If one isn't available or you don't feel comfortable doing that, you can get a ride instead.

Preparing ahead of Time

Discuss beforehand what time you expect to be ready, and have a plan for meeting your driver. A likely place is at the hospital discharge center. Another option is to call your ride when you're ready to come home or when you begin check out of, or are discharged from, the hospital. In some facilities, the receptionist will be willing to call your ride and provide updates while you're still in surgery or the anesthesia's wearing off. Be sure to have these items with you when you go in for surgery:

- Your ride's name and phone number
- A back-up contact or the number of a taxi company in case your first choice isn't able to come and get you
- A soft cushion to protect your sore abdomen from the seatbelt and bumpy ride home.

Transportation and Medical Tourism

If you're getting bariatric surgery as part of a medical tourism trip, a ride to and from the clinic or hospital should be part of the package. The hospital might have dedicated shuttles to take you around. If not, be sure to have a few different taxi numbers on you so that you can get back to the hotel and rest without worrying about how to get there. Call the numbers before your surgery so you know that the companies are still in business.

Packing for the Hospital

Packing your bags ahead of time reduces stress and prevents you from forgetting things. Your surgeon's office may be able to provide you with a standard packing list. It's likely to include these items.

What to Pack

- **Paperwork and Contact Information:**
  - Papers from the surgeon's office
  - Your insurance company's name, phone number and fax number and any contact names you have and a copy of your pre-approval letter for reimbursement
  - Personal contacts. Write down names and phone numbers of people for the hospital to contact in case of an emergency or for you to call if you need to or simply want to talk. Write each person's relationship to you.

- **Medications and Supplements:**
  - Prescription medications. Take enough for your expected hospital stay, plus enough for a couple extra days just in case you stay in the hospital longer than you expected. Be sure to have the medications in a powder or liquid form so you can still take them after the surgery even though you can't swallow whole pills.
  - Instructions for your prescription medications. For each, write down the time you take it, the dose, and whether you take it with food. These instructions can be helpful because you might be a little groggy after your surgery or a nurse might be administering your medications. Don't forget to write down any special instructions that your family physician or surgeon gave you for taking your medications around your time of surgery.
  - Pain medications. These may be prescription or over-the-counter. Pack the medications that your surgeon recommends.
  - Dietary supplements. As long as your surgeon has cleared each one, pack your dietary supplements in powder or liquid form, as well as instructions for taking them.
- **Comfortable Clothing:**
  - Bring loose-fitting clothes, with special attention to a loose-fitting waist. An elastic waistband will feel much more comfortable than a tight-fitting belt or zippered waistband after your surgery. Ask the hospital how many changes of clothes to bring; most likely, you will just wear one set to the hospital and wear a hospital gown for most of your time in the hospital.
  - Enough changes of underwear and socks—plus a couple extras—for the amount of time your surgeon estimates you'll be in the hospital
  - A warm sweater just in case you get cold
  - Wear a pair of comfortable sneakers to the hospital.
  - Pack a pair of non-slip or rubber-soled slippers.
- **Personal Items:**
  - Toothbrush and toothpaste
  - Hairbrush or comb
  - An extra hair band or scrunchie if you have long hair and need it tied back
  - Hand lotion and chapstick to prevent dryness
  - Hand sanitizer in case you want to wash your hands but are too tired to get up after surgery.
  - Shampoo and conditioner
  - Soap or shower gel
- **Entertainment:**
  - Reading material: magazines, books, a Kindle, or newspapers
  - Games: crossword puzzles or Sudoku books

- Music: a CD player and CDs or an iPod
- Video: a laptop with a DVD player and a couple of DVDs to watch
- Extra batteries and/or your battery charger(s): for your music player, laptop, cell phone, and Kindle
- Your cell phone. Charge it up before you go to the hospital.
- Pencil, pens, and paper
- The BariatricPal.com app for smartphone or Kindle! You can connect to the community and stay in touch while you're at the hospital!
- **Miscellaneous:**
- Continuous positive airway pressure, or CPAP, machine if you have sleep apnea. If you normally sleep with a CPAP machine, ask your surgeon whether you should take it to the hospital with you. The facility might be able to supply you with one so you don't have to lug your own.
- Reading glasses
- Your teddy bear, lucky horseshoe, or whatever else it is that gets you through the challenges in life
- A small rolling suitcase is ideal because it's big enough to fit the essentials and you don't have to lift it off of the ground. You won't be able to do heavy lifting when you're coming off of the sleeve surgery.

Leave a Few Things at Home!

Leaving the non-essentials at home lowers stress because you don't have to worry about losing them at the hospital. These are a few of the items that you don't need to bring:

- **Luxury Items:**
  - Dress clothes and shoes. You'll be in a hospital gown, and dress clothes and shoes will be uncomfortable anyway.
  - Makeup and other nonessential toiletries, such as eyebrow tweezers
  - A full range of shower and bath items. Save the luxurious bath for when you're home in the comfort of your own bathtub.
- **Valuable Items:**
  - Jewelry. All it does is draw attention to you and invite theft. Leave it at home.
  - Cash and unnecessary personal information that can get stolen

Above All, Relax!

Don't worry too much about forgetting things. The hospital will take care of the absolute essentials and will probably be happy to make up for anything you forget, such as a magazine or hand sanitizer. The focus now is for your surgery to go as well as possible.

Additional Packing Considerations for Medical Tourism

Medical tourism isn't as complicated as you may think. That's especially true if you've opted for an all-inclusive package deal or if your surgeon's clinic is used to working with foreigners. They'll guide you through the preparation so you can be sure that you've taken care of everything before getting on that plane. Most of your packing will be the same for Mexico or Venezuela, but there are extra items to consider. Your surgeon may supply you with a specialized list for tourists.

Extra Daily Essentials:

- *Extra clothing.* Don't count on doing a laundry while you're gone. You almost certainly won't have one available to you at a low cost in your hotel. You definitely don't want to find and use a Laundromat while you're trying to recover from the sleeve surgery! Keep in mind that you don't need a lot of extra clothes because you'll be in a hospital gown.

- *Extra underwear.* Yes, it's embarrassing, and no, it's not likely…but diarrhea is a definite possibility after getting sleeved. Don't worry about cleaning dirty underwear; instead, just pack a few extra pairs. They're light and small, so they're easy to pack.

- *Toiletries.* Double-check to make sure you have what you need. You can buy things like toothpaste and shampoo anywhere in the world, but sometimes it's nicer to have the brands from home that you're used to.

Special Items for Travelers:

- *A pocket dictionary.* This lets you get your point across quickly. You can use the occasional Spanish word instead of waiting for a Spanish-speaking healthcare professional to go and find an English-speaking colleague to translate.

- *A calling card.* Cell phone fees can be astronomical when calling home from another country. Ask your surgeon what most patients do when they want to call the U.S. You might end up using your hospital or hotel land line telephone with a calling card for only a few cents per minute.

- *Passport.* Check, double-check, and triple-check your passport. Make sure that it is current and that it good through at least six months after your planned return date. That's the standard recommendation of the U.S. Embassy, and it's a requirement to be able to enter Venezuela.

- *List of contacts.* Include your regular list of family members and friends; as well as the name, address, and phone number of your hotel; your medical contacts such as your primary care physician; your regular pharmacy; and the name, phone number, and fax number of the surgeon who will be taking charge of your aftercare.

- *Plane tickets, if you're going by plane.* Check for your outgoing and return plane tickets, if you have paper tickets. You might have e-tickets, also called paperless tickets, so you'll just need ID and a credit card to check in at the airport.

- *Money.* Major credit cards, debit cards, and bank cards are accepted nearly everywhere in the world, and you might not need much cash. Take more than one card, if you have them, in case for some reason one doesn't work. Extra cash can always come in handy, and most places will accept dollars instead of the local currency of Mexican pesos or Venezuelan bolivars if you're desperate.

Getting Help

Be prepared for anything. Always be aware of available resources when you're traveling in a foreign country, especially if you're traveling alone and planning to have a minor surgery. These are some things to consider:

- Know what to do and where to go if you lose your passport. Contact the nearest U.S. Embassy. Venezuela has one in Caracas, and U.S. Embassy locations in Mexico include popular bariatric surgery destinations, such as Monterrey and Tijuana.[12],[13]
- Write down the contact information of your hospital and hotel and keep it with you at all times. Have the name of the hospital and hotel, the name of your surgeon, and the address and telephone numbers of the hospital and hotel.
- Carry the company's contact information if you're getting your sleeve done as part of a medical tourism package.

The Last Few Hours Are Finally Here!

You're packed and ready for surgery! What exactly do you do on the day before surgery? What will happen when you get to the hospital? This section will prepare you for these final few hours before you get the sleeve gastrectomy.

Last-Minute Checks

You might as well go over your checklist once again to make sure your bags are packed and you've followed all of your surgeon's pre-surgery instructions. If you don't already know, find out where your ride should drop you off at the hospital the next day and where to check into the hospital. These extra tasks can help distract you from surgery.

Pre-Surgery Diet and Medications

General anesthesia, which puts you to sleep during surgery, increases the risk of food leaving your stomach and entering your lungs. Patients should fast for at least six hours before surgery to avoid this dangerous situation and also to reduce nausea and vomiting when you wake up from surgery.[14] Your surgeon is likely to recommend an overnight fast with nothing other than water after about 10:00 p.m.

Overnight Fast

The overnight fast not only makes the anesthesia procedure smoother, but it also prevents any food remaining in your stomach to interfere with your surgeon's view of your stomach. It's a common procedure before surgery.[15] You can only have water and not other beverages, such as the following:

- Diet drinks
- Tea or coffee
- Anything with caffeine

Medications

Each medication may have a different set of pre-surgery instructions, so read through them to make sure you are following your physician or surgeon's instructions correctly for each medication. If you're not sure, call your surgeon or the pharmacy. Blood thinners, such as warfarin (with the popular brand name of Coumadin) and Plavix, can increase bleeding during and after surgery. Your doctor will probably have you skip your dose on the day of surgery. If you're on insulin to control your blood sugar levels, you'll probably take a smaller dose than usual. That's because you won't be eating carbohydrates during the day, so your blood sugar levels won't spike as much as they usually do.

Don't Forget Your "Before" Pictures!

They're not absolutely necessary, but this is your last chance to catch yourself as a pre-surgery patient who's ready to leave obesity in the past! Your "before" pictures are the ones you get to contrast with your "after" pictures. You can pull them out of your wallet or even paste them on your refrigerator so that you always see them and use them as motivation to keep going when times get tough. They remind you that whatever you're going through is worth it so that you never have to take another "before" picture again. They're encouraging, and they give you the pride you deserve when you see how far you've come.

Checking into the Hospital

Hospital staff will take care of you from when you check in with the receptionist. You will meet with the surgeon, the anesthesiologist, and possibly other members of the surgical team, such as nurses, who will be there during the procedure. The surgeon or a nurse will perform some last-minute checks. You'll be asked to confirm that you haven't eaten since yesterday, that you've followed the liquid diet as instructed, and that you've met all of the other criteria. There might even be some silly-sounding questions, like "Are you here for

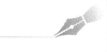

Tip

Chapter 3, "Vertical Sleeve Gastrectomy 101," identifies the members of your surgical team. The chapter also goes into detail about the surgical process—and everything that happens while you're unconscious under the anesthesia.

the sleeve gastrectomy?" These simple questions help prevent mistakes in surgery.

Then someone will wheel you to the holding area outside of the operating room in a wheelchair. You'll have an IV placed into you so that the anesthesiologist can deliver anesthesia during your surgery. You'll also be hooked up to things like a heart rate monitor and an oxygen monitor. These devices guide the anesthesiologist in giving you anesthesia during surgery and monitoring your well-being.

You will be wheeled to the operating table and lie on your back in a comfortable position with your head on pillows. The anesthesiologist will place a mask over your nose and mouth to breathe through. The mask delivers oxygen. The first part of the anesthesiology process is the induction process to calm you down. It might happen through an injection or through an endotracheal tube, or pipe that goes from the mask down your throat, to breathe through. You'll breathe in a gas that relaxes you and numbs pain. Next, you'll be put to sleep with an anesthetic through your IV tube. While you're asleep, the anesthesiologist will also deliver a muscle relaxing drug so that your muscles don't accidentally twitch as a reflex during surgery.

The next time you wake up, you'll have a vertical sleeve and only 85% of your stomach—hopefully the right combination to help you lose weight for life!

✍ Summary

☞ Now you know everything about preparing for the surgery. You know how to prepare your home, what to pack, and what else to bring if you're going abroad. You know what to eat the night before surgery, how you're getting to the hospital, and what will happen once you get there. In short, you're ready for the sleeve!

☞ The next chapter picks up when you wake up from the sleeve surgery and talks about recovering as quickly and easily as possible. There'll be bumps along the way, but a bit of preparation can smooth your journey.

Your Turn: Last-Minute Checklist

A checklist is always helpful when you're packing for an overnight stay. Here's what you might want to take to the hospital. Just check them off when they're in your suitcase or purse.

_____ Any paperwork from your insurance company or the hospital

_____ Passport if going to Mexico

_____ All of your prescription medications

_____ Change of underwear and socks

_____ Non-slip slippers or light sneakers

_____ Toothbrush and toothpaste

_____ Hairbrush or comb

_____ Lotion or hand cream

_____ Chapstick or lip balm

_____ Hand sanitizer

_____ Book, magazines, MP3 player, or any other entertainment

_____ Cell phone (fully charged)

Contact Information (name and telephone number):

_____ Your primary care physician

_____ Your ride home from the hospital

_____ Your insurance company

_____ The number and address of the nearest U.S. consulate (if you are going to another country for your surgery)

Your own items:

_____ Lucky rabbit's foot

_____

_____

_____

1   Schumann R, Jones SB, Cooper B, Kelley SD, Bosch MV, Ortiz VE, Connor KA, Kaufman MD, Harvey AM, Carr DB. Update on best practice recommendations for anesthetic perioperative care and pain management in weight loss surgery, 2004-2007. Obesity (Silver Spring). 2009;17(5):889-894.

2   Acetaminophen. Medline Plus, National Institutes of Health. Web Site. http://www.nlm.nih.gov/medlineplus/druginfo/meds/a681004.html. Updated 2012, 15 January. Accessed October 4, 2012.

3   Dugdale DC, Zieve D. Pain medications - narcotics. MedlinePlus, National Institutes of Health. Web site. http://www.nlm.nih.gov/medlineplus/ency/article/007489.htm. Updated 2011, May 22. Accessed October 4, 2012.

4   Corticosteroid (oral route, parenteral route). (2012). Mayo Clinic. Retrieved from http://www.mayoclinic.com/health/drug-information/DR602333/METHOD=print

5   Aspirin. Acetaminophen. Medline Plus, National Institutes of Health. Web Site. http://www.nlm.nih.gov/medlineplus/druginfo/meds/a682878.html. Updated 2011, 16 March. Accessed October 4, 2012.

6   Ibuprofen. Medline Plus, National Institutes of Health. Web Site. http://www.nlm.nih.gov/medlineplus/druginfo/meds/a682159.html. 2010, 1 October. Accessed October 4, 2012.

7   Salsalate. Medline Plus, National Institutes of Health. Web Site. http://www.nlm.nih.gov/medlineplus/druginfo/meds/a682880.html. Updated 2010, 1 September. Accessed October 4, 2012.

8   Naproxen. Medline Plus, National Institutes of Health. Web Site. http://www.nlm.nih.gov/medlineplus/druginfo/meds/a681029.html. Updated 2012, 15 June. Accessed October 4, 2012.

9   Dugdale DC, Zieve D. Diet – clear liquid. Medline Plus, National Institutes of Health. Web site. http://www.nlm.nih.gov/medlineplus/ency/patientinstructions/000205.htm. 2010, November 21. Accessed October 4, 2012.

10 Realize. How a sleeve gastrectomy works. Ethicon Endo-Surgery. Web site. http://www.realize.com/what-is-sleeve-gastrectomy-surgery.htm. Accessed October 5, 2012.

11 Catheline JM, Fysekidis M, Dbouk R, Boschetto A, Bihan H, Reach G, Cohen R. Weight loss after sleeve gastrectomy in super superobesity. J Obes. 2012;epub Jul 22.

12 Venezuela: Country Specific Information. U.S. Department of State. Web site. http://www.travel.state.gov/travel/cis_pa_tw/cis/cis_1059.html. Accessed October 6, 2012.

13 Mexico: Country Specific Information. U.S. Department of State. Web site. http://travel.state.gov/travel/cis_pa_tw/cis/cis_970.html. Accessed September 17, 2012.

14 Mayo Clinic Staff. General anesthesia. Mayo Clinic. Web site. http://www.mayoclinic.com/health/anesthesia/MY00100/METHOD=print. 2010, June 26. Accessed October 6, 2012.

15 Dugdale DC, Zieve D. Diet – clear liquid. Medline Plus, National Institutes of Health. Web site. http://www.nlm.nih.gov/medlineplus/ency/patientinstructions/000205.htm. 2010, November 21. Accessed October 4, 2012.

11
Recovering from Surgery

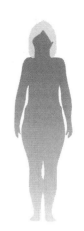

Congratulations! You're now a sleeve patient for life! No matter how much you've planned for getting the sleeve or how much weight you lost before the actual surgery, losing your stomach and finally getting the sleeve naturally feels like the true start of your weight loss journey and new lifestyle.

This is a very important period in your sleeve journey because what you do now affects your short-term recovery and long-term success with the gastric sleeve. This chapter will describe what to expect as you recover from the VSG and how you can improve your experience. The chapter covers:

- Your stay in the hospital
- The first few days at home
- Returning to normal activities and to work

This chapter takes you from being a sleeve rookie to a sleeve pro! By the end of it, you'll be well on your way to recovering from surgery and focusing on losing weight with the sleeve.

Your Stay in the Hospital

The sleeve gastrectomy takes about one[1] to two or more hours.[2] The procedure tends to be shorter if your surgeon is experienced; it is longer if you have an open gastrectomy instead of a laparoscopic one or if there are complications. You'll wake up about an hour or so after the procedure's finished and be closely monitored for a few hours. Next, you'll likely go to your hospital room where you'll be cared for by one or more nurses until you leave the hospital. Within days, you'll get to go home and recover!

Fully Regaining Your Consciousness as the Anesthesia Wears Off

The anesthesia will wear off, and you'll wake up about an hour or two after the surgeon has finished working on you. You probably won't remember much over the next few hours because you'll still be groggy from surgery. There'll be a lot of nurses bustling around, but you don't need to worry about anything.

The PACU

You're most likely to find yourself in a special room called the post-anesthesia care unit, or PACU, when you wake up from surgery. The PACU is a room for patients who just had surgery. It's a room that's equipped with a bunch of high-tech equipment to monitor vital signs such as blood pressure and heart rate. Some patients may be hooked up to IVs giving them medications, fluids, or nutrients.[3] You'll probably have an IV in your arm to provide fluids and prevent dehydration because by the time you wake up from surgery, you won't have had anything to drink for several hours. You might have a tube in your throat to help you breathe.[4]

A nurse or team of nurses will monitor you closely as you fully regain consciousness. They'll look at the machines you're hooked up to and check that everything's okay, and they might make some adjustments in your IV. Every couple of minutes or so, they'll ask you how you feel, and they can add pain medications or medications to reduce nausea if you are overwhelmed. They might ask you silly personal questions such as your name or address just to make sure that you're thinking clearly. The nurses might pay so much attention to you that they can even get annoying as you go from being mostly asleep to fully alert. That's a good sign, though: if you're awake enough to feel pestered, you're recovering pretty well!

The Humorous Side of the PACU

During your time in the PACU, you might not remember much of about your early conversations with your nurse. Many patients ask over and over again about their operation and seem to understand the answer. Then they'll ask again a couple of minutes later. You'll probably do the same. Once you're alert enough to stop repeating your questions and recognize that some of the other patients are repeating their own questions just like you were, you might find the behavior pretty funny – and realize how patient the nurses are to continue to cheerfully and enthusiastically answer each patient multiple times.

You Might Start to Feel Post-Surgery Pain

It's not just the anesthesia that wears off after surgery, but also the muscle relaxants and pain medications that your anesthesiologist gave you while you were unconscious. As you become more alert and have less medication to dull the pain, you will probably start to feel pain in your stomach area where the surgeon made the incisions to insert the laparoscopic tools or to access your stomach. You might feel pain right in your abdomen where the surgeon cut your stomach and sealed the sleeve. Shoulder pain is common after a laparoscopic sleeve gastrectomy because of the extra gas that might still be in your abdominal cavity. The pain will increase as your pain medications are wearing off. The nurse may give you medications to manage the pain.

Leaving the PACU

You'll stay in the PACU until you're fully awake and alert and your heart rate, breathing and blood pressure are stable. If you have obstructive sleep apnea, you'll be in the PACU for about three extra hours.[5] You'll be there until the nurse is sure that you're no longer under the influence of anesthesia. That's to make sure that you don't fall asleep and stop breathing without your CPAP machine. You'll probably go to the hospital room where you'll be staying for a few nights.

Staying Hydrated Right after Surgery

Preventing dehydration is important after surgery. The IV in the PACU will provide enough fluid to prevent dehydration, but you need to start drinking fluids when your IV is removed. You might not want to because you'll feeling nauseous or in pain, but nurses will continue to encourage you to drink.

Ice chips, or chopped or shaved ice, is a good choice for your first post-surgery food:

- It is pure water, so it helps prevent dehydration.
- It is solid, so you can't eat it too quickly. Wait until it melts in your mouth before swallowing.
- It helps you progress to taking small sips of regular water.

You can't avoid all discomfort after the sleeve surgery, but you can make your transition to a liquid diet easier by following a few tips:

- *Take small sips and drink slowly.* Small pieces of ice are perfect for forcing you to do both of these. Take very small spoonfuls and make sure they melt completely in your mouth before you swallow. When you progress to water, take very small sips.
- *Avoid very hot or cold liquids.* You don't want to irritate your sleeve. Ice is okay because it'll be melted and won't be that cold by the time you swallow it.
- *Sit up to make it easier for foods to go down.* A motion called peristalsis is pretty effective at pushing foods and beverages downward in your gastrointestinal tract.[6] That's why kids can swallow without choking while they're standing on their heads. However, some sleeve patients experience heartburn, and you can reduce your risk by eating and drinking in an upright position.
- *Avoid carbonated beverages.* This isn't just for the calories. You should even avoid diet beverages, including diet soft drinks and sparkling waters. The bubbles not only make you feel bloated and possibly nauseous, but it can also stretch the sleeve and lead to leaks later.
- *Keep sipping.* It's hard to drink a lot at this time, so focus on sipping your fluids continuously to make sure you get enough.

Each of these guidelines is actually good practice for the future. Eating slowly and mindfully, and avoiding carbonated beverages, will all help reduce the amount that your sleeve stretches in the future, too. It's a good habit to only eat in an upright position to prevent esophageal reflux, heartburn, or an unpleasant feeling of fullness. Eating only when seated at the table in an upright position is also a great habit to get into because it prevents you from mindless eating and drinking while you're preparing food or passing through the kitchen.

Benefits of Being in the Hospital

If you don't have serious complications, you'll be in the hospital or clinic for about two to seven days. Staying in the hospital lets you make rapid progress, so take advantage of the opportunities! These are some benefits of staying in the hospital:

- *Trained medical professionals are on hand if anything goes wrong.* More likely, you can voice your concerns and have trained medical professionals reassure you that nothing's wrong even though you are worried. You may feel nauseous or be vomiting or even a little dizzy from the anesthesia, and you'll almost certainly have some pain in your stomach or shoulder. During these first several hours, it's comforting to be able to describe each of your symptoms to a nurse, ask if they're worth worrying about and find out what caused them.

- *You don't have to worry about going to the bathroom.* You're definitely going to be tired and likely going to be in pain. It will be a lot easier to have a medical professional help you in the bathroom than to have to go by yourself or to ask your spouse or someone else to help you. It's far less embarrassing to have a nurse rather than a family member help you in the bathroom. Also, nurses are trained to support bariatric patients by using special equipment or teamwork as necessary. Hospital bathrooms are equipped with features including handrails to grab onto and high-seated toilets so that you don't have to bend your knees as far to sit on the toilet. In a hospital, an option if you are having trouble urinating is to use a catheter. This is an option if you just can't make it to the bathroom in the first few hours or days after surgery.

- *You don't have to worry about putting on a brave face for your kids.* Most parents don't want their children to see them when they're not at their best. You're going to be weak and tired after surgery. Staying in the hospital away from your children prevents them from having to see you in a weakened state at home. Also, it prevents you from feeling pressure to play with them or help out around the house.

- *It builds your confidence.* You might be a nervous wreck, or at least a little unsure of yourself, right after your surgery. After all, it's a life-changing experience and a permanent change to your body. It's nice to have nurses to depend on and the peace of mind that you're in good hands during this time. You can ask all of your little questions and get sound advice from your nurse without having to worry about feeling stupid or making a mistake that'll set back your recover. By the time you're discharged, you'll be better able to identify your signs and symptoms and know what to do about them.

- *It builds your family's confidence.* Your own emotions affect your family's reactions. If you're anxious and concerned, they will be too. If you are confident and reassuring from the moment you walk in the door at home, your family will feel much more comfortable. You can set the example so that they don't feel uneasy around you. Pay attention to how the nurses take care of you in the hospital. That'll give you some ideas of what to ask your family members to do for you. They're probably eager to help you out, but don't want to hurt you and don't know what to until you tell them their roles in your recovery.

In the Hospital

Your only job in the hospital is to recover. Follow your surgeons' and nurses' instructions so that you can be confident that you are laying the best possible foundation for your future with the gastric sleeve. You may not be feeling very energetic, and the days will probably pass faster than you think. This is what you can expect to fill your days when you're in the hospital:

- *One or more appointments with your surgeon.* Your surgeon will need to check your progress and permit your release from the hospital when it's time.

- *One or more appointments with your nutritionist or dietitian.* We'll talk about appointments with the dietitian later in the chapter.
- *Visits from your family and/or friends.* The hospital will probably have regular visiting hours when your family can come see you in your room or you can visit with them in a hospital lounge or another public place.
- *Carefully planned meals.* You'll be on a liquid diet and your nurse should automatically bring you your meals and snacks. Don't forget to keep some water near you at all times so you can stay hydrated.

Unplanned Time

It's normal to feel very tired after surgery, and a bit of down time in the hospital will help you recover. Surgery is tough on your body not only because of the actual surgical procedure and cuts, but also because of the barrage of anesthesia and medications from your surgery. Your down time is when you can take naps, read books, do crossword puzzles, watch DVDs, and do all the other activities you packed for yourself. As you feel stronger, you might start to take short walks in your room and the hospital halls during your free time.

Staying Active

Staying active can help you feel better and may even speed up recovery. Staying active can be as simple as standing up every few minutes during the day, walking around your hospital room, or going down the corridor. Slow walking is enough to increase your blood flow. Circulating blood is necessary for your surgery wounds to heal.

Pain medications

The first day and night may be very painful because the anesthesia will wear off and the pain from surgery will be in full force. You'll continue to have pain for several days or weeks, but the worst of it will be over within a couple of days. Nurses will continue to provide pain medications as you need them. Your surgeon may prescribe certain pain medications, such as opioids, or narcotics. These include codeine, vicodine, and oxycodone.[7]

Another common pain medication after bariatric surgery is ketorolac.[8] Like ibuprofen and aspirin, ketorolac is a non-steroidal anti-inflammatory drug, or NSAID used to treat pain.[9] Compared to normal NSAIDS such as ibuprofen and aspirin, ketorolac is only available by prescription. Using ketorolac can help you decrease the amount of narcotic painkillers that you need, but you shouldn't take it for more than a few days as your doctor recommends. Side effects of ketorolac may be similar to those that you are fighting after surgery, including diarrhea, nausea, and fatigue.

Recovering at Home

You'll be in the hospital for about two to seven days. As you progress, your surgeon will probably give you a closer estimate of when you can expect to go home. When you find that out, you should make plans or confirm your plans for getting home.

Getting Discharged from the Hospital

You need to get discharged before you leave the hospital. You will be eligible for discharge after your surgeon examines you and gives you the okay to leave. At a major hospital, the discharge station may be a large desk at the front of the bariatric surgery ward. In a smaller clinic, you might be discharged at the front reception desk.

It won't take too long to get discharged. You'll go through the usual medical checkout procedures, such as paying your co-pay or the full or partial amount of services depending on your financing plan. The receptionist should confirm your next appointment with the surgeon, and may also verify your next dietitian appointment if your dietitian's office is in the same medical facility. You may need to sign some paperwork or fill out some forms. If you're still having trouble walking far or being on your feet for a long time, a nurse might wheel you to the curb outside to wait for your ride in a wheelchair.

Some surgeons prevent patients driving themselves home for their own safety. The receptionist at discharge may require you to identify the person who is ready to drive you. That person might even need to come into the discharge area so that the receptionist can see him or her in person.

What to Ask Before You Leave the Hospital

Most of the steps of the discharge process are pretty clear, so you don't have to worry about remembering them. There are a couple of important things to be sure you know before you leave the hospital.

- *Find out the best phone number to use if you have questions when you're at home.* This is probably different than the general hospital number that you might use to make appointments or call for general questions. You might get a direct number to your surgeon or surgeon's staff so that you don't have to spend time on hold or going through telephone menus. You may be calling this number a lot over the next several days!

- *Get an off-hours number.* This doesn't necessarily need to be an emergency number, but it could be. Before you leave the hospital, make sure you know which number to call at any time of the day or night, and on weekends.

- *Be sure you understand your post-surgery instructions.* Your surgeon should have provided you with written instructions and gone over them with you. They should guide you through the entire recovery process, including your gradual return to regular physical activity, any changes in how to take your regular prescription medications and specific instructions for using pain medications.

- *Make sure you have your diet guidelines.* Instructions for what to drink and eat next several weeks should be written clearly. Ask about anything that looks confusing.

On the Ride Home

Keep resting as much as possible. To use that pillow that you put in the car or packed for yourself before surgery, place it under your seatbelt and over your abdomen to reduce stomach pain. The pillow reduces jarring and irritation from the seatbelt, especially when the car bounces or turns.

It's normal to get anxious when you leave the hospital and you're no longer under constant medical supervision, but try to stay calm. Your surgeon and hospital would not have released you if you didn't seem to be ready. And you're not completely on your own. You can still call the hospital or your surgeon if you have trouble or any questions.

Your First Few Days at Home

As soon as you're over your initial anxiety at being at home on your own, you might feel empowered. You will start, over these days and weeks, to feel capable of doing anything you set your mind to—including losing the weight you want by following the instructions for the sleeve. You will undoubtedly make mistakes along the way, but you can overcome setbacks by staying positive and focusing on your goals.

Some Pain Is Normal

As mentioned earlier in the chapter, your surgery wounds will be painful. The pain should be less intense than in the hospital by the time you get home, especially if your hospital stay was a little longer than average. However, you'll probably still feel pain in your laparoscopic incisions on your abdomen as well as deeper in your stomach where the surgeon cut away your large stomach pouch. They may feel like muscle soreness or a sharper pain.

These are some additional possible sources of discomfort:

- Your shoulder or neck may continue to ache for as long as there is extra gas in your abdominal cavity. That's the gas that was pumped in during the laparoscopic procedure if that's what you had.

- Nausea is possible because of the pain as well as the pain medications. You need to call your doctor if the nausea becomes so bad that you can't drink and you start to become dehydrated. That can happen within several hours[10].

Pain Medications

Your pain medications will be similar to those in the hospital. You can continue with your prescription opioid medications, if your surgeon recommends them, and/or with the prescription non-steroidal anti-inflammatory drug called ketorolac. At this time, your surgeon might suggest using less of the prescription medications and more over-the-counter options, which are typically milder and less risky. Examples include ibuprofen or aspirin, and acetaminophen, or Tylenol. Your surgeon will probably suggest taking pain medications only as

> **Tip**
>
> The earlier portion of this chapter, dedicated to your hospital stay, discusses the different types of common painkillers and which are most likely to be prescribed for treating your pain after the surgery. Chapter 6, "Are you a Good Candidate for the Sleeve?" discusses the possible side effects and complications after getting the vertical sleeve.

needed, and to take as few as possible to manage the pain. Limiting your painkillers to only when you really need them is healthier:

- It reduces the amount of chemicals in your body.
- It builds mental toughness.
- Some kinds of painkillers can be addictive.
- Some pain medications can slow the healing process after the VSG or increase your risk of having an ulcer.
- Pain medications can interfere with your regular medications, which may already be affected by your surgery and changes in diet.

Pain Management Strategies and when to Consult Your Surgeon

Unfortunately, minimizing your use of pain medications means that you'll be putting up with at least some degree of pain. These are a few strategies that can help you cope with the pain so it doesn't seem as bad. Practicing these strategies can help you get better at managing the pain. As you find yourself growing stronger, don't forget to tell yourself how proud you are of yourself. After all, it's a tough situation to be in, and you can handle it:

- *Distract yourself by focusing on something else*. This takes your mind off of the pain. You can turn to an old hobby or use your post-surgery recovery time as an opportunity to start a new hobby, such as blogging or sewing.
- *Talk yourself through it*. Reassure yourself either out loud or in your head that you're fine. Take inventory of your pain—try to identify exactly what hurts, how bad it is, and what's causing the pain. Then think about how bad it *could* be and how strong you are for not letting it bother you. The pain might not seem so bad once you've stared it in the face.
- *Go social*. Phone a friend, write some emails, or visit BariatricPal.com. People can keep you company, and you don't even have to hide the pain. Time can fly by when you're absorbed in your telephone or online conversations, and the sharp pain might subside before you need medication.
- *Get moving*. Activity can distract you and calm you. It also increases circulation, so you might feel less pain. Any activity that you do can be helpful. That might mean that you stand up and sit down a few times, using the edge of a table for support, or it might mean that you walk around the house for a few minutes. Doing arm circles and swinging your legs back and forth can be enough to reduce pain without needing to stand up if that's too much for you.
- *Use a heating pad and/or ice pack*. Place the heating pad on the area of pain, whether it's your stomach, shoulder, or neck. If you want, alternate with ice packs. Heat increases blood flow and is soothing. Ice is a natural painkiller and anti-inflammatory. Follow the instruction on the heating pad and ice packs so you don't get burned or risk frostbite.

Only use them for the recommended length of time stated on the label, usually 10 to 20 minutes, and wrap them in a towel instead of applying them directly to your skin.

- *Delay or reduce your pain medications.* Try to delay your next dose by a few minutes at a time and see if you can stretch that out for longer. You can also try a smaller dose. Of course, only consider changing your medication schedule and/or dose if your surgeon gives you permission.

Learning how to distract yourself and put your mind on other things is a valuable skill for the rest of your weight loss journey. Sometimes, you will feel hungry before it's time for a meal or snack. Your new mental discipline can help you accomplish other tasks instead of giving in to your hunger and going straight to the refrigerator.

> **Tip**
>
> Chapter 17, "What to expect in the First Year After VSG," talks about creating a call list of people to call when you can tell that you're about to slip off of the diet.

When to Consult Your Surgeon

Pain is unavoidable after surgery, and many sleeve patients experience additional side effects of the sleeve gastrectomy. Normal side effects may include gastroesophageal reflux and early satiety, or feelings of fullness, when you've only eaten a portion of your planned meal or snack. Most side effects are not serious, but some are:

- About 8[11] to 10%[12] of sleeve patients get more serious complications that may require medical attention.
- About 5%[13] of sleeve patients need to be readmitted to the hospital.
- About 3% of sleeve patients need a second surgery to correct a complication.

Call your surgeon if you have any of the following symptoms or suspect that you have a serious medical condition.[14]

Fever and Redness

A temperature of 101 or more degrees can be a sign of an infection. About one to six percent of sleeve patients get infections after surgery.[15] Infections can start at the incisions from surgery, and they may also appear red and become more painful.[16] An untreated infection can spread to the rest of your body. Sepsis is a more serious infection that can occur if conditions were not sterile during surgery; about two percent of sleeve patients get sepsis.[17] Another possible cause of fever is a blood clot, such as a pulmonary embolism, which blocks blood flow to your lungs and can be fatal if not treated. A fever might not need treatment, but you should consult your surgeon to check.

Shortness of Breath or Chest Pain

Shortness of breath can be a sign of a few different conditions that require attention:

- Pneumonia occurs in about three percent of sleeve patients[18] and is caused by an infection. You might also have chest pain and coughing.

- Pleural effusion occurs in about two percent of sleeve patients.[19] It's when fluid builds up in your lungs and makes it hard to breathe; you might also have a fever, cough, and hiccups. Your surgeon might take an x-ray if a pleural effusion is suspected.

- Blood clots may be another cause of shortness of breath. Blood clots are well-known complications of surgery, and other symptoms include painful, red, or swollen legs. A pulmonary embolism is a blood clot that affects your lungs.[20]

- Shortness of breath is a potential sign of a pulmonary embolism. Swollen legs can happen if a blood clot is blocking the blood flow to them. If you have swollen legs, you might need to go to the hospital and get an ultrasound so that your surgeon can see if there is a blood clot.

Nausea

Nausea is a common effect of anesthesia, and you'll probably feel nauseous in the hospital. Hospital nurses may give you anti-nausea medications in the hospital. Painkillers can cause nausea, too. You need to call your surgeon if your nausea gets so bad that you can't stomach fluids. You can get dehydrated if you go for more than a few hours without drinking fluids. Nausea occurs in about five percent of gastric sleeve patients.[21]

Vomiting

Vomiting can have a variety of causes, and some of them are serious. Repeated vomiting is not only a possible sign of a serious health condition, but it can also lead to dehiscence, or splitting of your surgery wounds, because of the force of vomiting. It's safest to call your surgeon if you vomit more than once and don't know the cause. These are some possible causes of vomiting after the sleeve gastrectomy:

- *As a side effect of taking narcotic painkillers on an empty stomach.* Your surgeon may be able to suggest a better pain medication schedule for you.

- *As a sign of an anastomotic leak.* Leaks and fistula occur in up to 20% of sleeve patients[22] and they can require another surgery. Other symptoms of leaks include fever, stomach pain, and a rapid heart rate.

- *Gastritis, or an inflamed stomach.*[23] This can lead to anemia. Your surgeon may recommend over-the-counter or prescription antacids. You might also need to reduce the amount of NSAIDs that you're taking until your gastritis gets better.

- *Eating too much.* You can vomit if you eat more than your sleeve can comfortably hold. This isn't a big concern when you're on the liquid diet during the first week or two

> **Tip**
>
> See Chapter 5, "VSG: Risks and Considerations," for an-depth discussion of the potential side effects and complications from the sleeve gastrectomy. The chapter goes into symptoms of potentially serious or mild complications and which patients are most likely to experience them. Chapter 13: Recovery and Your Post-Surgery Diet and the next one discuss your post-surgery diet and how to eat to protect the sleeve.

after surgery. It's more likely to become a problem when you start eating real foods. You can prevent overeating by limiting yourself to the amount of food on your diet plan and by eating only until you are full.

Sharp Stomach Pain

Sharp stomach pain that comes on suddenly or becomes worse can be a signal that something's wrong and you need to call your surgeon. Some post-surgery pain is normal as your surgery wounds heal, but the pain should gradually decrease. A sudden increase in pain or a noticeable change in the type of pain you feel can be a sign of these problems and may need medical attention:

- Gastritis[24]
- Anastomotic leak
- Splitting of surgery wound

In most cases, you do not have a medical emergency and your surgeon can take care of your problem fairly easily. The tried and true guidelines never go out of style, though: if you think you have a medical emergency, call 9-1-1. If you think you need emergency care, go to the nearest emergency room. It is always better to be safe than to risk a complication.

Keep Letting Your Wounds Heal

Your skin will have some visible marks where the surgeon made surgical cuts. You might have about two to five cuts that are each around an inch long.[25] Your surgery wounds will be slightly larger if you had an open procedure. A good amount of healing already took place in the hospital, and your job at home is to continue to care for yourself. Your hospital discharge guidelines might include instructions for your cuts. Most likely, you will need to keep them clean and dry to prevent infections and to allow the sides of the cuts to close properly. Just sponging off instead of taking a full shower helps ensure that the wounds stay dry.

Follow your surgeon's other instructions for care, too. You might have to change the dressings, or bandages, regularly, and there might be an antibiotic cream or ointment to put over the cuts to prevent infections. If you have stitches, your surgeon might need to take them out for you, although some kinds of surgical stitches are made out of materials that will eventually dissolve by themselves so you don't need to get the stitches removed.

Your surgery scars will eventually disappear or become nearly invisible, and they probably won't bother you. If they do, there are some treatment options that you can consider later on when you're closer to your goal weight and your body stops changing so much.

Relaxation and Recovery

The best thing you can do for yourself when you get home is to relax. Your job now is to recover as quickly and well as possible so that you can be healthier as you continue your weight loss journey. Relaxing doesn't come naturally to everyone. Here are a few tips:

- Don't do hard chores if they're not necessary. Resist the urge to vacuum or rearrange the furniture to scrub the floors underneath.

- Don't lift heavy objects. You'll heal faster if you don't lift anything heavy for a little while.

- If you have children, be sure to set some ground rules if you haven't already, or review them if you have. Your children should not be jumping at you or demanding to be picked up during this time.

- Loving spouses and caring family members and friends may also need gentle reminders not to hug you.

Taking a Break from Stress

Mental rest is as important as taking it easy physically. Surgery is a big deal for your body and your mind. It's not only the actual surgery that can be exhausting, but also the stress of planning for surgery and the relief of having it over – admit it, you were probably more than a little nervous before the procedure! If you're reading this book before getting it done, you're probably anxious about it. Of course that's normal.

After the surgery, give yourself a mental and emotional break as well as a physical break. Make a conscious effort not to get worked up about things that aren't that important. This may even be a good time to begin a new habit of setting aside time each day for yourself. Now, the time might be devoted to deep breathing and relaxation. Soon the time might evolve into your daily exercise time, starting with stretching and eventually developing into what will become your regular routine.

> **Tip**
>
> Chapter 16, "Getting and Staying in Shape with Exercise," discusses starting a safe exercise routine. It also gives some suggestions on fitting in your daily exercise and learning to love it.

Support Is Important, Too

Take advantage of your friends and family and let them help you. Almost all of us have close friends or family members who are not only willing but anxious to help by doing anything they can to make recovery easier. These are some of the simple but significant ways that your supporters can aid you:

- Check in on you during the day at regular intervals if you're home alone.

- Drop off your children at school and pick them up after school, as well as take them to any afterschool activities that they have.

- Babysit for a few hours to give you a little bit more quiet time.

- Lift something heavy for you, such as a full laundry basket or some bags of groceries.

- Run a few errands, as you shouldn't drive a car for a couple days after surgery until the anesthesia and pain medications are completely out of your system.

Asking friends and family members for help can seem a little awkward to you, especially if you're used to doing everything on your own or if you have a regular pattern in which everyone knows their own roles, so you don't really directly ask each other for help. They might not know exactly what to do to be helpful and might feel like it's not their place to offer because they worry that you'll be insulted. It's up to you to take the first step and ask for help. Both you and your supporters will be so glad you did. Once you start the conversation, the ice will be broken. You can let them know specific things they can do to help, and they will feel more comfortable asking what they can do.

Returning to Normal Activities and Work

When you first get home from the hospital, you'll be tired and you won't feel like doing much. That's okay because resting is exactly what is best for you at this time, and you can become more active as you get your energy back. Within a few weeks, you can be back in full swing with work and life.

Keep Moving but Don't Strain

A little light activity is good for you even when you're tired. It speeds up your blood flow so that more oxygen and nutrients are delivered to your surgery location and your wounds might heal faster. You can keep doing the same things at home that you were doing in the hospital: standing up and sitting down repeatedly, walking around your house, or even walking up and down the driveway.

Don't Lift Heavy Objects

It's standard advice after surgery to avoid lifting heavy objects or straining to manipulate them. You don't want to strain so much that you put pressure on your abdomen and risk splitting your sleeve. It's hard to define "heavy" because everyone has a different idea of what's "heavy." A good initial goal might be to limit yourself to lifting less than eight pounds, which is the weight of a gallon of milk. After that, you can increase your limit by no more than about one pound per day. These are some possible objects that are too heavy to lift or use. If you're not sure whether something's heavy, just err on the safe side and don't lift it:

- Boxes, suitcases, and bags of groceries
- Furniture
- Vacuum cleaners
- Strollers
- Children (even if they ask nicely for you to carry them!)

Keep Moving as You Progress to Normal Activities

- Any kind of light activity around that you can comfortably do without straining helps you heal faster, feel better, and progress more easily to your regular activities. Standing up frequently instead of sitting still is a great way to start.

- Other very light activities include walking around the house or down the driveway, easy chores such as folding clothes, and stretching.

- Next, you can work your way up to walking slowly, playing golf, and being able to play with children, without lifting them up, of course. Water activities, such as water aerobics and swimming, are great choices because they're low-impact, so they don't strain your joints.

- Be sure to get your surgeon's okay before getting into the pool because you don't want to get your incisions wet before they heal.

- In general, the more active you were before your surgery, the faster you can increase your activity levels after the surgery. You're also going to be able to do more activities sooner if your surgery was laparoscopic and you have not had any serious complications or severe side effects from the surgery. Usually, patients with a lower pre-surgery BMI can get back to regular activities faster.

As you read through the list of how to progress to getting back to your regular activities, keep in mind that any estimated timeline that you see for adding in new activities is just that: an estimate. You might be faster to feel comfortable doing some activities than other sleeve patients, and it might take you a little longer to progress to other activities. That's okay. The important part here is to listen to your body. Take your time adding in new activities and increasing the amount you do because you don't want to risk hurting yourself or having a problem with the sleeve. Immediately stop any activity that causes pain. If the pain doesn't stop when you stop the activity, call your doctor or surgeon for advice.

Going Back to Work

If you work, going back to work is a big milestone. It's one thing to recover from surgery and get used to your gastric sleeve in the comfort and privacy of your own home. It's quite another thing to go to work to fulfill your duties and responsibilities while dealing with your new stomach in public.

You can probably return to work within a few weeks of surgery if you didn't have complications. You'll probably have to wait a little longer if you're having sleeve complications or if your job requires you to be very active or lift a lot of weight. Don't rush your return to work no matter how eager you are to get back there. You are still recovering from surgery and don't want to put yourself at risk for any setbacks that can occur if you get too ambitious. Also, if you feel sick at work, be strong enough to let yourself come home and recover more fully.

> **Tip**
>
> Chapter 12, "Post-op Care," will have information about your return to work and what to expect from your colleagues and with your sleeve. You'll learn about handling medical problems at work, figuring out who your true work friends are, and how you can deal with the sensitive topic of eating. We'll talk about some of the different options for how much and exactly what you want to tell various people about your bariatric surgery.

✍ Summary

- ☛ This chapter took you from the operating room in the hospital to getting back to work and other regular activities. Now you know what to expect when you wake up from surgery, how your hospital stay will go, and what you can do at home to make your recovery from surgery as fast and smooth as possible.

- ☛ These days and weeks are important in laying the foundation for your future success with the sleeve. Patience during recovery can help you get through this time with the best possible results. Your wounds will heal faster if you don't try to rush anything, you'll be at lower risk for developing complications and your future weight loss should be easier.

Your Turn: Prepare for the Post-Surgery Challenges!

Shortly after getting the gastric sleeve, post-surgery pain and strong hunger may be two of the biggest challenges that you'll face. This form can help you prepare for these challenges so that you can overcome them more easily.

What do you expect the pain to feel like? How do you expect the hunger to feel?

List at least five things you can tell yourself when the going gets tough

e.g., It'll be worth it because …

I've worked so hard for it that I can't stop now…

It'll get better soon

....

....

....

....

....

List at least three activities you can do to distract yourself from the pain or hunger.

e.g., call my best friend Martha

Do the crossword puzzle in the newspaper.

....

....

....

....

....

A Glimpse into My Life with the Sleeve...Linda from Kentucky

Snapshot

59 years old

Starting Weight: 251 pounds

Current Weight: 167 pounds

Height: 5'7"

Mother, wife, and human resources director

Loves to quilt, crochet, and sew

Weight Problems Holding Her Back

I was not really a yo-yo dieter. About once a year I would go on Weight Watchers or count calories, and would lose a few pounds. However, I lost so slowly that I got discouraged and gave up after a couple of months. Other than the few pounds from each effort, my weight continued to creep up about five pounds per year. I was not able to engage in any but the lightest exercise, not even walking, due to severe hip and knee arthritis.

I never tried the high protein, low carb diets because they did not appeal to me, a sugar and carbohydrate freak. Of course, now high protein and low carbohydrate is my lifestyle!

I was most successful with Weight Watchers in 2003 when I lost about 35 pounds. At that point the arthritis was not as bad, so I was able to use a rowing machine, which helped me tone up and increase the weight loss. I maintained for a few months, and then when a stressful period at work began, I quickly turned to food and gained it all back.

Committing to the Unthinkable: Weight Loss Surgery

Aware only of gastric bypass and feeling it was far too drastic and dangerous, I did not even consider bariatric surgery until 2011. I was always certain that I did not want a bypass due to the invasive nature of the procedure and the problems with malabsorption and other complications. I was also afraid it would kill me! My husband suggested it to me as a possibility, and it bothered me that he would even suggest something so dangerous.

However, one of my primary responsibilities is health insurance in my position as Director of Human Resources for a bank holding company. Our insurance does not cover bariatric procedures. When one of our employees questioned me as to why, I answered that the bypass was far too dangerous and drastic. She responded that new and safer procedures were being done now and that the company should reconsider its position.

Unaware of these procedures, I did some online research and learned that there in addition to the bypass, there were other options, such as the band, the sleeve, and plication. This information planted the seed that weight loss surgery might be an option for me, and my interest grew. I continued to research and felt that this could be the answer, but I was very fearful in general and uncertain which procedure would be best for me.

I at first thought I would have the band, as I was very frightened and sickened by the thought of having most of my stomach removed. I just could not deal with the permanence of the procedure. More research turned up a lot of bad news regarding the band, leaving me more uncertain of which procedure, if any, to have.

In spite of my misgivings, I made the appointment to attend an informative seminar sponsored by a highly acclaimed bariatric practice nearby. My husband went with me, and we heard more positive things about the sleeve, and some positive about plication. The plication was a very new procedure with this practice and most others. I at that point decided I wanted plication, still very fearful of having most of my stomach removed.

I moved forward in the process and attended the all-day intake appointment. Every time I was asked which procedure I was planning and answered "plication", the staff members whispered behind their hands, "No! You want the sleeve!" When I asked why, I was repeatedly told that the results are just not as good as with the sleeve.

I swallowed my fear and decided to go with the sleeve.

Going Ahead with the Procedure

My insurance does not cover any bariatric procedures, so I paid for it myself. Although I could have financed the surgery outright, I chose to finance through Bliss, a company that deals only with surgeons with very good outcomes. The reason I chose Bliss is because they also offer additional insurance to cover complications, which I wanted for peace of mind.

Although there are several practices specializing in bariatric procedures in nearby communities, it was very easy to choose. One had outstanding complication and morbidity rates, and the surgeon was very forthright, charismatic and genuine in his desire to help people change their lives. His confidence was contagious. His personal assurance that this was the right thing to do, that I would be fine, that I would get excellent results, and that by putting myself in his hands I had mitigated 99% of the risk, gave me the confidence to proceed.

His practice had a nutritionist on staff, and I consulted with her once prior to the surgery. She would have been and is still available for consult had I needed or should I need assistance. However, the pre-op education and materials were very detailed and thorough. I read and reread the materials. I watched and rewatched the videos. I used the VST forum extensively, so I had a solid understanding of what I could eat when, so have not needed further consultation.

Relationships and Sharing Her Story with Others

My family and most of my friends have been very supportive. My husband has always been aware of the consequences of my weight on my health and realized the weight was threatening my independence. I was very anxious about telling my two grown sons, and was surprised and relieved when they expressed their support and understanding. I suppose they too had witnessed the effect of the weight on my health.

While I would not say they were unsupportive, two friends were very anxious and concerned over the surgery, and encouraged me to find another way. Now that it has turned out okay, they are truly supportive and often make positive remarks about my success.

I have not kept the surgery from anyone. I told all my coworkers and family, and I will tell anyone else if it seems appropriate. Such openness has led to one or two hurtful remarks. But I did have to laugh when it got back to me that the one of the IT staff, upon learning that my pet cat died, asked, "What? Did she starve it to death?"

A Few Bad Moments Despite the Overall Success

I had just the usual post-op stuff: immediately after the surgery, the pain was mild. I did use pain medications, but not very much. The worst pain was the gas pain in the shoulder, not in my abdomen. I did have days of constipation at first followed by a couple of weeks of very frequent, loose, nasty bowel movements. I was afraid to go back to work, but fortunately, the diarrhea subsided by the end of my three-week leave. I also had:

- *Days of gas pain in the left shoulder, so painful*

- *Days of frequent loose bowel movements*

- *Constant constipation due to the iron supplements*

- *Learning to deal with so many meds plus supplements*

- *The first time I overate and experienced excessive salivation*

The Good Moments Are Too Many to Count!

- *Cooking and sponsoring family dinners, which was a huge worry for me*

- *Wearing a clothing size that does not include an X*

- *Wearing clothes that show my shape, rather than hide my shape*

- *Moving and walking fast and with confidence*

- *Being able to get up and down off the floor*

- *Being able to do all the housework myself*

- *Touching my sides, sitting down, and feeling not one roll of fat*

- *Not being camera shy*

- *Not being ashamed when I run into people I haven't seen in a while*

- *My reflection in a door or window*

Still Waiting to Decide about Goal Weight and Plastic Surgery

I am not finished losing weight yet, so have not had any plastic surgery. Although I originally planned to have plastics, I am unsure at this point if I will. I started with a BM of 40, and have lost 70 pounds. I am unsure what my final weight will be. I have already concluded that my original goal will be too low. I still want to look and feel healthy, so I am leery of strictly targeting BMI.

I do have some loose skin on my arms and legs, and my butt is flat and saggy. My belly isn't too bad yet, but that is where the remaining weight is. I will decide if it is worth the cost, pain, scars, and risks when I reach my final weight. I am almost 60 years old, so vanity is not as large an issue for me as it would be for younger folks. If I have but one procedure, it would be a tummy tuck.

Weight Loss without Exercise but with a Careful Diet

I do not exercise due to continued arthritic pain in my shoulders, hands, hips, and knees. I will soon have a second total knee replacement and hope after the recovery that I will be able to use the rowing machine and stationary bike. My weight loss has been sufficient without exercise, but I have lost a great deal of muscle mass and strength, especially in my legs. I would really like to regain it.

Here is a typical day of eating at six months out:

4:30 a.m.	*Click caffeinated protein drink, made with equal parts 2% milk and water*
6:00 a.m.	*About 5 ounces of Muscle Milk to wash down medications and supplements*
8:00 a.m.	*11 ounces of Muscle Milk*
10:00 a.m.	*28 grams of dry roasted unsalted almonds*
11:20 a.m.	*4 ounces low-fat cottage cheese, plus dill pickle spears*
1:00 p.m.	*several cucumber slices*
2:00 p.m.	*10 slices pepperoni*
3:00 p.m.	*30 grams unsalted peanuts*
4:00 p.m.	*2 Laughing Cow cheese wedges with 8 Special K crackers*
6:00 p.m.	*Protein for dinner, usually with no or very low carbs*

I drink Crystal Light throughout the day. I can no longer stand the taste and feel of plain water, when before the surgery I drank it constantly. This has been the one disappointment.

Beforehand, I would have eaten a huge bowl of sweetened oatmeal for breakfast, a sandwich for lunch, a huge dinner (lots of carryout and fattening recipes) with fruits and sweets several times throughout the day.

Getting in a Few Treats, Sticking to the Diet on Special Occasions, and Dealing with Hunger

Whenever there is a special occasion, such as a birthday, family dinner or work luncheon, I simply eat a little of whatever is served, as I do not want to put others out or bring focus to what I can or cannot eat. I select a few things that appeal to me or that I feel will be well-tolerated. Husband and I order pizza once a week, but it must be thin crust and not greasy. I eat less than one full piece. For some reason, on any day I eat pizza, the next day I will wake up one pound lighter! Now that is living!

I do not have to avoid many foods, just white fluffy breads, highly spiced foods, and greasy foods. I have always had a problem with dry white meat such as chicken breast, so I avoid that. I also have trouble with hard boiled eggs because they are dry, so I don't eat those. I have for some reason been terrified to try lettuce so have not had a salad since the surgery.

So far my favorite recipes are the Mini Meatloaves from the website www.smells-like-home.com (which I learned about on the forum) and any of the "cupcake" recipes from www.emilybites.com (also learned about on the forum). My husband, while not sleeved but watching his weight, loves these recipes too.

Typically if I have a craving, I eat the food, just in tiny portions. I don't even crave greasy foods, which make me sick. I have recently found myself wanting sweets again, which were previously my poison and downfall, so I struggle to fight that tendency.

Unlike most sleeve patients, I have continued to experience hunger since day one post op. It is not as strong or persistent as pre-op, but it is real hunger. I have tried all the acid meds, and while they help just a little, I remain hungry! I wish I had lost the hunger, but on the other hand, I believe because I still get hungry I can still truly enjoy food, and I do.

Consistent Support from BariatricPal

On weekdays I visit the boards several times throughout the day. On weekends I often miss because I am never sitting down! The online community is my support group. I learned so much about the surgery pre-op from the members, and now that I don't really need their help and support, I visit to keep up with the other members and to offer support and encouragement wherever I can.

I visit online bariatric recipe sites, such as Emily Bites and The World According to Eggface. I also follow several bariatric patients on You Tube, which I find informative and inspirational. At first I searched You Tube for stories from folks in my age group. I did find a couple of such success stories of folks in my age group, and that too helped me decide that it wasn't too late to make the change. You may or may not want to know who those individuals are. There was a woman whose You Tube ID is "meggieprice", and a gentleman whose You Tube ID is "MyStu34". Both stories had a huge impact on my decision.

Tips from a Successful Sleever

- *Know what you are getting into!!*

- *Be aware that this is a life-long and life-changing commitment.*

- *It will affect relationships.*

- *Read, listen, study.*

- *Practice living the lifestyle before the surgery.*

- *Plan to succeed.*

- *KNOW that…*

  - *It will be hard.*

  - *There will be pain.*

  - *There are risks.*

  - *There are side effects.*

  - *There are limitations.*

- *KNOW you must endure through all of the above to succeed.*

1   Vertical sleeve gastrectomy. Medline Plus, National Institutes of Health. Website. http://www.nlm.nih.gov/medlineplus/ency/article/007435.htm. 2011, January 26. Accessed October 24, 2012.

2   Moy J, Pomp A, Dakin G, Parikh M, Gagner M. Laparoscopic sleeve gastrectomy for morbid obesity. American Journal of Surgery. 2008;196(5).

3   Bhimji S, Zieve D. General Anesthesia. MedlinePlus, National Institutes of Health. Website. http://www.nlm.nih.gov/medlineplus/ency/article/007410.htm. Updated 2011, January 26. Accessed October 24, 2012.

4   Schumann R, Jones SB, Cooper B, Kelley SD, Bosch MV, Ortiz VE, Connor KA, Kaufman MD, Harvey AM, Carr DB. Update on best practice recommendations for anesthetic perioperative care and pain management in weight loss surgery, 2004-2007. Obesity (Silver Spring). 2009;17(5):889-894.

5   Schumann R, Jones SB, Cooper B, Kelley SD, Bosch MV, Ortiz VE, Connor KA, Kaufman MD, Harvey AM, Carr DB. Update on best practice recommendations for anesthetic perioperative care and pain management in weight loss surgery, 2004-2007. Obesity (Silver Spring). 2009;17(5):889-894.

6   Dugdale DC, Zieve D. Peristalsis. Medline Plus, National Institutes of Health. Website. http://www.nlm.nih.gov/medlineplus/ency/article/002282.htm. Updated 2011, November 17. Accessed October 24, 2012.

7   Dugdale DC, Zieve D. Pain medications - narcotics. Medline Plus, National Institutes of Health. Website. http://www.nlm.nih.gov/medlineplus/ency/article/007489.htm. Updated 2011, May 22. Accessed October 25, 2012.

8   Schumann R, Jones SB, Cooper B, Kelley SD, Bosch MV, Ortiz VE, Connor KA, Kaufman MD, Harvey AM, Carr DB. Update on best practice recommendations for anesthetic perioperative care and pain management in weight loss surgery, 2004-2007. Obesity (Silver Spring). 2009;17(5):889-894.

9   Keterolac.. Medline Plus, National Institutes of Health. Website. http://www.nlm.nih.gov/medlineplus/druginfo/meds/a693001.html. Revised 2010, October 1. Accessed October 25, 2012.

10 Gagnon LE, Karwacki Sheff EJ. Outcomes and complications after bariatric surgery. Am J Nursing. 2012;112(9)26-26.

11 Pech N, Meyer F, Lippert H, Manger T, Stroh C. Complications, reoperations and nutrient deficiencies two years after sleeve surgery. J Obesity. 2012, April.

12 Pech N, Meyer F, Lippert H, Manger T, Stroh C. Complications, reoperations and nutrient deficiencies two years after sleeve surgery. J Obesity. 2012, May.

13 Hutter MM, Schimer BD, Jones DB, Ko CY, Cohen ME, Merkow RP, Nguyen NT. First report from the American College of Surgeons – Bariatric Surgery Center Network laparoscopic sleeve gastrectomy has morbidity and effectiveness positioned between the band and the bypass. Ann Surg. 2012;254(3):410-422.

14 Bhimji S, Zieve D. Vertical sleeve gastrectomy. Website. http://www.nlm.nih.gov/medlineplus/ency/article/007435.htm. Updated 2011, January 26. Accessed October 27, 2012.

15 Huang C-K. Single-incision laparoscopic bariatric surgery. J Minim Access Surg. 2011;7(1):99-103.

16 Pech N, Meyer F, Lippert H, Manger T, Stroh C. Complications, reoperations and nutrient deficiencies two years after sleeve surgery. J Obesity. 2012.

17 Pech N, Meyer F, Lippert H, Manger T, Stroh C. Complications, reoperations and nutrient deficiencies two years after sleeve surgery. J Obesity. 2012.

18 Pech N, Meyer F, Lippert H, Manger T, Stroh C. Complications, reoperations and nutrient deficiencies two years after sleeve surgery. J Obesity. 2012.

19 Pech N, Meyer F, Lippert H, Manger T, Stroh C. Complications, reoperations and nutrient deficiencies two years after sleeve surgery. J Obesity. 2012.

20 Pulmonary embolism. National Heart, Lung and Blood Institute. Website. http://www.nhlbi.nih.gov/health/health-topics/topics/pe/printall-index.html. 2011, July 1. Accessed October 26, 2012.

21 Hutter MM, Schimer BD, Jones DB, Ko CY, Cohen ME, Merkow RP, Nguyen NT. First report from the American College of Surgeons – Bariatric Surgery Center Network laparoscopic sleeve gastrectomy has morbidity and effectiveness positioned between the band and the bypass. Ann Surg. 2012;254(3):410-422.

22 Marquez MF, Ayza M, Lozano RB, Morales, M, Diez JM, Poujolet RB. Gastric leak after laparoscopic sleeve gastrectomy. Obes Surg. 2010;20(9):1306-1311.

23 Bhimji S, Zieve D. Vertical sleeve gastrectomy. Website. http://www.nlm.nih.gov/medlineplus/ency/article/007435.htm. Updated 2011, January 26. Accessed October 27, 2012.

24 Dugdale DC, Longstreth GF, Zieve D. Gastritis. Website. http://www.nlm.nih.gov/medlineplus/ency/article/001150.htm. Updated 2011, January 31. Accessed October 28, 2012.

25 Bhimji S, Zieve D. Vertical sleeve gastrectomy. Website. http://www.nlm.nih.gov/medlineplus/ency/article/007435.htm. Updated 2011, January 26. Accessed October 27, 2012.

12
Post-op Care

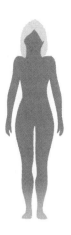

The last chapter discussed your very early post-surgery recovery phases in the hospital and when you first get back home. This chapter covers the medical care that you should continue to receive as you progress with the sleeve. Your postoperative care program, or aftercare program, is a long-term program to keep you healthy and support your weight loss success with the gastric sleeve. It may last for months or years after surgery. This chapter talks about these topics:

- Your post-surgery surgeon appointments
- Medical tests that you may have
- Other healthcare appointments in your post-surgery care program
- Support group meetings and other sources of support
- Staying positive and persistent during this time

By the end of the chapter, you'll know what to expect during your post-surgery care. You'll also know why each part is important so you stay motivated to keep getting the care you need. Each step you take with the vertical sleeve sets the stage for your future health and weight loss, so it's important to work with your medical team and get the best care.

Your Post-Surgery Care Program

The quality of your post-surgery care program can be an important influence in your weight loss success and health with the gastric sleeve. As you know, the aftercare program is an important consideration when choosing your surgeon and medical team. Chapter 7, *Planning for the Surgery and Choosing Your Surgeon*, mentioned that post-surgery care should be considered when choosing your surgeon and medical team. Following a comprehensive care program can have several benefits, such as:

- A lower risk of complications
- Better weight loss
- Lower risk of psychological problems
- Fewer food intolerances; that is, fewer foods that are difficult for you to eat because of the sleeve[1]

Your post-surgery care program is an all-encompassing program to support your well-being and weight loss. It is likely to include these components:

- Follow-up appointments with the surgeon
- Regular medical tests to monitor your nutrient status and health conditions
- Appointments with your dietitian for nutrition counseling and meal planning
- Meeting with a clinical psychologist or psychiatrist for your mental health
- Going to regular support group meetings

Your surgeon will probably encourage or require you to attend medical appointments for the several months following your surgery. In reality, your post-surgery medical care should last for life. You will always be working to avoid sleeve complications, following a careful diet, getting medical tests, and attending support group meetings. Aftercare started as soon as you got out of the sleeve gastrectomy surgery in the hospital, and it continues as you continue to recover and start to lose weight at home.

Aftercare Appointments with Your Surgeon and Medical Testing

Your surgeon will probably examine you at least once or twice in the hospital. Soon after surgery, the surgeon needs to check whether your sleeve looks right. Before you go home, your surgeon needs to give you a final examination to make sure you're ready to be discharged. In one of these appointments or in another appointment your surgeon should give you your post-surgery instructions and see if you have any questions or concerns.

Surgeon Appointments throughout Your Weight Loss Journey

You will continue to see your surgeon after you get discharged from the hospital. You may have a couple of appointments with your surgeon during your first few weeks after leaving the hospital. You might schedule these appointments before you leave the hospital after your sleeve gastrectomy. Then your appointments will become less frequent until they are monthly and eventually annually.

Typical Schedule of Surgeon Appointments

The American Society for Metabolic and Bariatric Surgery, or ASMBS, recommends the following appointments for bariatric surgery patients:[2]

- One to six times during the first six months
- One to two times during the next six months
- One to two times during the first year
- Annually for the rest of your life

You will need more appointments if you have nutritional deficiencies, if you don't lose weight as fast as expected, or if you develop complications with the sleeve.

Aftercare after Going Abroad for the Gastric Sleeve

If you got the sleeve in Mexico, Venezuela or another place that is too far for you to continue your aftercare program there, you'll probably have your aftercare appointments with a surgeon who's closer to home. Before surgery, your surgeon should have been able to help you plan for your post-surgery care. If you didn't already plan, you can still look around for a surgeon who will care for you. Try asking your own surgeon for recommendations or look around just as you would if you were searching for a surgeon for the actual sleeve procedure.

What Happens in Your Regular Appointments?

Your regular aftercare appointments won't take too long. Part of your visit will be like any other visit to a doctor. You will get weighed, which of course has a special meaning now that you're on your weight loss journey with the sleeve. Your surgeon should ask you how you are doing, and you should mention any concerns or symptoms. If you suspect a problem, your surgeon may do some tests, such as a radiological scan using a blue dye to diagnose an anastomotic leak.[3] Your surgeon may order routine tests, such as blood tests to check your cholesterol, blood sugar, or nutritional status. If you have had any tests done recently, you can go over them with your surgeon.

Medical Tests to Expect in Your Post-Surgery Care Program

Whether or not you have specific symptoms, you'll have regular medical evaluations done during the aftercare program. If your surgeon works in a large clinic or hospital with its own laboratory, you can probably get your tests done on the same days that you see your surgeon for post-surgery follow-up appointments. These are some of the tests you can look forward to:

Nutritional Assessments

The gastric sleeve puts you at risk for nutritional deficiencies because your food intake is so limited. We'll go over the specific vitamins and minerals in more detail later, but these are some of the more likely nutritional tests you'll get on a routine basis:[4]

- Iron
- Vitamin B12
- Vitamin D
- Folate
- Albumin (to measure protein)

Blood Tests for Chronic Health Conditions

These tests are some of the best parts of losing weight with the vertical sleeve. Many of your obesity-related chronic conditions will improve as you lose weight, and your blood tests will show it. If you had diabetes or pre-diabetes before the surgery, your blood sugar levels will probably come way down—you may even be able to get off blood sugar medications. The same is true for indicators of heart disease, such as total cholesterol, LDL cholesterol, and triglyceride levels.[5] All of these will probably drop too, and you may be able to get off of your medications for cholesterol and triglycerides.

> **Tip**
>
> Chapter 13, "Recovery and Your Post-Surgery Diet," Chapter 15, "The Sleeve Diet, Weight Loss and Your Health," discuss nutrients and nutrient deficiencies in more detail. You'll learn which nutrients you need to pay attention to, which foods they're in, why you might not be getting enough, and how to prevent deficiencies.

Nobody likes getting their blood drawn, but these results will definitely be good motivation for continuing your healthy diet, and we bet you'll start to look forward to your regular blood tests just so you can see the good news and be proud of yourself for being so good to yourself.

Blood Pressure

This is another one that's probably going to get near the healthy range as you lose weight and start to exercise. Obesity makes your blood pressure higher, and losing weight and lowering your blood pressure is healthy for your heart and kidneys. Your physician may eventually let you get off blood pressure-lowering medications.

Bone Density Scan

You probably won't get this one too often because it's pretty expensive, but it's a great test to see how healthy your bones are. When you lose weight fast, your bones can lose density and become a little weaker and more likely to fracture. Nearly 40 million Americans have osteoporosis, or weak bones, and many don't realize it until they break a hip after what should have been a minor fall.[6] You're most likely to get bone density scans every couple of years if you're an older woman, but your doctor might recommend one if your weight loss is very fast or you're not getting enough calcium and vitamin D.

Dietitian Appointments

A comprehensive aftercare program includes regular follow-up appointments with a dietitian, with appointments starting one to two weeks after surgery. Appointments become less frequent over time and you might meet the dietitian at one, two, three, six and nine months after surgery before switching to an annual schedule.[7]

Your dietitian can be the proverbial rock during your weight loss journey if you have the opportunity to work closely with him or her for any length of time. Your dietitian will help you make plan meals, set reasonable goals, and help you overcome any problems that may come up with your diet. The dietitian will also help you with the following topics.

Plan a Menu & Be Wise About Food Choices

There will be foods that you can and cannot eat on the sleeve diet. Following the rules is especially critical during the first few weeks after surgery. Your dietitian will let you know which foods and liquids are okay and which are not allowed during each stage of the sleeve diet as you progress from liquids to solid foods.

Food Lists to Menu Planning

You're changing your whole pattern of eating, and menu planning with the dietitian can prevent you from feeling overwhelmed. Even when you know which foods are okay from your food list, you need to know additional information to plan menus for entire days and have your meal plan as nutritious as possible:

- *How much* of each food to eat
- *When* to eat your meals and snacks
- *When* to drink your fluids
- *What* to eat within a day
- *How* to meet your nutrient requirements

Sticking to your diet is a lot easier when you know all of these things. You and your dietitian can work on planning daily and weekly meals and menus that are nutritious and low-calorie. At first, you'll probably rely on the dietitian to do most of the work. As you get more experience, you'll get better at planning your own meals.

Ideas and Recipes to Prevent Boredom

A list of foods can be very boring…until your dietitian shares new recipes for you to try. Dietitians are trained to be able to suggest to you interesting ways to use foods using simple recipes so you don't have to be a chef. Your dietitian can also give you ideas on what to contribute to a potluck dinner and what to choose when you're at a restaurant with friends.

Setting Goals and Troubleshooting

Part of your appointment time with the dietitian will include goal setting. Some of the goals that you set will have to do with weight loss, but others will be unrelated to the numbers you see on the scale. They'll be things such as stopping your meal when you are full or remembering to take your supplement every day. Dietitians can also help you troubleshoot if you're not hitting your weight loss goals or if you're having some problems with the sleeve that seem related to your diet. Your dietitian can assess your diet and point out a few problems with it that you might not have even realized. Minor changes can make a big difference in your weight loss results.

Post-Operative Nutritional Assessment

In addition to working with you on your diet and weight loss, the dietitian may help ensure that your nutritional status is good. There are some standard ways to do this.

- **Weight and Body Fat -** The dietitian should assess your nutritional status at each post-surgery appointment. Dietitians will monitor your weight, BMI, and percent excess body weight to make sure that you're losing weight as hoped and you're eating the right amount of calories at each stage of weight loss. You might also get your percent body fat measured. If you're not losing weight as fast as you expected, the dietitian can work with you to figure out how you can change your diet to hit your goals.

- **Checking Your Blood Tests -** They'll also review your blood tests to see how your nutrient status is. We've already talked about using blood tests to check your levels of protein and some vitamins and minerals. If you have abnormal results, the dietitian can discuss strategies such as healthy eating and dietary supplements to bring your nutrient levels back to normal.

- **Assessing Your Diet -** Each appointment, your dietitian will probably assess your diet by asking what you typically eat. When you have your diet assessed, the dietitian may notice that your intake of certain nutrients is low. For example, if you're not eating fortified grains or many vegetables or beans, you might have a low intake of folic acid. In that case, the dietitian may recommend that your doctor order a folate test to check your status. The dietitian might not even need tests to make some recommendations. For example, a fish oil supplement can be a healthy choice if you don't eat seafood. Your dietitian can also use dietary assessment to help you with some of the following:[8]

  - Figuring out why you have dumping syndrome, nausea, or vomiting

  - Suggesting times when you can drink more fluids

  - Help you increase your dietary variety

Additional Roles

Your dietitian's degree of involvement depends on how closely he or she works with the surgeon and what your clinic's standard protocol is. Some dietitians may fulfill additional more roles. Together, the two of you might work on the following issues:[9]

- Choosing foods that promote healthy weight loss because they are nutritious, low in calories and filling. Examples include egg whites, chicken breast, seafood, fat-free dairy products, vegetables, whole grains, and fruits.

- Avoiding foods that interfere with weight loss because they are high in calories and not very filling. Examples include refined carbohydrates, such as sugary foods and white bread, fried foods, and other high-fat foods.

- Reviewing your medications to make sure you're taking what you should.

- Psychological issues, such as emotional eating, getting social support, and improving your body image.

You'll meet with the dietitian pretty often at first, and gradually have less frequent appointments as you get further along in your weight loss journey. The exact frequency will depend on factors such as your insurance, your surgeon's recommendations, your own preferences, and your dietitian's regular procedure. You'll meet more often if you're having trouble following your meal plan, and you might meet less often if you're really nailing your eating, losing weight at the rate you want, and feeling confident about where you're headed. Appointments can be as frequent as every week, or you might feel comfortable going for longer without an appointment.

> **Tip**
>
> Chapter 9, "Pre-Surgery Preparations," and Chapter 10, "Final Preparation for the Sleeve Surgery," for more information on what a dietitian does and what you can expect during appointments. Chapters 13 and 14 have information on the post-surgery diet right after surgery and on the sleeve diet that you'll be following as part of your long-term lifestyle change for weight loss and management.

Nowadays, it's easy to email your dietitian some questions or an electronic food record and see if you can get some suggestions.

It's Okay If You Don't Have a Dietitian

Not everyone has the opportunity to meet with a dietitian so frequently, especially if you're self-pay or your insurance has stricter limits on your dietitian appointments. That's okay. Take advantage of any professional nutritional help you can get from a qualified nutritionist or dietitian, and be aware of the many other resources that can help you with your diet:

- Your surgeon or clinic probably has standard instructions for sleeve or bariatric patients. You might get allowed and prohibited food lists and serving sizes for each stage of recovery from surgery and your long-term sleeve diet. Clinic staff should be able and willing to answer your questions, no matter how detailed.

- This book is a fairly detailed guide to the sleeve diet that takes you right from the time you get out of surgery until you're well into the long-term sleeve diet for weight loss and eventually maintenance. This book lets you know the following:
  - Which foods you can and cannot have at each stage
  - How to make a meal plan
  - Choosing healthy foods
  - Eating proper serving sizes
  - Staying aware of nutrient deficiencies
  - Figuring out what to do when you have a reaction to a certain food

- BariatricPal.com is a social networking platform with thousands of members who are sleeve patients. You can benefit from their experiences. Sleeve patients are ideal sources of information when you have very detailed questions, such as about specific types or amounts of food or certain symptoms or health conditions. Surgeons may not be able to answer these questions with such accuracy. Another benefit of this online community is that people are online at all times of the day and night, so you're likely to be able to message or chat with community members whenever you need them.

- Other online sources are likely to provide what you need in terms of food lists and basic information. As discussed in Chapter 7, *Planning for Your Vertical Sleeve Gastrectomy and Choosing a Surgeon*, you'll soon learn which sites seem trustworthy and which don't.

Meeting with a Mental Health Professional

Meetings with a mental health professional are part of a comprehensive post-surgery care program. Not all surgeons require regular appointments after your sleeve surgery. That would mean that your only mandatory appointment with a clinical psychologist or psychiatrist would be your pre-surgery evaluation. Even if you're not obligated to meet with a psychologist as part of your requirements for completing your surgeon's aftercare, you should still have access to one in case you need it or want to take advantage of those services.

Dealing With Post-Operational Emotional Challenges

After getting the sleeve, you're likely to have some emotional and mental challenges. These are normal responses to the dramatic changes you're going through in your life. The sleeve experience can be draining even if you have a minimal amount of trouble with the sleeve and your weight loss is exactly as much as you hoped. It's a long, hard process, and all that effort is a mental strain. Even your visible results can be an emotional challenge—as delighted as you might be to get the body you want, looking like a whole new person can be stressful. In addition, your relationships with people can change when some people inevitably start to treat you differently than they used to when you were obese. They can be uncomfortable around you or make you feel abnormal for being a bariatric surgery patient.

How a Psychologist Can Help

A psychologist can help with these concerns. You might address them during a prescheduled appointment that was made before your surgery as part of your post-operation care program. Or you can make an appointment specifically to address your worries.

Strategies for Positive Thinking

The power of positive thinking sounds a little corny, but boy, does it work. You can easily get yourself in a self-defeating rut or cause yourself to fail if you fall into the trap of thinking negatively. On the contrary, positive thinking can keep you motivated and give you strength to succeed in your diet program. A mental health professional can teach you tricks for turning lemons into lemonade just by changing the way you react to a situation—without changing the actual circumstance. Some people are naturally positive, and the rest of us need a little practice to get into the habit. A psychologist can suggest ways to practice your positive thinking strategies.

Knowing Yourself a Little Better

Psychologists know how the mind works and how powerful it is. Some of us are naturally good at knowing ourselves, and some of us are not. Once you learn how to interpret what your mind is hinting at and learn an appropriate response to deal with your doubts or fears, you're going to be stronger than ever. For example, you might notice that your most powerful cravings for sweets come in the evening after dinner. Your psychologist might think through the situation with you and have you dig deep within yourself. You might, in fact, realize that you're not really craving sugar – instead, maybe you're in the habit of having dessert because you associate it with well-being from your childhood. A psychologist might suggest an alternative, such as writing up your daily food diary, which keeps you feeling safe but doesn't hurt your diet.

Detecting Signs of Depression

Extreme obesity can lead to depression, and bariatric surgery patients often have fewer symptoms of mild depression after losing weight than before surgery.[10] However, there is a small risk of depression after the sleeve surgery. These factors can contribute to depression:

- Realizing that your obesity was hiding an underlying issue. Now that you're losing weight, it's harder to hide behind your obesity and you have to confront the issue.
- Many life changes. You look different, feel different, have a different body, have different relationships with people, and have different physical abilities. All these changes can be overwhelming.

A psychologist can monitor you for depression and get you treated in its early stages. Treatments might include one-on-one therapy with the psych, extra group support sessions for sleeve patients, or both.

It's important to continue to see a psychologist or at least have access to one for years after your gastric sleeve procedure. Some sleeve patients develop more symptoms of mild depression by the end of five years than in their first year after the surgery.[11]

Setting Goals and Overcoming Barriers

Goal-setting is important whenever you're trying to accomplish something because it helps you stay focused. A psychologist can help you with setting more general goals than the ones you set for your weight loss or with the dietitian. You can learn strategies for setting realistic long-term and short-term goals. You can plan how you will achieve them and how you can evaluate your progress along the way.

Overcoming Troubles with Your Weight Loss

A mental health professional can help you address emotional or psychological problems that may be interfering with your weight loss. In fact, the American Society of Metabolic and Bariatric Surgery, or ASMBS, recommends psychological attention as part of your care plan if you're struggling with weight loss after bariatric surgery.[12] Psychological factors, such as not understanding how the sleeve works or inability to stick to the sleeve diet, can hamper your weight loss and can be addressed by a psychologist.

Even if you don't discuss many things that are directly related to how the vertical sleeve works or what you should be eating, your psychologist can be pivotal in your long-term weight loss success. Take advantage of the mental health professional services that you are entitled to from your insurance or through working with your surgeon, and you'll probably notice that you also approach other aspects of your life with a healthier and more productive attitude.

Connecting With Support Groups

Support groups are almost indispensible to effective postoperative care. They're so important to your success that before agreeing to do your sleeve procedure, your surgeon is likely to ask you to sign a contract stating that you will attend group sessions. You might be required to attend at least one meeting every week or two, and that might eventually turn into one meeting per month as you get further out from surgery and closer to your goal weight and lifetime maintenance. Most patients are encouraged to regularly attend bariatric surgery group support meetings for life.

How Support Groups Can Help

Why are support groups so effective at turning you into a success story? Meetings are educational and motivational, so you can learn what you need to know and have the motivation to do what you need to do to lose weight. These are a few ways that support groups can help:

- *Provide social support*. The sleeve journey can feel lonely even if your family and friends are very supportive. They can't understand exactly what you're going through.
- *Keep your spirits up*. The changes from the sleeve can be overwhelming. Group meetings are events that you get to look forward to because you can relax and just be yourself. Seeing others who are experiencing the same things as you and are managing to embrace it positively can motivate you to be just as upbeat.
- *Expose you to new ideas*. Many meetings will likely include guest presentations. You might hear from plastic surgeons, long-time bariatric patients, or dietitians. There's always an opportunity to learn about the latest developments in the bariatric world or new tricks for sticking to your diet.
- *Long-term success*. Some of the strategies you learn may come in handy years down the road as you continue to follow the sleeve diet and lifestyle.

Mindfulness and the Sleeve

You're likely to increase your mindfulness by participating in support group meetings. Mindfulness describes the ability to "be in the moment," or be aware of your feelings and surroundings. It lets you think more clearly so you can connect your current thoughts and actions to consequences in the future. These are some examples of how mindfulness can benefit you:

Choosing a high-protein, low-calorie egg white instead of a tempting high-sugar, high-fat, high-calorie piece of pie because you realize that your current craving will pass and you'll be better off later if you choose the egg white.

Choosing to exercise instead of watch TV because you can clearly recognize that you'll feel better after you work out and you'll lose weight faster, even though watching TV is more comfortable at this moment.

Support Group Meeting Locations and Leaders

Many surgeons, especially the ones who work in larger clinics and hospitals or who specialize in bariatric surgery, run their own support groups. Meetings will probably be held in the hospital building. If your surgeon doesn't have his or her own group, you will probably be directed to a nearby facility to attend meetings with other sleeve and bariatric surgery patients from the area.

Support Groups and Sticking to Your Diet

Only a fraction of bariatric surgery patients stick to their diets exactly as instructed. The rest may eat foods that aren't recommended, drink beverages while eating solid foods, have larger portions, or eat fewer meals and snacks than recommended. Poor eating behaviors can interfere with your short-term and long-term weight loss and increase your risk for complications, such as vomiting and dehydration.

Attending support group meetings can help you maintain your good nutrition habits or improve your bad habits in a variety of ways:

- The other group members and the group leader can suggest strategies to make following your diet easier. They might share recipes to make your nutritious diet more interesting, healthier options for satisfying cravings, and ways to remember to eat frequently and measure your portions.

- You can learn which foods are more and less likely to cause problems at various stages of your weight loss journey.

- Going to regular meetings can keep you motivated because you'll know that you'll be seeing the other group members each week or month. That'll give you a sense of accountability during the week or month as you're working hard to make the right choices and stay on track.

- Group meetings can help you track time. You might even start setting goals based on your next meeting. For example, you could set the goal of getting in an extra cup of water each day in the week before your next meeting.

Source[13]

Structure of Group Meetings

Your support group meetings will probably have a structured format. A typical meeting might last for one to two hours. A variety of people may lead these meetings, and the leader may switch from session to session. These are likely group leaders:

- Your surgeon or another surgeon from your clinic group
- Your clinical psychologist or another counselor
- A nurse or other bariatric healthcare professional
- A peer counselor, or sleeve or other bariatric patient who has been successful after his or her own surgery and is interested in helping other patients see the same results.

Typical Meeting Agenda

Often, the meetings start with a round of introductions. You might be asked to say your name and some basic information, such as where you are in the process of getting the sleeve or bariatric surgery. Attendees at the meeting might be:

- Thinking about it and gathering information
- Trying to choose a surgeon
- Getting ready for surgery
- Already sleeved and on the road to goal weight

If you're at a meeting with patients from different surgeons, you might tell each other who your surgeon is. After the introductions, there might be some sort of presentation by the meeting leader or an invited guest. For example, in one weight loss surgery meeting, the guest lecturer was a surgeon whose specialty was removal of excess skin for formerly obese patients who'd lost a lot of weight. In his presentation, he described the process of removing extra skin from the underarms and talked about who would be good candidates for the procedure.

After the main presentation, the floor will probably be opened up for questions about the presentation and then for general questions about anything related to the sleeve. Don't be afraid to ask any of your questions, even if they may seem embarrassing. Everyone else in the room has had to deal with embarrassing sleeve-related side effects in public. They've had the same experiences with diarrhea, vomiting and getting too full very fast—or if they haven't gotten the sleeve yet, they're worried about these things. They want to know just as badly as you do about how to prevent it—and a lot of the other patients will have excellent tried-and-true advice for you.

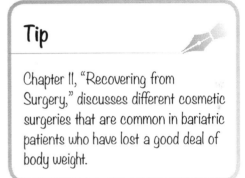

Tip

Chapter 11, "Recovering from Surgery," discusses different cosmetic surgeries that are common in bariatric patients who have lost a good deal of body weight.

The meetings can be excellent opportunities to make a few friends. Sure, just like with any other group, you'll like some people, be neutral about others, and maybe a couple will even rub you the wrong way. But you're coming in with shared experiences of years of obesity and a commitment to becoming healthy using bariatric surgery. That's some deep stuff, and it can be the basis for some amazing friendships.

Cognitive Behavioral Therapy

Some group sessions might be based on principles of cognitive behavioral therapy, or CBT.[14] This is especially likely if you have a psychologist leading your meetings. You might also use CBT techniques in individual sessions with your psychologist. CBT has been used in treating psychosocial disorders, such as depression and addictions, as well as for managing chronic diseases. As a bariatric surgery patient, you might be able to use CBT for the following:

- Increasing adherence to your diet
- Preventing vitamin and mineral deficiencies
- Sticking to the recommended amounts of exercise
- Improving your monitoring and management of diabetes and high blood pressure
- Improving your body image, self-esteem, and relationships with others

How does CBT work? It focuses on being able to control your thoughts and actions. You use a variety of methods to increase the likelihood that you'll perform the healthy actions you want. These might include learning more about the benefits of eating a varied diet, asking your family and friends to praise you for measuring your food, setting a timer so you remember to eat each meal or snack, and keeping only nutritious foods in the house.

Alternatives to Attending Support Group Meetings In-Person

In-person support groups are nice because you have the opportunity to meet people and get involved. Unfortunately, they're not always practical or possible for you. They may be too far from home or incompatible with your schedule.

Videoconferences and Conference Calls

Videoconferences and conference calls are increasingly common options for live meetings, and you don't have to drive to them. You can attend from your own home. You just need some basic equipment such as computer speakers and a microphone. A webcam is cool because it lets everyone who's at the meeting, either in person or from their own computers, see you, too. You'll need some sort of software, which is usually available for a free download, and instructions for installing the software will be easy to find and follow from the hosting company's website.

The group meeting's organizers can tell you how to "attend" the meeting. You might be able to access the meeting from the group's website, or you might need to log in to a conference-hosting service and/or make a telephone call. Skype is just one example of a company that offers meeting-hosting services.

Other Options

You can still get the social support you need even if your schedule simply doesn't allow you make it to a live meeting. Recorded videos of live meetings are available from a few sources. You can watch webcasts and webinars at any time, such as while your children are in bed or while you're walking on the treadmill. Often, you can even participate by sending in your questions before or after the actual event. Discussion forums provide additional support group options. You can participate in online conversations on your own time or schedule group live chat sessions with other forum members.

Staying Positive Post-Surgery!

The first few weeks after surgery can be tough. You might have stomach pain from your healing wounds, gastrointestinal symptoms, nausea, hunger, and anxiety about your future lifestyle. You might be tired of seeing your surgeon and dietitian so often, and of getting so many medical tests. Measuring your food, selecting appropriate foods, taking your multivitamins and getting enough water can all be burdensome.

The worst part might be that your weight might not even come off as fast as you'd expected because your focus during this time is on recovery, not weight loss. You might start wondering you even bothered to get the gastric sleeve in the first place.

Don't Give Up! It's Time for a Pep Talk!

Just don't let these thoughts get you down. These reactions are perfectly normal, justified, and allowed. After all, you prepared for the VSG for months. It's normal to get a bit down after any event that big, no matter how phenomenal the results are. Even gold-medal Olympians can feel a bit lost after the Games — they just dedicated at least four years of their lives to their dreams and suddenly feel let down after they finally win the Olympic gold. Like Olympians, you can get through this emotional low time and continue to work hard so that everything will eventually fall into place and be worth it.

Always Look Ahead

Don't even start wondering whether you *should* have gotten the sleeve or not. There's no going back once you have your vertical sleeve gastrectomy, so there's no point in wondering whether it was your best choice. The best thing you can do now is to look ahead.

Remind Yourself of the Important Things

There are some reminders that you can keep repeating to yourself to get yourself through this hard time:

- *You are not alone.* Nearly all sleeve patients go through the exact same challenges – and come out on top — and that can be a comforting thought to keep in the back of your head.

- *Things will get better. This period of trials and tribulations will eventually end.* Sure, you'll always face some challenges with the sleeve, but all this practice is letting you get better at dealing with them.

- *This is a lifelong journey.* The goal isn't to lose weight as fast as possible. It's to lose weight and maintain your weight loss for life. After a few years, you'll realize that won't matter exactly how fast you lose weight. It won't matter whether it takes you one year, three years, or five years to hit your goal weight. What *will* be important from this time is that you stuck to your program, made healthy choices to avoid health complications, and developed the skills you need to control your weight for life.

> **Tip**
>
> During this time, your support system is crucial. Chapter 11, "Recovering from Surgery," talks about different sources of support, both in your life and online, to turn to when you're starting to doubt yourself or you need a little extra encouragement or motivation.

Keep It in Perspective

These weeks may seem endless as you're going through them; later they'll seem like a flash. Now, keep reminding yourself why you got the sleeve, what your weight loss will mean to you and your family, and how proud you will be of yourself when you finally get into the swing of things as an experienced sleever.

Summary

- This chapter described a standard postoperative care program from the hospital to months or years after your gastric sleeve procedure. You should have regular appointments with your surgeon to be sure that you're healing well and preventing complications. You can expect to have certain medical tests regularly, too. The dietitian and psychologist can provide valuable support and information, so take advantage of these experts when you can! Support group meetings can serve a variety of roles from informative to supporting to motivational.

- These can be challenging times, so we ended the chapter with a little pep talk that can come in handy if you're feeling a little down on yourself. Many sleeve patients find that things get a lot better if you can just stick it out now.

- This chapter covered pretty much everything you need to know about your aftercare program—except for your diet. That's important enough to deserve a chapter on its own because a good post-surgery diet will speed your recovery from surgery and lay the foundation for steady weight loss and good eating habits in the future. In the next chapter, you'll learn all about your diet for the first several weeks after your vertical sleeve gastrectomy.

Your Turn: Keep Your Post-Surgery Appointments Straight!

List three things that you are most looking forward to in your first year after surgery.

*Example: I can't wait to go biking with my son for the first time! ....

You're going to have a lot of appointments after your surgery. This form can help you keep them straight so you know when they are, where they are and how to prepare. We recommend using this template for each of your appointments so that you always stay on top of your medical care.

Date of appointment: ....

Time of appointment: ....

Appointment with (Name) ...., (position or title) ....

Location of appointment (may need hospital name and specific building and room number)

....

Preparation required (e.g., fasting, bringing medical history or results from recent blood tests, diet log to show a dietitian, list of questions to ask): ....

Other notes (e.g., do you need a ride?) ....

1   Keren D, Matter I, Rainis T & Lavy A. Getting the most from the sleeve: the importance of post-operative follow-up. Obesity Surgery. 2011;21(12):1887-1893.

2   Mechanick JI, Kushner RF, Sugerman HJ, Gonzalez-Campoy M, Collazo-Clavell ML, ... Dixon J. American Association of Clinical Endocrinologists, The Obesity Society and American Society for Metabolic and Bariatric Surgery medical guidelines for clinical practice for the perioperative nutritional, metabolic and nonsurgical support of the bariatric surgery patient. Obesity. 2009;17:S1-S70.

3   Marquez MF, Ayza M, Lozano RB, Morales, M, Diez JM, Poujolet RB. Gastric leak after laparoscopic sleeve gastrectomy. Obes Surg. 2010;20(9):1306-1311.

4   Ziegler O, Sirveaux MA, Brunaud L, Reibel N, Quillot D. Medical follow-up after bariatric surgery: nutritional and drug issues. General recommendations for the prevention and treatment of nutritional deficiencies. Diabetes Metab. 2009;35(6 Pt 2):544-547.

5   Mechanick JI, Kushner RF, Sugerman HJ, Gonzalez-Campoy M, Collazo-Clavell ML, ... Dixon J. American Association of Clinical Endocrinologists, The Obesity Society and American Society for Metabolic and Bariatric Surgery medical guidelines for clinical practice for the perioperative nutritional, metabolic and nonsurgical support of the bariatric surgery patient. Obesity. 2009;17:S1-S70.

6   NIH Senior Health: Built with You in Mind. (n.d.). Osteoporosis: what is osteoporosis? National Institutes of Health. http://nihseniorhealth.gov/osteoporosis/whatisosteoporosis/01.html. Accessed October 29, 2012.

7   Snyder-Marlow G, Tayle D, Lenhard MJ. Nutrition care for patients undergoing laparoscopic sleeve gastrectomy for weight loss. J Am Diet Ass. 2010;110(4):600-607

8   Aills L, Blankenship J, Buffington C, Furtado M, Parrott J. ASMBS Allied Health nutritional guidelines for the surgical weight loss patient. Surg Obes Relat Dis. 2008;4(5Suppl):S73-S108.

9   Aills L, Blankenship J, Buffington C, Furtado M, Parrott J. ASMBS Allied Health nutritional guidelines for the surgical weight loss patient. Surg Obes Relat Dis. 2008;4(5Suppl):S73-S108.

10 Mechanick JI, Kushner RF, Sugerman HJ, Gonzalez-Campoy M, Collazo-Clavell ML, ... Dixon J. American Association of Clinical Endocrinologists, The Obesity Society and American Society for Metabolic and Bariatric Surgery medical guidelines for clinical practice for the perioperative nutritional, metabolic and nonsurgical support of the bariatric surgery patient. Obesity. 2009;17:S1-S70.

11 Strain GW, Saif T, Gagner M, Rossidis M, Cross-sectional review of effects of laparoscopic sleeve gastrectomy and 1, 3 and 5 years. Surg Obes Relat Dis. 2011;7(6):714-719.

12 Mechanick JI, Kushner RF, Sugerman HJ, Gonzalez-Campoy M, Collazo-Clavell ML, ... Dixon J. American Association of Clinical Endocrinologists, The Obesity Society and American Society for Metabolic and Bariatric Surgery medical guidelines for clinical practice for the perioperative nutritional, metabolic and nonsurgical support of the bariatric surgery patient. Obesity. 2009;17:S1-S70.

13 McVay MA, Friedman KE. The benefits of cognitive behavioral groups for bariatric surgery patients. Bariatric Times. 2012;9(9):22-28.

14 McVay MA, Friedman KE. The benefits of cognitive behavioral groups for bariatric surgery patients. Bariatric Times. 2012;9(9):22-28.

13

Recovery and Your Post-Surgery Diet

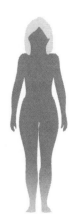

Of course food is at the center of your weight loss. You need to know what to eat, how much, and when. This chapter finally begins to dig into your sleeve diet, but we have to warn you that the post-surgery sleeve diet is an exercise in patience. We know that you've waited for so long for the surgery and prepared so carefully for weeks or months that all you can think about is losing weight as quickly as you can. Not so fast, though!

Recovery needs to be your focus for several weeks after surgery. During this time, minimizing side effects and preventing complications are far higher priorities than weight loss. The post-surgery diet helps you do this by gradually progressing from a liquid-only diet to a solid diet. These are the stages of the post-surgery sleeve diet:[1]

- Liquid diet
- Pureed diet
- Soft foods diet
- Regular sleeve diet

We'll cover the first three phases in this chapter and save the solid foods phase, or the regular sleeve diet, for the next chapter. That's the one you'll be on for the long term as long as you're not having complications from the sleeve.

This chapter covers the following topics:

- Why the post-surgery diet is absolutely critical for your health and weight loss
- What you can and cannot eat during each phase of the diet
- When to go on to the next stage
- What to do if you have a reaction to a specific food
- Food lists and sample meal plans for each phase

So are you ready to start eating for health and recovery? Here's how!

Yes, a Post-Surgery Diet is Important

You've gone through a lot so far in your sleeve journey, but it's not yet time to focus on losing weight even though you have the sleeve. For the next few weeks concentrate on recovering and setting a good base for the future instead of struggling with your weight. It's tough to change your mindset since you've gone through so much already in your fight against obesity, but it's absolutely crucial for your future success.

Why You Need to Follow the Post-Surgery Diet

It is necessary to follow the post-surgery diet as closely as you can. The old saying that cheaters only cheat themselves is absolutely true in this case. We're not talking just about stalling your weight loss temporarily if you cheat. These are possible effects of going off the diet by eating too much or eating the wrong foods:

- Interfering with weight loss for the long term. If you stretch your stomach sleeve, you'll feel less restriction when you eat, so you'll tend to eat more. That makes the sleeve, or your main weight loss tool, far less effective.

- Gastrointestinal symptoms, such as diarrhea, bloating, cramping and constipation

- Nutrient deficiencies

- Serious complications, such as leaking or infections

The post-surgery vertical sleeve diet has other benefits too:

- It lets you get used to eating smaller portions at meals and snacks instead of large meals.

- It builds on the food-planning and monitoring skills that you were working on before surgery.

- It helps you develop new skills, such as chewing your food slowly, eating only until you are full, and avoiding beverages at meals.

A Few Challenges to Expect

Avoiding these complications should be strong motivation to follow your diet properly even though this is a challenging time in your sleeve journey. Being prepared for the following challenges to your willpower can help you overcome them:

- *Slower weight loss than hoped*. You're not counting calories now; you're focusing on eating the right foods (or liquids) and preventing nutritional deficiencies. The goal now is to recover from surgery and lay the foundation for safe and healthy weight loss soon. Slower weight loss now is less glamorous but more likely to lead to long-term success. Don't let it frustrate you, and don't question yourself.

- *Slow progress*. Each stage will take at least a week and likely more to get through.[2] You'll only add in a few new kinds of food at a time. There may be times when a new food causes discomfort, and you'll have to delay your progression. Be patient and listen to your body, and remember that weight control is not a race. It's about losing weight and maintaining your weight loss, whether that takes 5 years, 10 years, or 20 years.

- *Change*. You'll get used to different eating patterns, such as small meals and snacks. You will be unable to eat many foods that you used to enjoy.

- *Hunger, especially when you're on a liquid diet*. The purpose of the sleeve is to make your stomach smaller so it fills up quickly, but it doesn't work so well when you're on a liquid diet because liquids empty quickly from your stomach. Another reason why you may be hungry is that it takes about 20 to 60 minutes for your hunger and satiety hormones to respond to food and tell your brain that you're

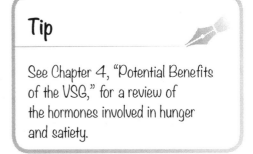

Tip

See Chapter 4, "Potential Benefits of the VSG," for a review of the hormones involved in hunger and satiety.

full.[3] This means that you should practice eating slowly and stopping before you're completely full. That can be a change from the past several years if you're like many obese patients, who are used to ignoring their fullness signals.

- *Crabbiness.* You'll be in pain and discomfort from surgery and possible side effects. You may be hungry. You may be stressed out about your health. You're still not close to your goal weight. You'll recognize that you're being uncharacteristically short-tempered but may not be able to control yourself.[4]

- *Mistakes.* Nobody's perfect, and neither are you. You'll inevitably eat something that's not on the diet, measure a portion wrong, or forget to take your multivitamin. The difference between successful weight loss and ongoing struggles is whether you get back on track.

- *The unexpected*. You might start to enjoy the tastes of healthy foods as you reduce sugar and fat in your diet. Junk food might not taste so good any more. You might notice that for the first time in a long time…you're full! Hours or a day might pass without fixating on food. That's when you can be confident that the sleeve will work for you.

Remind yourself that it's all about the end goal! Each trial that you successfully overcome will increase your confidence and your ability to stay on track. As long as you limit your intake to the recommended amounts, you *will* lose weight.

Kitchen Equipment to Get You Started

You don't need much, but a bit of kitchen equipment will help on your post-surgery diet. Having the right tools and utensils makes it easier to stick to your meal plan. These items are almost indispensible:

- *Measuring cups and measuring spoons*: From now on, "eyeballing" it will not work. Get into the habit of measuring each portion of everything you put into your mouth. If your meal plan calls for a quarter-cup of cream of wheat made with one tablespoon of milk, measure out a quarter-cup of cream of wheat and a tablespoon of milk. Even experienced chefs can underestimate portions and slow weight loss by accidentally taking in way too many calories.

- *Kitchen scale*: A kitchen scale can be invaluable for measuring foods that don't fit neatly into cups and spoons. Examples include meat and fish. Scales are also useful for measuring foods, such as dry cereal, that can settle during packaging, so their actual weight and volume isn't exactly the same as what's listed on the package. For solid food, weight is always more accurate than volume. Analog kitchen scales have the traditional dial that points to the weight of the food when you put it on the scale. Digital, or electronic, kitchen scales can be easier to use because they display the weight in ounces or grams on a screen for you. They can run on batteries or be electric.

- *Blender*: A full-size blender can handle pretty much anything you throw into it, and you may find yourself using it several times a day during the pureed foods phase. A hand blender can be a good option for the semi-solid foods phase. You don't have the hassle of cleaning the full-sized blender, and it may leave a few small chunks in your food.

- **Strainer:** When you're able to get your pureed food through a strainer, you can be confident that there are no chunks left. There are different grades of strainers with bigger or smaller holes to meet your needs. Strainers with smaller holes are better for early stages of your sleeve diet.

- **Storage bags and containers**: Storage bags and containers can store single servings of food. They help you plan ahead. You can use them to carry food with you when you know you won't be able to measure your portions when it's time to eat later. They're also useful for letting you make an entire, multiple-serving recipe. Before you serve yourself your single portion, pack up the rest of your recipe into single-serving portions in individual plastic storage containers or little bags to put in the fridge or freezer. Then you'll always have the right amount of food on hand.

> **Tip**
>
> **Checking Your Kitchen Equipment before Surgery**
>
> Chapter 10, "Final Preparation for the Sleeve Surgery," recommends taking some time before surgery to get your entire home and kitchen ready. This includes gathering the kitchen items that you'll need after surgery. The more preparation you do before surgery, the easier your recovery will be.

You may already have these items on hand. If not, you can get them at any kitchen supplies store or mass merchandiser and most grocery and drug stores. Many dollar stores have measuring cups and spoons that are perfectly adequate.

Phase 1 – Liquid Diet

You can't eat solid food right after surgery. Instead, you'll be on a liquid diet.[5] Most, but not all, surgeons recommend a clear liquid diet for one to two days after surgery. The full liquid diet, which is less restrictive, begins either after the clear liquid diet or right after surgery. It lasts until about 10 to 14 days after surgery if you have no complications and you're ready to progress, but you can be on it for longer.[6] Some patients can start to add pureed foods after seven days if their dietitian allows it.[7] Strict adherence to the diet can help you in the following ways:

- It provides some nutrients while letting your body recover from surgery.[8] A full liquid diet can provide enough calories and protein so that it is safe to stay on it for weeks at a time.[9]

- The remaining portion of your stomach is still healing from the sleeve gastrectomy. Your surgeon fashioned your remaining stomach into a tube, or sleeve, and the seam of the sleeve needs to heal. Solid foods can prevent the seam from sealing up properly and can cause a leak, which requires another surgery. Infection is another risk.

- It reduces nausea.

What Do I Look for When Purchasing Measuring Cups and Spoons?

Some of us have been baking cakes and bread for as long as we can remember. For many more of us, gourmet cooking means defrosting a bag of frozen vegetables to serve with Chinese takeout. If that describes you, buying anything for the kitchen might seem beyond your abilities—or you might not even want to buy kitchen items because you're afraid that the next step is to make complicated recipes. But these worries aren't necessary. It's easy to get the measuring utensils that you need, and they're only going to help you lose weight—not tie you to the kitchen!

This is some basic information to help you get what you need:

- A standard full set of measuring cups includes a ¼-cup, a ⅓-cup, a ½-cup, and a 1-cup measure. They'll probably come together in a single package.

- A full set of measuring spoons has a ¼-, ⅓-, ½-, and 1-teaspoon measure, plus a 1-tablespoon spoon. They'll probably come together as a single product. Most measuring spoons that come in sets have holes on the other end of their handles. A single ring goes through each spoon so that the spoons are all attached and you won't lose them.

- A glass measuring cup is useful for measuring liquids and sometimes solid foods. It usually has a capacity of 2 cups, and each ¼ cup is marked from the bottom (0) to the 2-cup fill line near the top. The cup might also have metric markings up to 500 milliliters. Since the glass is clear, you can see from the side exactly how much fluid or food is inside the glass. Compared to other kinds of glass, heat-resistant won't crack when it's hot, so you can put hot liquids in it or microwave it. Pyrex is the most familiar brand name for heat-resistant kitchen glassware.

- Except for your glass measuring cup, it doesn't matter what your measuring cups and spoons are made from. Metal, such as stainless steel, is most common; some people prefer plastic because they like the way it feels, and it doesn't get hot. Metal utensils with plastic handles are easy to grasp and to clean.

- If you're a newbie in the kitchen, it's fine to just buy some inexpensive sets to start with. You can upgrade them if you want.

Need to know what the measurements mean? Chapter 15, "The Sleeve Diet, Weight Loss, and Your Health," has a handy chart for you!

- A liquid diet reduces your risk of discomfort, such as reflux, or regurgitation, heartburn, and gastrointestinal symptoms.

- A well-chosen liquid diet provides the nutrients your body needs to support healing from surgery.

- It prevents dehydration.

Foods on a Clear Liquid Diet

The clear liquid diet is described this chapter. You can't have any solid foods. Here's a reminder of the liquids that you can and cannot have.[10]

Allowed	Not Allowed
✓ Water	✗ Any solid or semi-solid food
✓ Broth	✗ Nectar
✓ Popsicles	✗ Canned fruit
✓ Gelatin	✗ Milk
✓ Tea	✗ Protein shakes
✓ Coffee	✗ Meal replacement beverages
✓ Sports drinks	✗ Juice with pulp
✓ Pulp-free fruit juices	✗ Cream (e.g., in coffee)

Table 20: Liquids You Can and Cannot Have

Foods on a Full Liquid Diet

The full liquid diet continues to promote recovery.[11] This diet can be nutritious enough for you to stay on it for weeks at a time if necessary, so there's no reason to rush through it. Be sure that your stomach tolerates each addition. Here's a run-down of some common options on the liquid diet.

Water - Water is calorie-free, it naturally helps reduce your appetite, and it's convenient. Staying hydrated promotes recovery, gives you energy, and helps you lose weight. Here are some tips to increase your water intake:

- Always have some water available!
- Keep bottles in the car and in your office.
- Keep a water bottle or pitcher of water and a glass on your desk so you remember to drink throughout the day.
- Jazz up your water if you don't like it plain. Try adding a sprig of fresh mint (you can buy a bunch at the grocery store) or use a slice of lime or lemon to fresh it up—just make sure you don't eat the mint leaf or get any lemon seeds in your water while you're on a liquid diet!
- Try ice water—some people find it more refreshing when it's ice cold.

Juice - Apple, grape, orange, and other juices and nectars are allowed on the diet. Fruit juices help you meet your daily requirements for potassium, which helps lower blood pressure and vitamin C, an antioxidant vitamin that is necessary for wound healing. Just be sure to choose 100 percent juices instead of juice drinks with added sugars. Sugar does not provide essential vitamins and minerals.

Broth or Bouillon - Clear soup, such as chicken, beef, and vegetable broth, doesn't have many nutrients, but it can provide some variety in the liquid diet when most of the rest of your liquids are sweet. These are some options for this diet phase:

- Flavored cubes that you dissolve in boiling water
- Flavored powder that you dissolve in boiling water
- Ready-to-heat broth or bouillon in cans or cartons
- Thin cream soups without any chunks (e.g., cream of tomato soup)
- You may be able to have pureed, watered-down soups, but be certain they don't have any pieces of food in them. Ask your surgeon or dietitian because different health care providers have different recommendations.

Reduced-Fat Milk or Soy Milk - Skim, or non-fat, milk, 1% low-fat milk, and calcium-fortified soy milk provide protein and calcium. Protein is necessary for your wounds from surgery to heal, and it helps suppress hunger. Calcium is necessary for bone health. We'll talk about calcium and other nutrients in more detail in *Chapter 15, "The Sleeve Diet, Weight Loss and Your Health."* Flavored milk and soy milk products, such as chocolate, vanilla or strawberry, are higher in sugar and calories than regular milk and unflavored soy milk.

Sugar-Free, Diet, or Light Beverages - These are usually calorie-free or very low in calories, with about 5 or 10 per cup. Check the nutrition label to make sure, though, because some "light" or "reduced-calorie" beverages might have 50 or more calories per cup. That's at least half the calories of full-sugar soft drinks or juice drinks. These are some good options:

- Crystal Light
- Sugar-free Kool-Aid
- Diet Snapple (without caffeine)
- Powdered, sugar-free flavored water mixes. These are handy because you can carry them in a pocket or purse and add them to water no matter where you are.

Avoid caffeinated beverages, such as coffee and energy drinks, and carbonated options, such as diet sodas. Caffeine can increase your stomach acid secretion and risk for ulcers, and carbonated beverages can make you feel overly full and possibly even stretch the size of your sleeve.

Gelatin and Popsicles - These treats can make you feel as though you're cheating on your diet, but you're not:

- Sugar-free options are very low in calories.
- Powdered gelatin is easy to make yourself, but it needs to chill for a few hours before you can eat it.
- Ready-to-eat gelatin in single-serving cups is easy to carry with you. It can be in the baking aisle, with powdered gelatin, or in the refrigerator section.

Protein Shakes - Getting enough protein each day can be challenging after surgery, but it's necessary for minimizing your lean tissue mass and speeding wound healing after surgery. Protein shakes can help while you're on the liquid diet since they're not rough on your stomach. Another benefit of many types of protein shakes is that they're fortified with vitamins and minerals that can be tough to get from your liquid diet after surgery. Sugar-free or low-carbohydrate shakes can be lower in calories. They're also less likely to lead to blood sugar spikes. Ask your surgeon or dietitian which brands are recommended and which nearby or online stores sell them.

Protein Supplements – Protein supplements, such as powders and powdered egg whites, can help you get to your recommended minimum of 65 to 75 grams of protein each day. You can dissolve them in water, juice, or milk, so they're easy to work into the liquid diet. Choose sugar-free varieties if you're opting for flavored protein powder.

Table 21 is a summary table of what you can and cannot have on a full liquid diet.[12]

Allowed	Unlikely – Ask Surgeon	Not Allowed
✓ Everything on the clear liquid diet	? Cream of wheat	✗ Bread, pasta, rice
✓ Butter, margarine, oil, cream	? Applesauce	✗ Nuts, beans, seeds
✓ Protein shakes	? Pureed potatoes	✗ Meats, poultry, fish
✓ Low-fat milk or soymilk	? Watery oatmeal	✗ Cheese
✓ Protein shakes and meal replacements		✗ Fruit
✓ Protein powders (protein supplements)[13]		✗ Vegetables
✓ Sugar, honey and syrups		

Table 21: Summary of what you can and cannot have on a full liquid diet

Liquids to Avoid

Not all liquids are allowed after the sleeve surgery because they can irritate, delay healing, or increase your risk for long-term struggles with the sleeve. Also, remember to avoid any liquid that you suspect is irritating your sleeve even if it's officially on your "allowed" list.

- **Acidic Juices -** You know how painful the acid from citrus fruits can be if you have ever bitten into an orange when you had a cut in your mouth. It hurts! Acidic juices, such as tangerine, orange, and grapefruit juice, can cause the same pain to your surgery wounds. Tomato juice, vegetable juice, and tomato soup are also high in acid and should be avoided if they bother you.

- **Carbonated Beverages[14] -** Your choices are already limited, and a refreshing diet soft drink or bottle of flavored or unflavored bubbly water may be tempting. But, carbonation can make you feel full and nauseous pretty fast. Worse, the bubbles can lead to stretching of the sleeve, which will reduce the restrictive effects of the surgery or increase your risk of having a leak by stretching the sleeve before the seam is fully healed.

What's the Scoop on Sodium?

What Is the Difference between Natural Sugars and Added Sugars, and How Do They Fit into My Diet?

Natural sugars are found naturally in many kinds of foods, and added sugars are added during food processing or preparation. They're usually added to make foods taste sweeter. Added sugars are what you probably think of first when you think of sugar. They include the following:

- white and brown sugar
- honey
- molasses
- corn syrup and high-fructose corn syrup

There are a bunch of different kinds of natural sugars. These are the most common:

- Lactose, or "milk sugar," is in milk and other dairy products.
- Fructose, or "fruit sugar," gives a sweet taste to fruit. It's also in vegetables. Of course, fructose counts as an added sugar when manufacturers add fructose (or high-fructose corn syrup) to other foods to sweeten them.
- Glucose is in many foods, including breads, cereals and other grains, fruit, vegetables, and dairy products.

Are Added Sugars or Natural Sugars Better for Weight and Health?

All kinds of sugars, whether they are natural or added, are carbohydrates. They have four calories per gram, and they're not very filling. Chemically and nutritionally, added sugars and natural sugars have the same effect on your body.

But…

Added sugars can harm your diet more than natural sugars.

- Added sugars are often in high-calorie foods that don't fit into the sleeve diet. Examples include ice cream, baked goods, sweets, and sugary beverages.
- Natural sugars are in many healthy foods, including fat-free yogurt, whole grains, fruits, beans, and vegetables.

Bottom Line

Avoiding foods with added sugars is a simple, effective strategy to help you lose weight.

Source[15]

- **Caffeinated Beverages -** Caffeine is a diuretic, which means it makes your body lose water. Normally it's not a big problem and doesn't even affect your hydration levels. After the sleeve surgery, though, it's already difficult to drink enough fluids to stay hydrated. Too much caffeine can also irritate the lining of your stomach and delay healing. A stomach ulcer is another risk of caffeine. These are common sources of caffeine:

  - Hot and iced coffee and coffee drinks, such as mochas and lattes
  - Some hot and iced tea, including some types of diet Snapple
  - Energy drinks
  - Dark chocolate
  - Hot chocolate, chocolate-flavored ice cream, and other chocolate flavored products likely only have small amounts of caffeine.

Calories and the Liquid Diet

Weight loss is all about eating fewer calories than you burn. You may be surprised to learn that calories can add up pretty fast on the liquid diet even though you're not eating solid food. Drinking a lot of high-calorie liquids can prevent weight loss. These are a few high-calorie fluids to limit or avoid because of their calories even though they're technically permitted on a liquid diet.

- **Cream or Cheese Soup -** Unlike broth and bouillon, soups with cream or cheese bases can have over 200 calories per cup. That's 400 calories in a 2-cup can, which is a standard size. Cream of mushroom soup, cream of chicken or tomato soup, clam chowder, and broccoli cheese soup are high in calories. Broth and bouillon can take just as long to eat and be just as satisfying while having only 10 to 20 calories per serving.
- **Diet Shakes -** Diet shakes, nutritional supplement shakes, liquid meals, and protein shakes, such as Ensure and Boost, can have 200 to 400 calories per serving. They're allowed on your liquid diet and are high in essential nutrients, but discuss them with your dietitian to see exactly how they fit into your meal plan. Some shakes are high in sugar and aren't that high in protein, fiber, or essential vitamins and minerals. These will just add calories without making you feel full.
- **Hot Beverages with Cream and Sugar -** Black coffee and plain tea are nearly calorie-free, but coffee and tea with cream and sugar are higher in empty calories; that is, calories without extra nutrients. Cream and creamers contain unhealthy saturated or trans fats. Each 8-oz. cup of sweetened coffee with cream or creamer can have 80 to 200 or more calories; the same is true for tea with sugar or honey.
- **Fruit Drinks and Other Sugar-Sweetened Beverages -** Fruit drinks have about 120 calories per cup, which is the same amount of calories as 100% fruit juices. But, fruit *drinks* are almost pure added sugars, and they don't have the natural nutrients in fruit *juices*. They also have artificial flavors and colors. They're basically the same as

fruit punch. Instead, choose 100% fruit juice for its nutritional benefits or sugar-free beverages for their taste.

- **Whole Milk -** It has all the protein and calcium of fat-free milk, but each cup of whole milk has 150 calories. A cup of fat-free milk has 80 calories. Whole milk is high in unhealthy fats.

"Solid Liquids" Are Not Liquids

Some foods seem like liquids, especially if you really, really want them to be. But they're not. A liquid has to pour freely as you're eating it. Unless your surgeon or dietitian specifically tells you that you can have some of these "solid liquids," they're not allowed on a liquid diet. Don't sneak them in and interfere with your future success with the sleeve:

- *Ice cream*: Ice cream melts into a liquid, but it's a food, not a liquid. Avoiding ice cream right now is better for your health anyway. It can have 300 to 600 calories per cup and tons of saturated fat (a kind of fat that raises your cholesterol levels) and sugar.
- *Yogurt:* It's high in protein, calcium, and probiotics (healthy bacteria that live in your gut and may boost your immune system. But it's not a liquid. You eat it with a spoon.
- *Pudding*: Pudding's one of those "recovery" foods that we think of when someone's healing and needs a simple comfort food. But it's not a liquid, so save it for the next phase of your sleeve diet. Hot chocolate is a better way to get your chocolate fix during the liquid phase, and a vanilla or banana-flavored protein shake can substitute for your pudding craving.

Hydration with the Gastric Sleeve

Water makes up more than half of the body weight of the average middle-aged adult.[16] You may not have thought about hydration before the surgery, but dehydration is among the most common complaints of bariatric patients after surgery.[17] It can occur within hours if you don't drink enough water or get your fluids from other sources. Why do you need water?

- It is necessary for maintaining a normal body temperature, for every metabolic reaction in your body, for digestion and absorption of nutrients, and for using them.[18]
- It prevents signs and symptoms of dehydration, such as dark yellow or a small amount of urine, less sweating than usual, headaches, nausea, confusion, and dizziness.
- A lot of people who regularly get tired and feel a headache coming on in the late afternoon can avoid these symptoms by drinking more fluids on a daily basis.
- It naturally helps you feel less hungry.
- It's calorie-free.

Getting enough water is always important, and you need even more when you're recovering from surgery so that the incisions in your stomach can heal. You need a minimum of 1.5 liters, or six 8-ounce cups, of fluids per day. That includes the amount of fluid you have at meals plus water and other liquids that you drink throughout the day.

You won't be having water and other beverages with your meals or just before or after meal times. Fluids would speed up the passage of food through your sleeve so you don't feel full for as long after a meal.[19] Instead, you need to take in your water throughout the day in between meals. Getting a cup or two of water in between each of your meals and before you go to bed at night should let you meet your water requirements without too much trouble.

Nutritional Supplements: Vitamins and Minerals

Without supplements, you're at high risk for nutrient deficiencies after the sleeve gastrectomy. If you weren't already taking vitamin and mineral supplements before your surgery, you'll probably start taking them during your liquid diet stage.[20] Your dietitian will tell you which ones you need and exactly what quantities to look for on the label when you're buying the supplement.

Most Common Vitamin and Minerals of Concern

Post-surgery, you're more likely to experience deficiencies of certain vitamins and minerals than others because of their different food sources, rates of absorption, and amounts needed. These are some of the vitamins and minerals to watch for:[21]

- *Calcium*: Calcium is necessary for maintaining your bone mineral density so that your bones stay strong as you get older. A restricted diet can cause osteoporosis and bone fractures (broken bones) later on.

- *Vitamin D*: You need vitamin D so that your body uses calcium properly. Your skin can make vitamin D when you're out in the sun, but many of us aren't out in the sun for long enough to make enough vitamin D, so we need to get it from our diet or supplements.

- *Vitamin B-12*: This vitamin works with folic acid to keep your heart healthy and prevent anemia.

- *Iron*: This mineral is necessary for preventing anemia, which can make you tired and susceptible to infections. It's an even bigger deal for menstruating women, who lose a significant amount of iron each month from blood losses in menstrual cycles.

- *Vitamin A*: This vitamin can become deficient on a very low-fat diet because you need to eat fat for your body to be able to absorb it. Your diet will be low in fat after the sleeve, putting you at risk for deficiency.

- *Thiamin (Vitamin B1)*: This is a vitamin that you need for metabolism. Severe deficiency is very rare, but it is possible if you have periods of vomiting. Slightly low status is likely in sleeve patients.[22]

- *Vitamin K*: Like vitamin A, vitamin K can only be absorbed when you have fat in the diet. Deficiency is rare for most people, but after the sleeve, you may need supplements.

- *Zinc:* This mineral is necessary for a strong immune response and for proper metabolism. It's in a lot of high-protein foods, but you can become deficient because of your low food intake on the vertical sleeve diet and because absorption depends on your dietary fat intake.[23]

- *Folic acid (Vitamin B9):* This vitamin is not only good for your heart and for preventing anemia but also for preventing neural tube birth defects. Women who might get pregnant *must* get enough folic acid to lower the risk of having a baby with spina bifida or a similar condition. The VSG doesn't affect folic acid absorption, and you're only likely to be deficient if you stop taking your recommended supplements.[24]

Multivitamin and Mineral Supplement

Having most of your vitamins and minerals in a single formula can save you a lot of trouble. A standard daily supplement usually has about 50 to 100 percent of the daily value of most vitamins and minerals, such as the B vitamins; vitamins A, C, D, E, and K; and many minerals, such as zinc, copper, iron (for women), and chromium.

Form of Supplementation

You won't be able to take your vitamins and minerals in regular pill form for at least a few weeks after your surgery. That's because swallowing those whole pills can aggravate the sleeve and lead to leaks or delayed healing. You can get your vitamins and minerals using liquid or powdered multivitamin and mineral supplements instead of large pills or capsules. Another option is to use a pill grinder to grind up your regular hard pills so you can sprinkle the powder on your food.

Vitamin and mineral supplements continue far beyond the liquid diet phase. You'll probably be on them for life because your diet is so restricted. Soon, though, you'll be able to swallow whole pills so you won't have to stick with liquid or powdered dietary supplements.

Sample Menus for Phase 1 – Liquid Diet

Here is a sample daily menu for your post-surgery clear liquid diet, which lasts for only one to two days. Basically, you'll be sipping on as many clear fluids as you can handle. There's another sample menu for the full liquid diet, which can last for a week or two. On the full liquid diet, your focus should also be on getting enough protein.[25] During both diets, be sure to drink plenty of water throughout the day to prevent dehydration (Sample Meal Patterns[26])

Meal or Snack	Sample Day on the Clear Liquid Diet	Sample Day for the Full Liquid Diet
Breakfast	½ cup sugar-free gelatin ½ cup fruit juice	8 ounces fruit juice mixed with 20 grams unflavored protein powder ½ cup gelatin sprinkled with 10 grams unflavored protein powder
Snack 1	½ cup gelatin	8-ounce protein shake
Lunch	8 ounces (1 cup) beef-flavored broth ½ cup apple juice	12 oz. low-fat milk with 10 grams sugar-free, chocolate-flavored protein powder

Meal or Snack	Sample Day on the Clear Liquid Diet	Sample Day for the Full Liquid Diet
Snack 2	½ cup decaffeinated diet iced tea	½ cup gelatin 8 ounces fruit juice
Dinner	½ cup vegetable-flavored broth ½ cup gelatin ½ cup fruit juice	8 ounces (1 cup) cream of chicken soup without chunks and with 10 g protein powder
Snack 3	1 sugar-free popsicle ½ cup of fruit juice	8 ounces low-fat milk and 10 grams protein powder

Table 22: Sample Meal Patterns for phase 1 – Liquid Diet

Phase 2 – Pureed Diet

Getting to the pureed diet phase is a big step. Transitioning to pureed foods means that your sleeve is healing well and that you're not having any serious setbacks. Successful completion of the liquids phase should give you confidence that indeed you *can* stick to the sleeve diet! In the pureed foods phase, you get to add real foods back into your diet! You'll have to select your foods very carefully, but your diet will be far more interesting and satisfying than the liquid diet. The purposes of this phase are to continue to allow your body to recover from surgery and to lose a little more weight. This phase will last until about three or four weeks after surgery.

Tips for Success in Phase 2

You're more experienced and stronger than you were in phase 1, but you're not yet fully recovered from surgery. Also, you're still getting used to the sleeve, and it's still early in your weight loss journey. It is as important to follow Phase 2 properly as it was to follow the liquid diet. These guidelines may help.

Be Patient

Many sleeve patients dislike the liquid diet because it's boring and it's not very filling. It's natural to be excited about phase 2, especially if you're not experiencing sleeve complications. Don't go overboard with your new options though. Instead, add in only one new food at a time and don't eat it again for another few days if you think it causes you trouble. Be prepared to go back to your liquid diet for a day or two if you have symptoms like a sore throat or nausea. The key to this stage of your post-surgery diet is patience. You're still at risk for nausea or stretching the sleeve if you eat the wrong foods or eat too much.

Pureed Foods – Not Chunky!

The pureed diet is true to its name. If the food isn't naturally smooth, such as pudding, you need to puree it before eating it to avoid little chunks irritating your sleeve seam. During this phase, you'll get a lot of use out of your blender or hand blender. You may use it multiple times per day and even more than once in a single meal!

Approaching Meals and Snacks

The size of your sleeve is only about 100[27] to 300[28] milliliters, or about 3 to 10 fluid ounces. That's not much. Your original stomach was more than 1,000 milliliters, or 4 cups (32 fluid ounces). You may not have noticed the small sleeve size during the phase 1 liquid diet because fluids pass through quickly and easily. As you add in non-liquefied foods during phase 2, you may notice a new sensation—fullness.

Fullness is a good and normal feeling that should come after a meal. As mentioned earlier, you'll probably have to learn to feel fullness, since you may be used to ignoring fullness. Sooner or later, though, you're likely to experience early satiety—an intense feeling of fullness that comes on well before you finish the food that you had planned. You won't be able to comfortably eat more, and at that point, the meal or snack will be over even though you have food left over.

It's hard to predict when early satiety will happen, so it's best to act as though you're always expecting it:

- Eat your protein first so that you're still likely to meet your protein requirements even if you do have to leave some food uneaten.

- Eat your vegetables and fruits next, because they provide important nutrients and health benefits.

- Get used to it. You have no control over it, so there's no point in being upset about it. Just pack your food away for another time and go about your day.

Foods on a Pureed Foods Diet

On a pureed foods diet, you can have all of the liquids from Phase 1, plus a few additional foods. Everything needs to be pureed or of a pureed texture. These are some examples of foods for a pureed diet.[29] [30] Remember, everything needs to be perfectly smooth. You can try putting it through a strainer if you're not sure whether it qualifies as "pureed."

Cottage Cheese – Cottage cheese may become one of your staples. Fat-free and 1% low-fat cottage cheese are high in protein and low in fat. Small-curd cottage cheese might be okay, or you can puree small-curd or large-curd cottage cheese to make it perfectly smooth.

Yogurt - Yogurt is another high-protein choice. It's also a great source of calcium, and it provides probiotics, which are healthy bacteria that can boost your immune system. Fat-free yogurt is lowest in calories and least likely to cause an upset stomach. You can also limit your calories, and carbohydrates, by choosing plain yogurt or, if you prefer a flavored yogurt, reading the label to make sure that has no added sugars. Instead, it should be sweetened with a calorie-free sugar substitute, such as aspartame or sucralose (brand name Splenda) instead of added sugars like corn syrup or sugar. Another thing to keep in mind is that you can't have a yogurt with fruit chunks in it during Phase 2.

Tofu - Tofu is another good source of protein, and fortified tofu has calcium. Only the silken, off-white kind of tofu is acceptable on a pureed foods diet. Veggie burgers and other meat substitutes, such as tofu meatballs and sausages, aren't okay for right now.

Peanut Butter - Creamy peanut butter isn't quite as high in protein as cottage cheese or yogurt, but it's still a good source. Plus, it's full of other beneficial nutrients, such as healthy fats, vitamin E, fiber, and magnesium. Its thickness and sticky texture can be welcome when you're limited to pureed foods, which are often watery. Chunky peanut butter is not okay for this phase of the sleeve diet.

Pudding - Chocolate, banana, and vanilla pudding are just a few options that can be treats during this phase of recovery. Ready-made puddings are often in single-serve containers. If the entire 4-ounce (one-half cup) container is too big for your tiny sleeve, be prepared to store the rest for another meal.

Mashed Bananas - Make sure to remove the strings when you peel your banana and to puree it thoroughly so that it doesn't still have chunks when you eat it. Bananas are high in carbohydrates. They're naturally sweet and are sources of dietary fiber, potassium, magnesium, and vitamin C.

Cooked Fruits - Some kinds of cooked fruits are okay on a pureed foods diet. Smooth applesauce and pureed and peeled cooked or canned peaches, apples, and pears are good choices if you puree them well. If you're making your own from fresh, peel them first. Stay away from stringy or fibrous fruits, like canned mandarin oranges, and avoid fruits with small seeds, like raspberries. Your dietitian can give you a more detailed list of which fruits are okay for now. Also avoid fruit jams, which are not only high in sugar and low in nutrients but can harm the sleeve.

Pureed Potatoes - Peeled, cooked, pureed potatoes and sweet potatoes, or yams, are likely allowed on your pureed foods diet. If they're still too thick after you puree them, try adding some water and pureeing them a little more. Very stringy yams should be avoided.

Soft Hot Cereal - Fortified cream of wheat and farina are nutritious choices for this phase, but you might need to stay away from oatmeal, even though it's healthy, because of its chunks. Let the cereal cool down before you eat it because your stomach wounds may still be sensitive to very hot and very cold temperatures.

Soup - You can add some cream and thin soups to your diet now in addition to the broth and bouillon that you had on the liquid diet. Be absolutely certain that

> **Tip**
>
> **Learning from Others' Experiences**
>
> If you want to compare your own experiences to those of other sleeve patients, you might want to log onto BariatricPal.com. Experienced members there can share memories of their own Phase 2 recovery diets. They can tell you about which foods worked for them and which didn't. Just keep in mind that everyone's journey is slightly different.

they have no chunks. It's safer to strain your recipe or the can of soup before eating it to get it smooth enough. Cream soups are high in calories and fat, so they won't be part of your regular diet when you get to the semi-solid food stage and beyond.

Your dietitian or surgeon might have slightly different recommendations for what you can and cannot have in Phase 2. Some sleeve patients, for example, can have pureed canned tuna within 2 to 4 weeks after surgery.[31] Your dietitian may also recommend a specific order to introduce food in so you start with the ones that are least likely to cause problems.

Your healthcare team and your body should be your guides. Some foods might not agree with you even though they're on the approved list. On the other hand, you might find that you are able to progress faster than average with other foods. Some people are very sensitive to spicy foods, and you might need to avoid things like chili powder and curries until you are certain that your surgical wounds have healed completely.

Allowed	Not Allowed
✓ Phase 1 liquids	✗ Raw and cooked vegetables
✓ Pureed, reduced-fat cottage cheese	✗ Meat
✓ Fat-free yogurt without chunks	✗ Bread and cold cereal
✓ Hard or soft silken tofu	✗ Most grains, such as rice and pasta
✓ Pureed cream and thin soups	✗ Nuts, seeds, and beans
✓ Pureed watery potatoes and sweet potatoes	✗ Raw fruit
✓ Mashed bananas	✗ Fruit with seeds or peel
✓ Some cooked, peeled fruits	✗ Fruit jam
	✗ High-calorie, unhealthy choices (e.g., ice cream and butter)

Table 23: Foods Allowed/Not Allowed in Phase2

Stage 2 Includes Some High-Calorie Foods That You Won't Be Eating Later

At this point, you're still eating some high-calorie foods and beverages, such as cream soups and protein shakes. These foods are okay now because you're still focusing on getting the nutrients you need to promote healing from surgery, but soon they won't be allowed. When you get to the soft foods stage and your long-term solid foods diet, you'll depend almost entirely on highly nutritious foods and calorie-free or low-calorie beverages to meet your needs.

Developing Good Eating Habits for Life with the Gastric Sleeve

Phase 2, the pureed foods diet, is a good opportunity to start practicing the eating patterns that you'll be following in the future. You're not yet eating the full range of solid foods that you'll be eating in a couple of months, but you should be following the same general guidelines as you will for your weight loss journey. These are some of the behaviors that will help you lose weight and prevent side effects.

Eating Slowly

This is important to your success because it lets you feel full before you've eaten as much food. Start in Phase 2 by taking small bites from a shallow spoon and setting the spoon down in between each bite. Savor each bite and chew it thoroughly before swallowing—as you should do anyway on a pureed diet to be sure that you're not swallowing any chunks! Then, pause for a few seconds before filling up your spoon and lifting it to your mouth for the next bite. Remembering to do this will take a lot of effort at first, but it will soon become habit. Another benefit of eating slowly is that you will concentrate more on eating and be able to enjoy your food more!

Eating Protein First

This is important for making sure you meet your requirements each day, even if you have early satiety as described above. Eating your protein food first at a meal has additional benefits. First, protein is a filling nutrient. It helps you stay full for a little longer after you eat so that you don't get hungry for the next meal as soon.[33] Plus, it helps to stabilize your body's blood sugar levels so you have more energy and don't have wild swings:

> **Tip**
>
> Chapter 15, "The Sleeve Diet, Weight Loss and Your Health," has a list of protein foods and the amount of protein in a serving.

- Choose high-protein foods first when you're selecting foods for a meal or snack.
- Eat your protein food first at each meal.
- Make your protein intake a priority by focusing on it early in the day.

Focusing on Fullness

You ate a lot more than you needed to during those years of fighting obesity. This might have been because you ignored your biological hunger and fullness signal, and instead ate for other reasons, such as pleasure, comfort, or habit. Now you're going to only eat what you *need* to, based on hunger. It will take you a while to learn to recognize the signals that you're full. It can take 20 or more minutes for your brain to recognize that you're full, and the signals can be very faint at first. To give yourself time to get full and retrain your brain to recognize fullness, you might have to pause in your eating before you feel full.

Making Healthy Food Choices

It's not your main focus yet, but you can start thinking about making healthy food choices. It's not a big deal; it's as simple as making little decisions such as these:

- Choosing cottage cheese instead of mashed potatoes because you feel that you need the protein more than the carbohydrates
- Choosing pureed carrots instead of cream of wheat because you want the vitamin A
- Choosing yogurt instead of a protein shake because you know it will keep you full for longer

Measuring Your Portions

Portion control is essential for success in losing weight and keeping it off. Measuring your portion sizes is the only sure way of making sure you're in control of how much you're eating. Continue to use your measuring cups and spoons to stay in control.

Staying Hydrated

Keeping up your fluid intake to prevent dehydration remains a challenge for many sleeve patients.[34] It's even harder in Phase 2 than Phase 1 because, in Phase 2, you shouldn't be drinking fluids with your meals or snacks. Instead, it's best to separate your intake of food and beverages by at least 30 minutes.[35] Stay focused on making it a priority to drink plenty of water each day, with a goal of one to two cups between meals. The deeper you can get this habit engrained in your mind, the easier it'll be to maintain the pattern when you move on to solid foods and are depending on the small sleeve to fill up quickly and stay full for longer so you can suppress hunger and lose weight.

Sample Menus for Phase 2 – Pureed Foods Diet

Here are two sample menus for your pureed foods diet. Each has five small meals or snacks and is designed to be high in protein to meet your needs.[36] You can switch servings of similar foods as long as you watch your portion sizes and choose high-protein options first. Don't forget to drink plenty of water to stay hydrated between meals.

Meal or Snack	Day 1 Sample	Day 2 Sample
Breakfast	2 tablespoons cream of wheat made with fat-free milk 1 scoop protein powder in one-half cup of fruit juice 2 tablespoons cottage cheese	½ cup cottage cheese ½ medium, mashed banana
Snack 1	1 tablespoon protein powder in ½ cup fat-free milk	½ cup cooked carrots
Lunch	8 ounces of vegetable soup ½ cup fat-free cottage cheese	8 ounces of beef broth with 20 grams of unflavored protein powder ½ cup cream of wheat
Dinner	1/4 cup mashed potatoes made with fat-free milk and 2 tsp. olive oil	¼ cup mashed sweet potatoes ¼ cup silken tofu
Snack 2	1 tablespoon peanut butter ½ cup applesauce	½ cup sugar-free vanilla pudding with 10 grams protein powder

Table 24: Sample Menus for Phase 2 – Pureed Foods Diet

Phase 3 – Soft Foods Diet

Your wounds from surgery are much closer to being healed within three or four weeks after the VSG. You may be ready to progress to Phase 3, the soft foods, or semi-solid foods, phase if you're not experiencing complications with the sleeve and you're able to tolerate all of the foods in the pureed foods diet. You can choose from a much wider variety of foods in Phase 3. The phase will probably last until about eight weeks after surgery.

Tips for Success in Phase 3

- *Stay Patient* - You're much stronger now than you were before, but you don't want to risk any setbacks at this point. Adding foods too quickly or eating foods that aren't allowed can lead to a leak or gastrointestinal discomfort. As you did in Phase 2, only add in one new food at a time, and be prepared to go back to the pureed or even liquid diet for a few days if you can't tolerate the new food.

- *Be Ready for Change* - Phase 3, the soft foods diet, is a transition period in a few ways. Physically, it's a bridge between the post-surgery recovery period and the time when you're back to your full range of normal activities. Mentally, phase 3 is when you shift from recovery mode to weight loss mode. You'll also be focused on a variety of food groups, not just protein. Your diet patterns during Phase 3 will reflect these changes, and by the end of Phase 3, your diet will be very similar to the diet you'll follow long term.

- *Keep Watching Your Portions* - Continue to measure the serving size of each food and beverage at every meal and snack. That helps keep your calories in check so you lose weight as expected. Also, larger meals increase your risk of developing a leak, experiencing nausea and vomiting, and stretching your stomach.[37] A larger stomach makes the surgery less effective by reducing the amount of restriction that you feel. You can further reduce your risk of vomiting by eating slowly.

Foods on a Soft Foods Diet

The increased range of allowed foods can make your diet healthier and more interesting than before. This phase is more variable than the previous stages, and your surgeon and dietitian may have some specific foods that are or are not recommended for you. Follow their advice if it is different from this list. You can eat some, but not all, of the foods from the previous phases. We'll go over that a little later after listing the following standard foods on a semi-solid diet.

- *Canned Tuna and Other Chunk Proteins* - Canned tuna and other chunk proteins, such as canned chicken and imitation crab meat, are very convenient. They are high in protein, low in fat, and ready-to-eat, and you can be confident that they have no bones.

- *Ground Meat* - Cooked extra-lean ground beef, turkey, and chicken are high in protein and iron and are good choices for a semi-solid diet. If you ever start to worry whether the meat is finely ground enough, you can puree it yourself before cooking it or wait until it's cooked before putting it through a strainer.

- *Eggs* - Eggs are high in protein and ideal for a soft foods diet because they don't have anything crunchy or fibrous in them. Soft-boiled and scrambled eggs are especially good choices. Egg whites contain all of the egg's protein, and they're fat-free and cholesterol-free. Yolks, in moderation, can be part of a healthy diet too.

- *Cooked Vegetables* - Vegetables are so healthy that they should be your top priority after protein. Canned vegetables are the safest choices when you're first introducing them back into your post-VSG diet because they're thoroughly cooked and very soft. You can also use fresh and frozen vegetables as long as you cook them well, peel them, and avoid seeds. Canned green beans; frozen peas; and peeled, chopped, and boiled carrots are great choices. Avoid stringy and fibrous vegetables, such as broccoli, cabbage and spinach, which may irritate your sleeve.

- *Cooked Grains* - Well-cooked white pasta and white rice are okay for most people on a soft diet, and fortified choices are rich in B vitamins and iron. To be on the safe side, you can blend them in water after cooking them to make them thinner and smoother. Bread and cold cereal aren't yet okay on this diet.

- *Fresh Fruit* - Ripe, soft, peeled pears and nectarines and melon may be tolerated on a soft foods diet. Avoid fruits with seeds, such as raspberries and strawberries, which can irritate your esophagus and sleeve. Also avoid dried fruit. Just like citrus juices, citrus fruits, such as oranges and tangerines, can be irritating because of their acid. Hold off on them until later in your weight loss journey.

- *Beans* - Canned beans are high protein and soft enough for a semi-solid diet, but they often cause gassiness. If your surgeon or dietitian recommends them, start with only a tiny portion, such as a tablespoon, and wait for at least a day to see if you tolerate them well. If you can't tolerate whole beans, you might be able to get away with hummus, or dip, made with garbanzo beans or chick peas.

- *Low-Fat Cheese* - It's high in protein and a good source of calcium. You can use it to add flavor to foods by melting it on meat, adding it to your scrambled eggs, or sprinkling shredded cheese on soup.

Foods from Phases 1 and 2 while in Phase 3

By the time you're in Phase 3, the soft foods stage, you can easily physically tolerate all of the liquids from Phase 1 and the pureed foods Phase 2. But, that doesn't mean that all of those options are part of your semi-solid foods diet. Phase 3 is about promoting weight loss as you transition to making healthy selections.

It's Time to Stop Drinking Your Calories

Fluids were your only sources of calories during the Phase 1 liquid diet, and your food choices were so limited during Phase 2 that you probably depended on protein shakes and other beverages with calories to meet your nutrient requirements. In Phase 3, the semi-solid foods stage, it's time to reduce these choices. High-calorie beverages decrease the effectiveness of the VSG because they don't fill you up as much as real foods even though they give you extra calories. This is especially true for sugar-sweetened beverages. Milk can remain in your diet because it's so healthy, but you'll still need to monitor your portion size. Water, tea, coffee, and diet drinks are low-calorie or calorie free.

Choosing Healthy Options

All of the foods from Phase 2 are allowed during Phase 3, but some are better choices than others during Phase 3. Nutritious, high-protein foods, such as fat-free yogurt and cottage cheese, should be regular parts of your diet. On the other hand, cream soups are choices to limit or avoid because they're not high in the nutrients you need.

Sample Menus for Phase 3—Semi-Solid or Soft Foods Diet

A typical Phase 3 diet includes four or five small meals each day, with water or other non-caloric liquids in between them.[38] This meal pattern looks very similar to the meal pattern you'll be following on the full solids diet, or Phase 4. Remember to separate your liquids and solids by at least 30 minutes to avoid dumping syndrome, increase fullness, and decrease the risk of stretching your sleeve. If the meals are too big for you to handle, stop eating. It's okay if you don't finish your food.

These are two sample menus for the Phase 3 diet. They're designed to provide about 70 to 80 grams of protein and 1.5 liters of water. You can swap foods from these suggested menus as long as you swap similar foods, such as green beans for carrots, and keep the emphasis on protein foods. Your surgeon and dietitian might have additional sample menus or suggest specific foods to include or exclude; listen to their advice!

Meal or Snack	Day 1 Sample	Day 2 Sample
Breakfast	½ cup cottage cheese 3 tablespoons farina made with 1 percent low-fat milk and sprinkled with protein powder 1 tablespoon smooth peanut butter	3 tablespoons banana mashed with 1 tablespoon protein powder ½ cup plain fat-free yogurt sprinkled with cinnamon and a sweetener packet ¼ cup protein shake
Snack 1	1 cup fat-free plain yogurt	1 cup (8 ounces) sugar-free protein shake
Lunch	2 ounces canned tuna ½ cup applesauce ¼ cup cooked pasta	1 ounce canned chicken breast 4 tablespoons canned green beans 3 tablespoons fat-free cottage cheese

Meal or Snack	Day 1 Sample	Day 2 Sample
Dinner	2 ounces lean ground turkey ¼ cup pureed peas ½ cup silken tofu	2 ounces cooked white fish with no bones ½ cup vegetable soup with 2 tablespoons protein powder 3 tablespoons well-cooked pureed pasta 1 tablespoon peanut butter
Snack 2	½ cup chocolate pudding 1 soft-boiled egg	8 ounces fat-free milk 1 tablespoon peanut butter ½ cup cooked Cream of Wheat

Table 25: Sample Menus for Phase 3 – Semi-Solid or Soft Foods Diet

Handy Food Lists

We've just gone over an awful lot of information. You can read it at your leisure and go back to it when you need to look something up. For the times when you just need to know what you can eat in your current phase, these food charts can help. There's one for each of the first three stages. You can just put them up on your refrigerator or use them as shopping lists.

Phase 1: Liquid Diet Foods for 1 to 2 Weeks after Surgery

- Water
- Caffeine-free tea or coffee
- Diet juice drinks (e.g., Crystal Light or sugar-free Kool-Aid)
- Fruit juices, nectars, or ciders (avoid citrus juices)
- Gelatin
- Popsicles, especially sugar-free
- Protein shakes (full liquid only)
- Protein powder
- Non-fat (skim) or 1 percent low-fat milk (full liquid only)
- Calcium-fortified soy milk (full liquid only)
- Broth or bouillon

Phase 2: Pureed Foods until 3 or 4 Weeks after Surgery

- Phase 1 plus…
- Fat-free cottage cheese
- Cream soups
- Creamy peanut butter

- Pudding
- Yogurt without fruit chunks
- Canned fruit
- Applesauce
- Mashed bananas
- Silken tofu (the soft kind)
- Creamed soup
- Pureed potatoes with water
- Cream of wheat and farina

Phase 3: Semi-Solid or Soft Foods until about 6 to 8 weeks after Surgery

- Phases 1 and 2 plus…
- Canned tuna or chicken
- Extra-lean ground beef, chicken, or turkey
- Eggs, egg whites, or fat-free, cholesterol-free egg substitute
- Rice
- Pasta
- Fresh fruit
- Cooked vegetables (not broccoli, asparagus, celery)
- Low-fat or fat-free cheese
- Imitation crab meat or fresh crab meat
- Fish—be very careful of bones

Summary

☛ This chapter took you through your post-surgery recovery diet from surgery to 4 to 8 weeks after surgery. You should be proud of yourself for making it from the clear liquid diet all the way through the soft foods diet. It means you've been diligent about sticking to the plan and making the best decisions. You've done everything you can to set the scene for successful weight loss with the gastric sleeve.

☛ The next chapter covers the sleeve diet that you will be following for years as you lose weight and keep it off. You'll learn what you can eat and start to understand how to put together your own healthy meal plans. You'll keep practicing your new eating skills as you try to lose weight and get healthy.

Your Turn: Getting Some Practice in Monitoring Your Diet and Yourself

The sleeve diet is all about you and your long-term lifestyle changes. The period of your post-surgery recovery and diet is an ideal time to practice thinking about your food intake and how you feel while you eat. The more you practice, the more natural it will become. For this worksheet (Table 26), choose a single day and fill out the answers to the questions below for each meal and snack.

Meal or Snack	What did you eat?	How hungry were you before the meal or snack? How hungry and satisfied were you afterwards?	Record other notes here. Did you have any trouble with sticking or obstruction? Did you enjoy the food? Did you chew it well?
Sample	Half-cup of cottage cheese, quarter-cup applesauce	Starving before. Still hungry afterwards, but hunger died down later.	No troubles. Had cooked apple yesterday and felt nauseous, but today's applesauce was fine.
Breakfast			
Snack 1 (if applicable)			
Lunch			
Snack 2 (if applicable)			
Dinner			
Snack 3 (if applicable)			

Table 26: Monitoring Your Diet and Yourself

1   Aills L, Blankenship J, Buffington C, Furtado M, Parrott J. ASMBS Allied Health nutritional guidelines for the surgical weight loss patient. Surg Obes Relat Dis. 2008;4(5Suppl):S73-S108.

2   Aills L, Blankenship J, Buffington C, Furtado M, Parrott J. ASMBS Allied Health nutritional guidelines for the surgical weight loss patient. Surg Obes Relat Dis. 2008;4(5Suppl):S73-S108.

3   Smeets AJ, Westerterp Plantenga MS. The acute effects of a lunch containing capsaicin on energy and substrate utilization, hormones and satiety. 2009;48(4):229-34.

4   Kalm LM, Semba RD. They starved so that others be better fed: remembering Ancel Keys and the Minnesota Experiment. The Journal of Nutrition. 2005;135:1347-1352.

5   Snyder-Marlow G, Tayle D, Lenhard MJ. Nutrition care for patients undergoing laparoscopic sleeve gastrectomy for weight loss. J Am Diet Ass. 2010;110(4):600-607

6   Aills L, Blankenship J, Buffington C, Furtado M, Parrott J. ASMBS Allied Health nutritional guidelines for the surgical weight loss patient. Surg Obes Relat Dis. 2008;4(5Suppl):S73-S108.

7   Snyder-Marlow G, Tayle D, Lenhard MJ. Nutrition care for patients undergoing laparoscopic sleeve gastrectomy for weight loss. J Am Diet Ass. 2010;110(4):600-607

8   Snyder-Marlow G, Tayle D, Lenhard MJ. Nutrition care for patients undergoing laparoscopic sleeve gastrectomy for weight loss. J Am Diet Ass. 2010;110(4):600-607

9   Dugdale DC. Diet – full liquid. Medline Plus, National Institutes of Health. Web site. http://www.nlm.nih.gov/medlineplus/ency/patientinstructions/000206.htm. Updated 2010, November 21. Accessed October 9, 2012.

10 Dugdale DC. Diet – clear liquid. Medline Plus, National Institutes of Health. Web site. http://www.nlm.nih.gov/medlineplus/ency/patientinstructions/000205.htm. Updated 2010, November 21. Accessed October 9, 2012.

11 Aills L, Blankenship J, Buffington C, Furtado M, Parrott J. ASMBS Allied Health nutritional guidelines for the surgical weight loss patient. Surg Obes Relat Dis. 2008;4(5Suppl):S73-S108.

12 Dugdale DC. Diet – full liquid. Medline Plus, National Institutes of Health. Web site. http://www.nlm.nih.gov/medlineplus/ency/patientinstructions/000206.htm. Updated 2010, November 21. Accessed October 9, 2012.

13 Snyder-Marlow G, Tayle D, Lenhard MJ. Nutrition care for patients undergoing laparoscopic sleeve gastrectomy for weight loss. J Am Diet Ass. 2010;110(4):600-607

14 Aills L, Blankenship J, Buffington C, Furtado M, Parrott J. ASMBS Allied Health nutritional guidelines for the surgical weight loss patient. Surg Obes Relat Dis. 2008;4(5Suppl):S73-S108

15 Gropper, S.S., & Smith, J.L. (2008). Advanced Nutrition and Human Metabolism (5th ed.). Wadsworth Publishing: Belmont, California.

16 Panel on Dietary Reference Intakes for Electrolytes and Water, Standing Committee on the Scientific Evaluation of Dietary Reference Intakes. Dietary reference intakes for water, potassium, sodium, chloride and sulfate. National Academies Press. Web site. http://www.nap.edu/catalog.php?record_id=10925. 2005. Accessed October 10, 2012.

17 Aills L, Blankenship J, Buffington C, Furtado M, Parrott J. ASMBS Allied Health nutritional guidelines for the surgical weight loss patient. Surg Obes Relat Dis. 2008;4(5Suppl):S73-S108

18 Myklebust, M., & Wunder, J. Healing foods pyramid: water. University of Michigan Health System. Retrieved from http://www.med.umich.edu/umim/food-pyramid/water.htm. Updated 2010. Accessed October 10, 2012.

19 Snyder-Marlow G, Tayle D, Lenhard MJ. Nutrition care for patients undergoing laparoscopic sleeve gastrectomy for weight loss. J Am Diet Ass. 2010;110(4):600-607

20 Snyder-Marlow G, Tayle D, Lenhard MJ. Nutrition care for patients undergoing laparoscopic sleeve gastrectomy for weight loss. J Am Diet Ass. 2010;110(4):600-607

21 Aills L, Blankenship J, Buffington C, Furtado M, Parrott J. ASMBS Allied Health nutritional guidelines for the surgical weight loss patient. Surg Obes Relat Dis. 2008;4(5Suppl):S73-S108.

22 Saif T, Strain GW, Dakin G, Gagner M, Costa R, Pomp A. Evaluation of nutrient status after laparoscopic sleeve gastrectomy 1, 3 and 5 years after surgery. Surg Obes Relat Dis. 2012;8(5)542-47.

23 Ziegler O, Sirveaux MA, Brunaud L, Reibel N, Quillot D. Medical follow-up after bariatric surgery: nutritional and drug issues. General recommendations for the prevention and treatment of nutritional deficiencies. Diabetes Metab. 2009;35(6 Pt 2):544-547.

24 Ziegler O, Sirveaux MA, Brunaud L, Reibel N, Quillot D. Medical follow-up after bariatric surgery: nutritional and drug issues. General recommendations for the prevention and treatment of nutritional deficiencies. Diabetes Metab. 2009;35(6 Pt 2):544-547.

25 Snyder-Marlow G, Tayle D, Lenhard MJ. Nutrition care for patients undergoing laparoscopic sleeve gastrectomy for weight loss. J Am Diet Ass. 2010;110(4):600-607

26 Snyder-Marlow G, Tayle D, Lenhard MJ. Nutrition care for patients undergoing laparoscopic sleeve gastrectomy for weight loss. J Am Diet Ass. 2010;110(4):600-607

27 Aills L, Blankenship J, Buffington C, Furtado M, Parrott J. ASMBS Allied Health nutritional guidelines for the surgical weight loss patient. Surg Obes Relat Dis. 2008;4(5Suppl):S73-S108.

28 Snyder-Marlow G, Tayle D, Lenhard MJ. Nutrition care for patients undergoing laparoscopic sleeve gastrectomy for weight loss. J Am Diet Ass. 2010;110(4):600-607

29 Snyder-Marlow G, Tayle D, Lenhard MJ. Nutrition care for patients undergoing laparoscopic sleeve gastrectomy for weight loss. J Am Diet Ass. 2010;110(4):600-607

30 Aills L, Blankenship J, Buffington C, Furtado M, Parrott J. ASMBS Allied Health nutritional guidelines for the surgical weight loss patient. Surg Obes Relat Dis. 2008;4(5Suppl):S73-S108.

31 Snyder-Marlow G, Tayle D, Lenhard MJ. Nutrition care for patients undergoing laparoscopic sleeve gastrectomy for weight loss. J Am Diet Ass. 2010;110(4):600-607

32 Snyder-Marlow G, Tayle D, Lenhard MJ. Nutrition care for patients undergoing laparoscopic sleeve gastrectomy for weight loss. J Am Diet Ass. 2010;110(4):600-607

33 Protein: moving closer to center stage. (2012). The Harvard School of Public Health Nutrition Source. Web site. http://www.hsph. harvard.edu/nutritionsource/what-should-you-eat/protein-full-story/index.html. 2012. Accessed October 11, 2012.

34 Aills L, Blankenship J, Buffington C, Furtado M, Parrott J. ASMBS Allied Health nutritional guidelines for the surgical weight loss patient. Surg Obes Relat Dis. 2008;4(5Suppl):S73-S108.

35 Snyder-Marlow G, Tayle D, Lenhard MJ. Nutrition care for patients undergoing laparoscopic sleeve gastrectomy for weight loss. J Am Diet Ass. 2010;110(4):600-607

36 Snyder-Marlow G, Tayle D, Lenhard MJ. Nutrition care for patients undergoing laparoscopic sleeve gastrectomy for weight loss. J Am Diet Ass. 2010;110(4):600-607

37 Snyder-Marlow G, Tayle D, Lenhard MJ. Nutrition care for patients undergoing laparoscopic sleeve gastrectomy for weight loss. J Am Diet Ass. 2010;110(4):600-607

38 Snyder-Marlow G, Tayle D, Lenhard MJ. Nutrition care for patients undergoing laparoscopic sleeve gastrectomy for weight loss. J Am Diet Ass. 2010;110(4):600-607

14

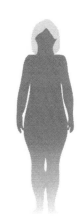

Losing Weight with the Sleeve Diet

The last chapter talked about laying the foundation for successful weight loss with the sleeve. The chapter progressed from your liquid diet through the pureed food diet to the soft foods diet. It's time to enter the solid foods stage when you are comfortable with the foods in Phase 3, the soft foods diet. Now it's finally time to focus on rapid weight loss and nutritious choices!

This chapter covers Phase 4, the solid foods diet. Phase 4 is the long-term food plan that can take you to your goal weight and beyond. In fact, you'll stay on Phase 4 of the sleeve diet for as long as you want to control your weight and maximize your nutrient intake. On Phase 4, you continue to add new foods slowly and gradually.

This is what you'll find in this chapter:

- Foods that you can have during this phase
- Foods to be cautious of
- A few tips for success with the sleeve diet
- Meal patterns and sample menus for the sleeve diet

Overview of Phase 4—The Solid Foods Diet

It's more accurate to call the solid foods diet a lifestyle instead of a phase. As long as you have no setbacks, you'll be following this diet for the long-term. Occasionally you may have trouble with solid foods and temporarily need to go back to a soft or pureed foods diet until you feel better, but those times should be rare and short. In general, the solid foods diet is your daily diet for life. These are the goals:

- Lose weight and then maintain your goal weight.
- Prevent complications with the sleeve.
- Prevent nutritional deficiencies.
- Eat a healthy overall diet.

Your Focus Shifts to Weight Loss and Health

It's finally time to focus on weight loss! Even though you've been wanting to lose weight for years and you've been preparing for months to lose weight with the gastric sleeve, you hadn't had the chance, until now, to focus on weight loss. Before surgery, your energy went toward organizing your medical team and other logistics; the first several weeks after surgery, you concentrated on making food choices aimed at a swift recovery and reducing your risk of future complications.

Full-Speed Weight Loss Ahead!

You now have control over the amount of weight you lose. Most VSG patients can expect to lose about one to two pounds per week by following the sleeve diet's food choices, meal patterns, and portion sizes. You'll regularly see and feel changes in your body when you lose weight at this rate. You'll be even healthier, and more likely to stick to the diet, when you select nutritious foods. We'll go over how to make nutritious choices a little later.

It Takes about One to Two Years or More to Hit Your Goal Weight

As you know by now, the gastric sleeve isn't a quick fix for obesity. It's a lifelong approach to managing your weight. It can take a year, two years or more than that to hit your goal weight. That may seem like a long time, but it's hardly anything compared with the years and years that you struggled with obesity. And, you'll feel better, look better, and be healthier long before you hit your final goal weight.

How long might it take for you to lose the weight? Here's the formula:

- Take your pre-surgery weight (A).
- Subtract your goal weight (B). (A-B).
- That number, (A-B), is C.
- Take your expected rate of weight loss (D). It might be one pound per week, for example.
- Divide C by D. (C/D).
- That's how many weeks it might take to hit your goal weight.

Here are a few examples:

- If you're 5'10" and your starting weight is 362 pounds (BMI of 52), you are about 188 pounds over a goal weight of 174 pounds (BMI of 25). If you lose one pound per week, it will take about 3.5 years to hit your goal weight.
- If you're 5'4" and your pre-surgery weight is 279 pounds (BMI of 48), you're about 134 pounds over a goal of 145 pounds (BMI of 25). If you lose two pounds per week, it will take about 67 weeks, or 15 months, to lose your excess weight.
- If you're 5'8" and your starting weight is 295 pounds (BMI of 44), you're 131 pounds over a goal of 164 pounds (BMI of 25). If you lose one and a half pounds per week, it'll take about 20 months, to hit your goal.

All sleeve patients have their own best rates of weight loss, so don't try to compare yourself to others. As long as you're eating healthily and following your surgeon's and dietitian's advice, you can be confident that you're doing the right thing.

Continuing to Protect Your Gastric Sleeve while Losing Weight

You will always be at risk for developing complications with the gastric sleeve. Examples of complications that can develop even after surgery is long behind you include dumping syndrome (with symptoms such as nausea, vomiting and diarrhea), leaks, staple line disruptions, and gastroesophageal reflux disease.[1] You can lower your risk of these effects by following these tips — which you'll continue to see in this chapter because they're important both for your safety and for your weight loss:

- Separate solids and liquids by at least 30 minutes.
- Have only the recommended portions of food.
- Stop eating when you're full—remember, your stomach is way smaller than it used to be, and you don't want to stretch it.
- Only try one new food at a time, and wait for a day or two to make sure you are tolerating it well.
- Chew slowly and thoroughly to prevent anything sharp from irritating your sleeve.

Shifting to Healthier Eating Habits

A wonderful thing about the VSG is that it gives you the chance to start over. You remove all the foods from your diet, and only add them back in over the course of several months. This long process can help you retrain your taste buds and develop new habits – habits such as automatically reaching for the nutritious choice instead of the junk. While you are learning to love healthy foods, you may also notice that foods can taste sweeter after the VSG.[2] Some patients even find that they lose their sweet tooth after the surgery.[3] It can take a while to happen.

The other major shift, beside in your taste buds, is in how much you eat. The sleeve diet includes learning a whole new set of serving sizes. Gone are the days of overloading a huge plate, wolfing it down, and going back for more. Now, you will measure out your food, chew each small bit slowly, enjoy your meal and leave the table—without reaching into the fridge for a post-meal snack!

Foods on the Solid Diet

During Phase 4, you add foods one by one until you're eventually able to eat nearly all healthy foods on your gastric sleeve diet. If you're like many sleeve patients, there'll probably be one or more foods that don't agree with you. There's nothing to worry about; just avoid the trouble foods and choose other healthy alternatives to keep your diet interesting and nutritious.

Food Lists for the Solid Diet

These are lists of some common foods that will probably become pretty regular in your diet. Pay attention to the serving sizes—remember to measure carefully, because they're probably a lot smaller than you're used to having. Don't forget that you can always stop eating before you finish your food if you feel full, and you don't have to eat the entire serving. Your sleeve is only a fraction the size of your original stomach, and you don't want to stretch it or feel sick from eating too much.

Protein Foods—The Base of Your Diet

These are high in protein, low in carbohydrates and fat and high in other essential nutrients. They're the cornerstones of your diet because they'll help you reach your daily protein needs. You should choose them first at most meals. The general serving size is about two ounces, or one-quarter cup.

These foods are almost pure protein:

- 2 ounces of lean meat
- 2 ounces of skinless chicken or turkey breast
- 2 ounces of extra lean ground beef, chicken, or turkey
- 2 ounces of soy-based meat substitute, e.g., soy crumbles
- 2 ounces of fish or shellfish
- ½ cup reduced-fat cottage cheese
- 1 egg, 2 egg whites or ½ cup of fat-free, cholesterol-free liquid egg substitute (or the equivalent in dried egg white powder)
- 2 ounces of canned flake meat or fish, such as chicken, tuna, or crab
- 1 one-ounce slice of deli meat (high in sodium, though, so don't choose too often

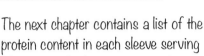

Tip

The next chapter contains a list of the protein content in each sleeve serving of common foods, so you can plan your diet to contain enough protein.

These foods have some carbohydrates and/or fat, but they're great choices because of their extra nutrients:

- 1 ounce of low-fat cheese, 2 tablespoons of grated cheese, such as parmesan, or ¼ cup of shredded cheese, such as cheddar or jack.
- ½ cup of yogurt (fat-free, no sugar-added or plain)
- ½ cup of pudding (fat-free, no sugar-added, calcium-fortified)
- 1 tablespoon of creamy (smooth) peanut butter—it's a small serving size because it's so high in calories.
- 4-6 almonds, cashews or pecans or about 2 tablespoons of peanuts, walnuts, or other nuts. (Chew them well and avoid them until you're sure you're comfortable on the solid foods diet.)
- 1 ounce of dry tofu (e.g., veggie burger) or 2 ounces (one-quarter cup) of silken tofu
- ½ cup of cooked beans. Add beans to your diet very slowly. You might start with just 1 or 2 tablespoons and gradually work up to ½ of a cup after a few days or weeks if they don't make you gassy.
- ¼ cup of hummus, or garbanzo bean dip.

Vegetables: Great Choice for Weight Loss and Life

Vegetables are low in calories and high in fiber, making them perfect for reducing hunger without interfering with your weight loss. When you can handle them, it's a good idea to include a serving or two with most meals and snacks so you can take advantage of their vitamins and minerals. Start with cooked vegetables, and be very patient as you add raw vegetables back into your diet. Always make sure you chew them thoroughly. The serving size for vegetables is bigger than for other groups because they're so low-calorie and healthy:

- ½ cup of cooked vegetables, such as cooked, canned or frozen carrots, green beans, broccoli and cauliflower florets, zucchini, or green peas.
- 1 cup of raw vegetables, such as peeled cucumbers, carrot sticks or lettuce
- ¼ cup of tomato sauce or salsa
- 6 ounces (¾ cup) of tomato or vegetable juice

Carbohydrate Foods: Fruits

Full of vitamins, minerals, and antioxidants, fruits deserve their reputation as healthy sweet treats. You may be surprised to learn that they have no protein and they contain carbohydrates in the form of sugars. Why are fruits good choices? They're pretty filling because they're fat-free and high in fiber. As you progress from Phase 3 of the sleeve diet, or the soft foods diet, you can start to incorporate more raw fruits into your diet. Ask your nutritionist about adding specific types of fruit back into your diet and how to prepare them. Seeds and scratchy peels can irritate your sleeve if it's not completely healed. Be sure to chew your fruit very thoroughly.

- ¼ cup of cooked, peeled fruit or canned fruit (in its own juice, not in heavy syrup)
- ½ cup of grapes (Avoid grapes until you're deep into the solid foods phase because their skins are difficult to chew thoroughly and they can get lodged in an unsealed sleeve seam.)
- ½ of a regular fresh fruit, such as a medium apple, orange, pear, or peach.
- 1 piece of small fruit, such as an apricot or plum
- ½ cup of canned mashed pumpkin

Carbohydrate Foods: Choose Nutritious Grains and Starches

Somehow carbohydrates have gotten a bad reputation, but that's not entirely fair. Carbohydrate foods are very healthy if you choose the right ones and stick to the suggested serving sizes. Fortified whole grains, such as whole-wheat, whole grain multi-grain and oats, are usually the best choices because of their fiber, antioxidants, and essential vitamins and minerals.

- ½ slice of regular bread or toast
- 1 slice of low-calorie bread or toast
- ½ of an English muffin
- ¼ of a bagel
- ¼ cup of cooked grains, such as rice or pasta, or hot cereal, such as cream of wheat, farina or oatmeal.

- ¼ cup of cooked starchy vegetables, such as potatoes, acorn squash, sweet potatoes, or butternut squash.
- ½ cup of puffed cereal, or one-quarter cup of bran cereal or granola
- 4 crackers, e.g., 4 saltines, four Ritz crackers or 4 quarters of a graham cracker (1 large graham cracker)
- ¼ cup of canned or cooked corn

Choose High-Fat Foods Wisely and Measure Your Portions

Fat is necessary for absorbing certain nutrients, and nutritious sources may have other health benefits as long as you limit your intake. Some sources of fats, such as oils, salad dressings, and avocados, are great choices. In contrast, butter is a poor choice because of its high amount of unhealthy saturated fat. High-fat foods are very high in calories, so always measure your serving size of these "extra" foods to avoid eating more calories than you intend. These are some healthy choices for fat:

- 1 teaspoon of olive oil or vegetable oil, such as canola or sunflower—yes, that's a *teaspoon*, not a tablespoon. A teaspoon is only one-third of a tablespoon.
- 1 teaspoon of mayonnaise
- 1 teaspoon of trans fat-free margarine
- 1 tablespoon of low-fat mayonnaise (such as Miracle Whip), salad dressing, cream cheese, sour cream or tahini (sesame seed paste).
- 2 tablespoons of mashed avocado or guacamole—avocados are high in heart-healthy monounsaturated fats, which made the Mediterranean diet famous, as well as vitamin C, vitamin E, and dietary fiber.

Foods to Postpone

Some foods are nutritious, but it's better to postpone them until you're well into Phase 4, the solid foods diet. These foods may be particularly hard, or difficult to chew, or have small pieces that can get into your sleeve. You should not eat them until you're certain that you're completely healed from the gastric sleeve surgery. These are some examples:

- Nuts and peanuts
- Seeds, such as sunflower and pumpkin
- "Sneaky" foods that may have nuts, seeds, dried fruit in them. Multi-grain bread with nuts and raisin bran are two examples.
- Popcorn
- Celery – it's very fibrous and the strings can get into the sleeve. Asparagus and broccoli stalks are also fibrous.
- Citrus fruits and pineapple – beside being acidic, they have pulp that can be irritating.

Foods to Avoid

The long-term gastric sleeve diet allows for a variety of healthy foods as you gradually widen your choices, but there are some foods that you should limit or avoid on the sleeve diet because they're unhealthy, high in calories, and/or low in nutrition. Other foods may be healthy choices, but some patients have trouble tolerating certain ones.

Sugary Foods

Sugary foods are high in calories and not very filling. Letting them creep into your diet can derail your weight loss. They can also cause dumping syndrome. These are some high-sugar foods to avoid:

- Fruit juice
- Sugar-sweetened fruit drinks and fruit punch
- Other sugar-sweetened beverages: lemonade, ice tea with sugar, coffee beverages
- Chocolate and other flavored milk
- Sugar-sweetened flavored soy milk
- Sugar-sweetened flavored yogurt
- Regular frozen yogurt and ice cream
- Canned and frozen fruit in syrup
- Sugary breakfast cereal
- Pastries and doughnuts
- Cakes, cookies, and pies
- Jams and jellies
- Sugar, syrup, honey, and molasses
- Dried fruit

Need a Sweet Treat?

There may be times when you want something sweet and decadent. Frozen whipped topping, better known by the brand name Cool Whip, is a great treat. Regular Cool Whip has **100 calories and 8 grams of sugar** per ½ cup. Fat-free Cool Whip has **60 calories and 4 grams of sugar** in a ½-cup, and sugar-free Cool Whip has **80 calories and 0 grams of sugar.**

A ½-cup of rich ice cream can easily have more than **200 calories and 22 grams of sugar.**

Which do you think is a better choice—ice cream or whipped topping?

Foods that You Can't Tolerate

Everyone has a different set of foods that they can tolerate. Some patients have to avoid certain foods, even though they're nutritious, because of symptoms of vomiting or regurgitation. You're more likely to tolerate a wider variety of foods when you follow the post-surgery diet progression very carefully and have a good post-surgery care program.[4] These are some foods that might unexpectedly cause symptoms:

- Red meat
- Poultry
- Salad
- Vegetables
- Bread
- Rice
- Pasta
- Fish

Yes, this list is pretty broad, but you're not going to have trouble with *all* of these foods. More likely is that you'll have trouble with only one or two foods in just one or two categories

Other Poor Choices

Other foods and beverages may be poor choices because they are unhealthy or because they can cause complications with the gastric sleeve. These are few examples of foods and beverages to avoid or at least limit.

- *Carbonated beverages*: These can make you feel unpleasantly full and give you dumping syndrome, especially if you choose sugar-sweetened ones. Both regular and diet soft drinks can lead to a leak in your sleeve or to stretching the volume of your sleeve so you don't feel as restricted later in your weight loss journey.
- *Alcoholic beverages*: Alcoholic beverages are bad for anyone watching their weight because of their extra calories without many essential nutrients. In fact, alcohol is doubly bad for weight loss because it lowers your resistance so you're more likely to eat more calories from other foods while you're under the influence. As if that weren't enough, alcohol is particularly bad for gastric sleeve patients. Your body's ability to metabolize alcohol changes because your stomach sleeve is smaller than a regular stomach. Drinking the same amount of alcohol as someone with a larger stomach leads to higher levels of blood alcohol.[5]
- *Tough meat*: Dry, stringy, tough meat can wreak havoc on your sleeve. Think about what happens when you swallow an unchewable piece of meat—it goes into your sleeve and can easily irritate it. Avoid tough meats as well as sausage and ground beef with gristle.[6]

- *Foods high in saturated fat*: Saturated fat isn't an essential nutrient, and it's unhealthy for your heart because it raises your blood cholesterol levels. It's bad for weight loss because it's high in calories, and it's often in high-calorie foods, such as cakes made with shortening, full-fat cheese, and fatty meats, such as steak and bacon.

- *Fried foods*: At best, fried foods contain extra calories that slow down weight loss; for example, a cup of steamed onion rings has 92 calories, while a cup of onion rings fried in 1 tablespoon of oil has 212 calories. Fried foods often have breading; a cup of breaded and fried onion rings has over 300 calories. At worst, fried foods are sources of trans fats, which are even worse for your health than saturated fats. To top things off, fried foods are often high in refined carbohydrates. (Think about doughnuts, fried chicken with thick breading, and French fries.) Why take something healthy and delicious and fry it?

- *Caffeine*: Caffeine's actual effects on your sleeve and weight loss aren't clear. It may increase your risk of ulcers, but there isn't much evidence either way.[7] Caffeine is a trigger for heartburn for many people. There is a reason to avoid caffeine that's very relevant to the gastric sleeve. Too much caffeine can harm your bones—and gastric sleeve patients are already at risk for weaker bones because of low nutrient intakes.

Tips for Phase 4

As you transition from Phase 3, the semi-solid or soft foods diet, to Phase 4, solid foods, there are a few things you can do to lower the chances of side effects from new foods.

- *Start with the solid foods that seem easiest and gradually work your way to a full diet.* There are no hard-and-fast rules for the order to introduce foods, but a little judgment can help you guess at the best foods to choose. For example, for your first raw fruit, you might choose cut ripe cantaloupe, which is soft, instead of a hard apple. Or you might go with oatmeal, a soft food, before moving to dry breakfast cereal.

- *Have only tiny quantities of new foods.* Add, for example, only a single bite of a cracker with your meal just to make sure that you can tolerate it before having a whole serving of crackers the next day.

- *Chew your food well.* Solid foods are solid—and you need to chew them thoroughly before swallowing them so that they don't make you nauseous or sick. Eating slower reduces your risk of complications with the sleeve.[8]

- *Be sure to follow your recommendations for protein, getting about 60 to 120 grams per day.*[9] This amount of protein can reduce the amount of lean muscle mass that you lose as you are losing body fat. If you don't get enough protein, your body will break down your muscle and your metabolism will slow down. You can increase your protein intake by choosing protein first at each meal, and by loading the front of your day with protein.

- *Aim for at least five servings of vegetables and fruits.* Eat them after your protein so that you don't risk filling up on grains before you get to your vegetables and fruit.

- *Drink only when it's at least half an hour before or after a meal or snack.* Liquids aren't very filling, and they can stretch your sleeve and lead to leaks. The recommended minimum is 1.5 liters (six or seven cups) per day. You can meet this by continuing to drink throughout the day in between meals.

Help with Meal Planning on the Sleeve Diet

Now you know which foods you can eat and what the regular serving size is. That's necessary, but it's not quite enough information for you to put together a full meal plan. You need some guidelines on which foods to choose to make up a varied and healthy diet for weight loss. You also need to know how big each meal should be. This next section will guide you through the general meal plan so you can start to plan your own menus. The more you practice, the faster and easier meal planning will be for your daily and weekly menus.

Sample Menus

Here are three sample menus for two different days. You'll notice that they have a variety of different foods so that you get a variety of nutrients and don't have to be bored with your eating. Each of these days has three small meals and three snacks; don't forget to drink your water in between your eating times! [10]

Sample Meal Patterns

Meal or Snack	Day 1 Sample	Day 2 Sample
Breakfast	1 packet of plain instant oatmeal made with fat-free milk (cinnamon and/or artificial sweetener optional) ½ medium banana 6 almonds	2 scrambled egg whites or one-quarter cup of liquid egg substitute made with skim milk and 1 tsp. canola oil 1 ounce low-fat cheddar cheese melted into eggs 1 slice of toast spread with 2 teaspoons trans-fat free margarine ½ of a medium orange
Snack 1	1 cup cucumber sticks (peeled) ¼ cup hummus	½ apple 1 tablespoon peanut butter
Lunch	½ whole grain English muffin 1 ounce turkey breast slice 1 ounce low-fat cheese ½ cup applesauce	½ cup canned tuna in water 1 cup of salad made with greens and other raw vegetables 1 tablespoon of salad dressing ½ whole-wheat bagel

Meal or Snack	Day 1 Sample	Day 2 Sample
Snack 2	4 crackers 1 hard-boiled egg	½ cup yogurt
Dinner	2 ounces chicken breast ½ cup cooked carrots ½ cup cooked brown rice (or white if you're just starting the solid foods diet)	Burger made with 3 ounces of extra lean ground beef, turkey or chicken or soy crumbles 1 light whole-wheat hamburger bun ½ to 1 cup cooked cauliflower 1 tablespoon light mayo (Miracle Whip)
Snack 3	½ cup chocolate pudding	12 ounces milk

Table 27: Sample Meal Patterns for Phase 4

Making Your Own Daily Menu from a Standard Meal Pattern

But what happens if you want to make your own meal plans? After all, you're going to be on this diet for years, and you don't want to get bored! A good meal plan meets your nutrient needs and has tons of flexibility so that you can pick and choose the foods you feel like eating each day. It has to be sleeve-friendly and lead to weight loss, too. Each day should include:[11]

- 60 to 120 grams of protein
- At least five servings of fruits and vegetables
- 130 grams of total carbohydrates
- 20 grams of fat
- At least 1.5 liters of fluid (drunk between meals and snacks)

You'll come close to your protein, carbohydrate and fat recommendations if you get these servings:

- 6 to 10 proteins
- 2 to 3 fruits
- 3 to 5 vegetables
- 5 to 7 grains
- 3 to 6 healthy fats (remember, these are *small* serving sizes!)

One-for-One Swaps

One way to make your own food plan is to make one-for-one substitutions. That means exchanging a fruit for a fruit, a grain for a grain, a protein for a protein, and so on. So, if you decide you want fish and peas instead of chicken and carrots, take a look at the food lists. On the protein list, you'd just swap one serving (2 ounces) of fish for one serving (2 ounces) of chicken. From the vegetable list, you'd switch ½ cup of peas for ½ cup of carrots. That's pretty simple, right? Just by substituting, you can make your diet completely personalized.

Are you ready to give it a try?

Table 26 a basic plan that'll keep up your protein intake and provide a balanced diet. Aim for about one cup of food at each meal, and one-half cup of food per snack. Remember to drink between meals, but not immediately before or after or during them.

Meal or Snack	Meal Pattern	Sample Day Based on the Patten
Breakfast	2 protein 1 grain	1 hard-boiled egg ½ cup whole-grain breakfast cereal 1 cup fat-free milk
Snack 1	1 protein 1 grain 1 fat	2 ounces canned tuna in water with 1 tablespoon light mayo 4 saltine crackers
Lunch	1 protein 2 vegetables 1 fruit	½ cup cottage cheese 1 cup cooked green beans ½ cup diced melon
Snack 2	1 fruit	1 plum
Dinner	1 protein 1 grain 1 vegetable 1 fat	2 ounces chicken breast grilled with 1 teaspoon olive oil ½ cup whole-wheat pasta
Snack 3	1 protein	1 cup yogurt (no sugar added)

Table 28: Basic Meal Plan (to help keep up you protein intake and provide a balanced diet)

The plan has plenty of flexibility. If you want fruit for breakfast, for example, have your "lunch" serving of fruit at breakfast. Or, if you want a sandwich for lunch, have your "snack 1" serving of grain at lunch. In that case, you might consider having one of your "lunch" servings of vegetables at "snack 1" so that your lunch doesn't get too big.

Strategies for Reducing Hunger

If the meal plan leaves you feeling hungry, try adding some vegetables because they're filling and low-calorie. Increasing your protein intake can also help. Protein is slow to digest, so it staves off hunger for longer. Be sure that you're drinking enough water throughout the day; sometimes your body can misinterpret thirst signals for hunger signals. Also, talk to your nutritionist or dietitian for strategies for reducing hunger.

Do You Need Help with the Measurements?

We've talked a lot about serving sizes and the importance of measuring them. The last chapter talked about measuring cups and spoons as some of the indispensible kitchen tools for success on the sleeve diet. If you don't have any cooking experience, though, the various measurements may be foreign to you. This is a conversion table so you can get a handle on your serving sizes. Knowing how to convert lets you read recipes and instructions from any source and measure them using your own set of cups and spoons.

Here's a conversion table of the most common measurements so that when you see them in a recipe or diet plan, you'll know exactly how much to take.

Converting Volumes

Unit	Equals	Also Equals:	In Metric
1 teaspoon (1 tsp.)	1/3 tablespoon (1/3 tbsp.)		5 milliliters (5 mL)
1 tablespoon (1 tbsp.)	3 tsp.	½ fluid ounce (½ fl. oz.)	15 ml
2 tbsp.	1/8 cup	1 fl. oz.	30 ml
4 tbsp.	¼ cup	2 fl. oz.	60 ml
8 tbsp.	½ cup	4 fl. oz.	120 ml
16 tbsp.	1 cup	8 fl. oz.	240 ml
2 cups	1 pint	16 fl. oz.	480 ml (about ½ liter)
4 cups	1 quart	32 fl. oz.	960 ml, or just under 1 liter
1 liter		33 fl. oz	1000 ml

Keep this chart handy toward the beginning of your sleeve journey when you're first starting to measure everything. If you measure all of your foods diligently, you'll soon find that converting becomes so natural to you that you feel as though you could do it in your sleep.

Keeping Your Menus Nutritious and Adequate

As you choose your foods, choose a variety so that you get a full range of nutrients. Also, remember to take your daily supplements as recommended by your surgeon or dietitian. Another caution is that the above meal patterns are for a very, very low-calorie diet. For most sleeve patients, that's okay. You're under the supervision of your medical team and you got the sleeve because you wanted to lose weight rapidly.

You should be aware that a diet with so few calories is considered an extreme diet and it has risks, such as nutritional deficiencies and loss of bone mineral density. As long as you work closely with your dietitian and surgeon and continue to follow their instructions for eating and taking your dietary supplements, the benefits of losing healthy amounts of excess weight should greatly outweigh the risks.

Some General Guidelines for Making the Sleeve Diet a Success for You

The VSG is still a relatively new technique, so surgeons and patients are still learning a lot about it. Nonetheless, there are already some pretty good ideas about the best ways to make the sleeve diet successful. Following these guidelines can reduce your risk for complications while making it easier to stay on the diet and lose weight.

Tips for Success on the Sleeve Diet

We've already talked about many of these tips. They're at the foundation of your success, and we suggest putting this list on your fridge so you see it often when you're ready to eat or drink:

- *Take small bites.* Using a small teaspoon instead of large soup spoon is an effective strategy. Another tip is to cut your food into small pieces. Focus on spearing a small piece of food with your fork instead of piling it on.

- *Chew each bite 30 times before swallowing.* This helps ensure that you're not letting hard pieces of food get into the sleeve. You don't have to count to 30 for each bite for the rest of your life, but try it for several meals until you get into the habit. Pretty soon, it'll feel natural.

- *Stop eating when you're full.* That keeps you from overeating. Because you may need to retrain yourself to recognize hunger signals, for the first several weeks or months you may need to stop eating *before* you think you're full.

- *Eat your protein first.* It's an essential nutrient for maintaining lean body mass, and you need to get enough of it. Choose it first at meals and be sure to get a high-protein breakfast and morning snack.

- *Separate solids from liquids.* Eat solid foods at least 30 minutes apart from when you drink liquids. This helps you take full advantage of the sleeve because solid foods stay in the sleeve for longer when you don't have fluids with them. If you drink beverages while you're eating solid food, food can pass through the sleeve faster so you don't feel full for very long after a meal. Drinking fluids with meals can lead to indigestion and reduced satiety after a meal.[12]

- *Don't get over-ambitious.* Only eat the foods that are in your allowed foods list, and introduce new foods gradually. Eating other foods can cause long-term trouble with the sleeve. Always stop to think how you feel before you eat more. It's better to stop eating if you feel full than to force yourself to continue eating your planned meal. Also be careful to avoid trouble foods if you discover them.

- *Measure all of your food so that you don't overeat.* Keep your meals and snacks small by measuring each portion and choosing only the type and amount of foods that are on your plan. A typical plan includes about three small meals and snacks each day.

- *Don't "munch."* Munching means eating and drinking bits of foods here and there. You might take a few tastes while you're in the kitchen cooking, grab a couple of nuts from the bowl on the secretary's desk, or have just a few tastes of your spouse's meal when you're out at dinner. Everything you eat counts, and these small bites of food can really add up to interfere with your weight loss. A single one-inch square piece of brownie and a tablespoon of peanut butter each have about 100 calories. Eating the crumbs while you're scraping the pan of brownies and licking the knife after you spread your peanut butter are just two examples of mindless munching that can add hundreds of calories without you even noticing it. To avoid this, only eat foods that you measure and plan, and only eat them at the table. Don't eat in your car or while in the kitchen.

- *Don't accidentally drink your calories.* That's one of the quickest ways to derail your weight loss and make the sleeve less effective. Soft drinks, juices, sweetened coffee and tea, and other beverages with calories can add hundreds of calories to your day and not make you feel full and satisfied. Fat-free milk and vegetable juice are likely to be the only caloric beverages that your dietitian recommends. Fat-free milk has 80 calories and eight grams of protein per cup. Tomato and mixed vegetable juice have about.50 calories per cup and provide servings of vegetables.

- *Stay hydrated.* The goal of 1.5 liters of fluid per day is just a minimum, and you need extra if you sweat heavily or the weather's especially hot or dry. With some practice, you can make habit out of drinking water and other non-caloric beverages in between meals and snacks to stay hydrated and prevent headaches and fatigue related to dehydration.

The Benefits of Eating Slowly

Many of the above guidelines are geared toward helping you eat more slowly, which promotes success on the sleeve diet. Eating slowly has a variety of benefits:

- *It lets you get full before you eat as much.* Remember how we mentioned that it takes a while for your brain to realize that you're full? If you wolf down your food, you might finish your food and go back for more because you still feel hungry. Eating slower gives your stomach a chance to send fullness signals to your brain before you've eaten too much.

- *It's more pleasant.* Eating slowly gives you a chance to savor your food. Before surgery, your idea of enjoying food might have been to see how much you could eat and how fast. After getting the sleeve and slowing down your eating, you might start to notice the flavors and appreciate them. You might feel a healthier satisfaction from the act of eating.

- *It reduces your risk of complications.* Eating too fast can make you vomit, feel nauseous, or have diarrhea. Eating too fast can stretch your sleeve if you overeat, so losing weight will be harder.

- *It helps you lose weight.* Eating slower not only helps you eat less, but it also helps you stick to your diet because you're more likely to be able to stay on a diet when you enjoy it. Eating less and sticking to the plan make an effective combination for weight loss!

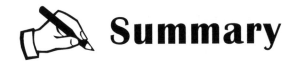 **Summary**

☛ This chapter is a key to your success with the sleeve. It covered the basics of the sleeve diet that you'll be following for the long-term. You know what you can eat and the serving sizes. The chapter provided a few sample meal plans and a basic menu that you can tweak to create varied menus for yourself day after day.

☛ This chapter mentioned making nutritious choices, but you might not yet know how to do that.

☛ The next chapter provides an overview of basic nutrition and gives some guidelines on selecting a balanced and healthy diet. By the end of the next chapter, you'll be an expert nutritionist!

Your Turn: Practice Making Some Menus!

This chapter provides a template for your daily menus. We came up with two sample menus based on the template, but you're going to need more menus than that if your meal plan's going to stay interesting! Why don't you try making your own menu based on the template? In Table 29 below, you can see the template in the left column. In the column on the right, write in foods and their serving sizes that match up with the template.

Meal or Snack	Meal Pattern	Sample Menu	Your Own Menu
Breakfast	2 protein 1 grain 1 fat 1 fruit	½ cup cottage cheese 1 slice reduced-calorie whole-wheat bread 1 tablespoon peanut butter ½ apple	
Snack 1	1 protein 1 grain 1 fat	½ whole-grain bagel 1 ounce low-fat cheese	
Lunch	1 protein 2 vegetables 1 fruit 1 fat	1 ounce low-sodium deli meat ½ cup cooked green beans 1 cup salad with 1 tbsp. salad dressing ½ orange	
Snack 2	1 fruit	1 apricot	
Dinner	1 protein 1 grain 1 vegetable 1 fat	2 ounces grilled chicken with 1 tsp. olive oil ½ cup cooked zucchini with 1 tsp. olive oil	
Snack 3	1 protein	1 cup fat-free yogurt, no sugar added	

Table 29: Create Your Own Menu – Template 1

Now, try a different meal pattern. Like the first one, this meal pattern meets the general recommendations for serving from each group. Having an alternative meal pattern to work with gives you even more options for menus so you never have to get bored.

Meal or Snack	Day 1 Sample	Sample Menu	Your Own Menu
Breakfast	2 protein 2 grain 1 fat 1 fruit	2 packets instant oatmeal 1 tablespoon peanut butter 1 cup fat-free milk ½ grapefruit	
Snack 1	1 protein 1 grain 1 fat	1 hard-boiled egg 1 cup red pepper strips 2 tablespoons guacamole	
Lunch	1 protein 2 vegetables 1 fruit 1 fat	½ cup cooked kidney beans ½ cup cooked orange squash 1 cup of cut melon 1 tablespoon ground flaxseed	
Snack 2	1 protein 1 grain	1 cup fat-free yogurt 1 ounce whole-grain cereal	
Dinner	2 protein 1 grain 1 vegetable	2 ounces grilled salmon ½ cup brown rice ½ cup brussels sprouts with 1 tsp. olive oil	
Snack 3	1 protein	½ mashed banana	

Table 30: Create Your Own Menu – Template 2

1   Rosenthal RJ. International Sleeve Gastrectomy Expert Panel consensus statement: best practice guidelines based on experience of > 12,000 cases. Surgery for Obesity and Related Diseases. 2012;8(1):8-19.

2   Snyder-Marlow G, Tayle D, Lenhard MJ. Nutrition care for patients undergoing laparoscopic sleeve gastrectomy for weight loss. J Am Diet Ass. 2010;110(4):600-607

3   Jacques J. Nutrition and the sleeve gastrectomy patient: from micronutrients to dietary patterns. Bariatric Times. 2011.

4   Keren D, Matter I, Rainis T & Lavy A. Getting the most from the sleeve: the importance of post-operative follow-up. Obesity Surgery. 2011;21(12):1887-1893.

5   Maluenda F, Csendes A, Aretxabala X, Poniachik J, Salvo K, Delgado I, Rodriguez P. Alcohol absorption modification after a laparoscopic sleeve gastrectomy due to obesity. Obes Surg. 2010;20(6):744-8.

6   Realize. Bariatric surgery recovery expectations. Website. http://www.realize.com/bariatric-surgery-recovery-expectations.htm. 2012, August 1. Accessed October 16, 2012.

7   Aills L, Blankenship J, Buffington C, Furtado M, Parrott J. ASMBS Allied Health nutritional guidelines for the surgical weight loss patient. Surg Obes Relat Dis. 2008;4(5Suppl):S73-S108.

8   Snyder-Marlow G, Tayle D, Lenhard MJ. Nutrition care for patients undergoing laparoscopic sleeve gastrectomy for weight loss. J Am Diet Ass. 2010;110(4):600-607

9   Ziegler O, Sirveaux MA, Brunaud L, Reibel N, Quillot D. Medical follow-up after bariatric surgery: nutritional and drug issues. General recommendations for the prevention and treatment of nutritional deficiencies. Diabetes Metab. 2009;35(6 Pt 2):544-547.

10   Snyder-Marlow G, Tayle D, Lenhard MJ. Nutrition care for patients undergoing laparoscopic sleeve gastrectomy for weight loss. J Am Diet Ass. 2010;110(4):600-607

11   Snyder-Marlow G, Tayle D, Lenhard MJ. Nutrition care for patients undergoing laparoscopic sleeve gastrectomy for weight loss. J Am Diet Ass. 2010;110(4):600-607

12   Snyder-Marlow G, Tayle D, Lenhard MJ. Nutrition care for patients undergoing laparoscopic sleeve gastrectomy for weight loss. J Am Diet Ass. 2010;110(4):600-607

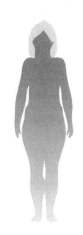

15

The Sleeve Diet,
Weight Loss
and Your Health

The last chapter included the essentials of the sleeve diet. After reading it, you know what to eat and how much to eat. You saw some sample menus and practiced making your own sleeve diet menu. The chapter gave several tips for success with the sleeve diet. The information in that chapter is enough to let you develop and follow a weight loss plan, but there's more to healthy eating than that. We mentioned healthy choices several times but didn't go into much detail. So, what are healthy choices? This chapter serves as a basic nutrition lesson and covers these topics:

- Calories, energy, and weight control.
- Protein, fat, and carbohydrates: their roles and choosing the best ones
- Vitamins and minerals and which ones you need to monitor as a sleeve patient
- Water: why you need it and how to get enough
- Making sense of nutrition labels
- Keeping condiments from sabotaging your diet
- Alcoholic beverages and how they can harm your weight loss and health

As you read through this chapter, you'll probably notice that a lot of it is common sense. As you probably already know, lean proteins, vegetables, whole grains, and fruits are healthier choices than sweets and fried foods. But there may be some surprises, such as learning that some high-fat foods are extremely healthy.

If you're not interested in all of the details right now, you can just skim this chapter. It may come in useful later when you're trying to select the healthiest options from among specific foods.

Calories and Weight Loss

You've already heard a lot about calories—it's impossible to avoid them! Calories come up almost everywhere, from nutrition labels on food packages to weight loss guides to calorie counts on restaurant menus. We've mentioned them many times in this book because they're the single most important factor in weight loss. Calories are units of energy. Your body converts food into usable energy, measured in terms of calories.

These concepts are critical:

- You must burn off, or expend, more calories than you consume, or eat, in order to lose weight.
- Your body weight will be stable if you eat the same number of calories that you burn off.
- You will gain weight if you eat more calories than you burn.

Weight Change	Energy Balance	Calories in versus out	Eating versus
Lose weight	Calorie (or energy) deficit	Calories in < calories out	eat < burn
Maintain weight	Calorie (or energy) balance	Calories in = calories out	eat = burn
Gain weight	Calorie (or energy) excess	Calories in > calories out	eat > burn

Table 31: Calorie Balance & Weight Change

There's no getting around the concept of energy balance. Sleeve or no sleeve, you must eat fewer calories than you burn if you want to lose weight. This is called creating a calorie deficit. You can create your calorie deficit by eating less, exercising more, or doing both. The sleeve is a tool to help you eat less because it restricts your food intake and may make you less hungry.

3,500 Calories per Pound of Body Fat

A pound of body fat is worth about 3,500 calories. What does that mean? For each pound of body fat that you want to lose, you have to create a calorie deficit of 3,500 calories. This means that you must expend 3,500 calories more than you consume.

To lose one pound per week, you need to burn off an extra 3,500 calories per week or have an average deficit of 500 calories per day. To lose two pounds of fat per week, you have to burn off 7,000 calories or have an average daily calorie deficit of 1,000 calories. Let's break down some numbers:

Calorie expenditure: An obese man who weighs 240 pounds and is 5 feet, 9 inches tall needs about 2,700 calories per day, before adding in any exercise that he may do. That's according to the Harris-Benedict equation, which is a famous and impressively accurate equation to estimate daily calorie needs.[1]

Calorie intake: Many sleeve diet plans have you eating only about 1,000 or 1,200 calories per day. The ones in the previous chapter are within that approximate range.

At an intake level of 1,200 calories per day, the man would be creating a calorie deficit of 1,500 calories per day—or an average weight loss of three pounds per week! You can see that a very low-calorie diet, such as the one you follow with the gastric sleeve, will lead to substantial weight loss.

As you lose weight, your energy needs, or metabolic rate, will decrease. Your weight loss will slow down if you don't make any changes, but you can make up for your slower metabolism—and improve your health—by increasing your physical activity.

Do You Have to Count Calories?

Now that you can see how your calorie intake affects your weight loss, you can see the importance of the calorie content of the foods and beverages that you select. Luckily, calorie-counting isn't necessary if you stick to the meal plan by having the recommended number of servings and proper portion sizes. Your dietitian and surgeon probably won't ask you to count calories as a guide to your diet intake, but they may encourage low-calorie choices. Whenever possible, compare the calorie content per serving of food when you are at the grocery store or about to prepare a meal, and choose the option with fewer calories. That will help you lose weight faster.

Nutrient-Dense versus Empty Calories: How Do They Affect Weight Loss?

When it comes to your weight, a calorie is a calorie is a calorie. Eat 3,500 calories too many, and you will gain a pound of body fat. Cut out 3,500 calories from your diet or burn off an extra 3,500 calories from exercising more—or any combination of eating less and exercising more—and you'll lose a pound. That's true no matter where your calories come from, whether it's junk food or healthy food.

So does it matter where your calories come from when you are talking about controlling your weight? In theory, it shouldn't. A calorie is always a calorie. In reality, though, getting your calories from healthy foods is a much better choice. Compared to junk food, healthy foods don't just provide more nutrients and protect you against heart disease, diabetes, and high blood pressure.

Healthy foods also help you control your weight! That's because they're usually more filling than junk food. That means you can get just as full from eating fewer calories of a healthy food than junk food. Think about these examples. Would you be less hungry after eating:

- 1 cup of cucumber sticks and 1 cup of fat-free yogurt or 2/3 ounce of potato chips (both are about 100 calories)?

- 1 packet of instant oatmeal, 2 scrambled egg whites and ½ apple or 1 ounce of cheese and 2 strips of bacon fried in 1 tablespoon of butter (both are about 200 calories)?

- 2 ounces of grilled chicken breast, ½ cup cottage cheese, 1 cup of cauliflower, and ½ cup rice or steak (both are about 300 calories)?

How can you tell the difference between healthy food and junk food? Well, the U.S. Department of Agriculture and Department of Health and Human Services use a term called "nutrient-dense" to describe foods that are high in nutrients. These are the foods you should focus on. "Empty calories" come from foods that don't have health benefits—they are "empty" of essential nutrients. Foods with empty calories are foods with saturated fat, trans fats, added sugars, refined grains, or high amounts of sodium.

In the following table are some nutrient-dense foods and foods with empty calories. Your diet should be based mostly on the left column. You can see that most, but not all, of the nutrient-dense foods are low in calories. For example, nuts, pe anuts, and avocados are high in calories and fat. But, they have important nutrients such as dietary fiber, heart-healthy fats, and vitamin E, so they make good choices—in moderation and if you chew them very, very well so they don't aggravate your sleeve.

Nutrient-Dense Foods (Choose These)	Empty Calories (Limit These)
• Lean meats (e.g., extra-lean ground beef and sirloin tip)	• Fatty cuts of meat, such as fatty steak, bacon, and sausage
• Tofu and soy products	• Fried foods, including French fries, onion rings, fried chicken, and banana chips
• White-meat poultry (e.g., chicken and turkey breast) without the skin	• Unenriched refined grains (e.g., unenriched white bread, pasta, and rice and refined, sugary breakfast cereals)
• Seafood, including fish and shellfish	
• Reduced-fat milk, yogurt, and cheese	• Full-fat dairy products
• Egg whites	• Sweets, such as candy, ice cream, and milk chocolate
• Beans, lentils, split peas	
• Unsalted nuts, peanuts, seeds	• Sugar-sweetened beverages
• Avocados, vegetable oil, olive oil	• Baked goods, such as pies, cookies, sweet rolls, and cakes
• Fruits	
• Vegetables	• Processed snack foods, such as crackers and potato chips
• Whole grain products such as oatmeal, whole-wheat bread and pasta, and brown rice	• Prepared foods, such as fast foods
	• Salty, fatty, or sugary sauces; dressings; gravies; and other condiments

Source[2]

Protein, Fat, and Carbohydrates

Proteins, fats and, carbohydrates are called the macronutrients because you need larger amounts ("macro") of them compared to the small amounts ("micro") that you need of the micronutrients, or vitamins and minerals. Protein, fat, and carbohydrates are similar because they each provide calories, or energy. They are different, though, because of their different roles and how they affect your health. Here's an overview of each of them.

Protein - All proteins are made of amino acids. When you think about protein metabolism, start with the proteins in food. Your body breaks down these food proteins into amino acids and then into even smaller components. Then your body rearranges these components and assembles them into amino acids and proteins that come together to form tissues and organs and structures. Proteins are not only part of your regular muscles but also your bones, skins, lungs, heart, and blood vessels. Proteins are necessary for a strong immune system to fight infections, for carrying nutrients and oxygen around your body, and for pretty much every reaction that occurs in your body.[3]

Protein as an Energy Source - Proteins from food provide energy. Each gram of protein has 4 calories. Your body is very good at using protein for energy, but it's healthier to get your energy from carbohydrates and fat. This lets you leave protein free for its other essential functions, such as preventing your body from breaking down your muscles for energy. The idea of using carbohydrate and fat instead of protein for energy is known as "protein sparing."

Complete and Incomplete Proteins and Vegetarianism - Proteins can be complete or incomplete. *Complete*, or high-quality, proteins have each of the essential amino acids, or amino acids that you need to get from your diet. *Incomplete* proteins are missing one or more of the amino acids, but you can get all of the amino acids you need by eating a variety of foods. These are some good sources of protein:

- Complete proteins include all proteins from animal sources, such as meat, poultry, fish, eggs, and dairy products. Soy is another complete protein.
- Incomplete proteins include most other plant-based proteins. Legumes, or beans, split peas, and lentils are highest in protein. Nuts, grains, vegetables, and seeds are also sources of protein.

A common myth is that vegetarians can't meet their protein needs. That's not true. Vegetarians can meet their protein needs, and it's not that hard. If you're a lacto-ovo vegetarian, the most common kind, you eat eggs and dairy products. Those are sources of complete protein, so you can meet your needs. You can still get enough protein if you're vegan and you avoid all animal products. Soybeans, veggie burgers, tofu and other soy-based products provide complete protein. You can also meet your needs by combining proteins. In protein combining, you eat a variety of sources of incomplete protein to make them complete. These are some examples of complete proteins:

- Beans and rice
- Crackers and hummus
- Bean and pasta soup
- Peanut butter and whole-grain bread

How much protein do you need while you're losing weight? A good rule of thumb with the sleeve is to aim for at least 60 to 120 grams of protein per day, at least toward the beginning of your weight loss journey. That's a range of 240 to 480 calories. If your daily total calorie intake is 1,200 calories, that means that 20 to 40 percent of your calories would be coming from protein. That range puts you near the national recommendations from the U.S. Department of Health and Human Services to get 10 to 30 percent of your calories from protein.[4] The average American gets 98 grams per day of protein and eats 2,507 calories, putting the average national protein intake at 16% of total calories from protein.[5]

Getting this much protein can be challenging when your total intake is so low, but you can do it if you make protein your priority, as already discussed in earlier chapters. Choose high-protein foods when you can. Make it a habit to eat your protein first, both at meals and in your daily meal plan. That means that you should eat your servings of protein foods first at meals so that you can be sure to get them in before you fill up. Also, start your day off strong with protein. Include at least two servings of high-protein foods at breakfast to give yourself a good start for the day.

Protein Content of Common Foods - We keep talking about keeping your protein intake high. Just after surgery, protein is necessary for your body to heal the wounds from the gastrectomy. As you lose weight, you need protein to maintain your lean muscle mass so you stay strong and keep your metabolism up. You need about 60 to 120 grams of protein per day,[6] but more than one-third of sleeve patients don't continually get enough protein throughout their first year with the gastric sleeve.[7]

These Charts Can Help You Translate Grams of Protein into Food

These handy charts/tables can help you make sure you get enough protein each day. Tables 32-34 contains foods that are divided into categories based on their protein content.[8] They're in the same categories as in the previous chapter's food list for the Phase 4 diet. Foods are listed alphabetically within each category.

- High-protein foods are nearly pure protein with very little carbohydrate or fat.
- Medium-protein foods have a high amount of protein and also some carbohydrates and/or fat.
- Low-protein foods mostly have carbohydrates and/or fat, but they provide some protein.
- Foods without protein aren't listed in this table. They include pure fats, such as oil and butter, fruit, fruit juices, many vegetables, juices, and most condiments.

Food	Sleeve Diet Serving Size	Protein per Serving, Grams
Beef, ground, extra lean	2 ounces	11
Beef, sirloin, lean only	2 ounces	16
Chicken breast, skinless, roasted	2 ounces	18
Chicken, canned	2 ounces	11
Chicken, ground, raw	2 ounces	13
Cod, fresh	2 ounces	11
Cottage cheese, fat-free or low-fat	½ cup	14
Crab, canned	2 ounces	10
Egg	1 large	6
Egg white	2 large	12
Egg substitute, fat-free substitute	½ cup	6
Halibut	2 ounces	10
Protein powder, unflavored/sugar-free	10 grams	5-8

Food	Sleeve Diet Serving Size	Protein per Serving, Grams
Salmon, fresh	2 ounces	11
Tuna, canned light in water	2 ounces	11
Turkey, ground	2 ounces	15
Turkey breast, deli meat	1 ounce	7
Turkey, white meat, skinless, roasted	2 ounces	16

Table 32: High-protein foods

Medium-Protein Foods

Food	Sleeve Diet Serving Size	Protein per Serving, Grams
Almonds	2 tablespoons (6-8)	3
Beans, canned or boiled (e.g., pinto, kidney, garbanzo, navy)	½ cup	7
Cheese, hard, fat-free	1 ounce	9
Cheese, hard, low-fat	1 ounce	7
Cheese, hard, regular (e.g., Swiss or cheddar)	1 ounce	7
Lentils, cooked	½ cup	9
Milk	8 ounces (1 cup)	8
Peanuts	¼ cup	3
Peanut butter	1 tablespoon	3
Pecans	2 tablespoons (6-8)	1
Seeds, sunflower	2 tablespoons	3
Soybeans, roasted	1 ounce	9
Tofu, silken, hard or soft	½ cup	6-10
Walnuts	2 tablespoons	4
Yogurt, fat-free	8 ounces (1 cup)	8-12
Yogurt, Greek, fat-free	8 ounces (1 cup)	23

Table 33: Medium-protein foods

Low-Protein Foods

Food	Sleeve Diet Serving Size	Protein per Serving, Grams
Bread, reduced-calorie	1 slice	3
Bread, white	½ slice	3
Bread, whole-wheat	½ slice	3
Cauliflower, cooked	½ cup	2
Carrots, cooked	½ cup	1
Corn, canned or cooked	½ cup	3
Green beans, cooked	½ cup	1
Oatmeal, dry	1 packet	2
Pasta, cooked, enriched white	½ cup	3
Pasta, cooked, whole-grain	½ cup	3
Rice, cooked, brown	½ cup	3
Soybeans, raw (green) – edamame	1 ounce	4
Spinach, cooked	½ cup	1

Table 34: Low-protein foods

These charts/tables can help you choose high-protein foods. They can also help you monitor your protein intake so you know that you're getting enough. If you're not getting enough protein, your dietitian can help you with strategies, such as having an extra high-protein snack or including a protein supplement in your diet. Many members of BariatricPal.com, an online community dedicated specifically to the gastric sleeve and weight loss, can give you their own tried-and-true tips for increasing protein intake.

Fat - Fat is a great source of energy—which unfortunately means that it's very high in calories. A single gram of fat has 9 calories, or more than twice the amount of calories in a gram of protein or carbohydrate. That's why a high-fat diet is often linked to obesity, and it's why following a low-fat diet is a recommendation to help people lose weight.

You Need Fat for Nutrient Absorption - Fat isn't all bad though. You need it to be able to absorb nutrients from your diet. That's a special challenge after you get the sleeve, and many sleeve patients are at risk for vitamin deficiencies because of a very low-fat diet. Vitamins A, D, E, and K are the vitamins most likely to be affected by your fat intake, and these deficiencies are somewhat common amount sleeve patients.[9]

Not All Fats are Equal - There are a few different types of fat. They all have 9 calories per gram, but they are definitely not created equal in terms of their effects on your body and health, especially your heart health.[10] In general, solid fats, such as butter, shortening and animal fat, are unhealthy. Liquid fats, or oils, are usually healthier. Often foods with unhealthy fats are low in other nutrients, and foods with healthy fats are high in other essential nutrients. *Table 35* helps you see the different types of fat, the general recommendations for healthy intake, and which foods they are in.

Type of Fat	Effects on Your Body and Recommendations	Food Sources
Saturated Fat	• Raises your levels of LDL cholesterol • Increases your risk for heart disease. • Keep your intake to a maximum of 7% to 10% of total calories, or 9 to 14 grams per day on a 1,200-calorie diet.	• Butter • fatty meats, such as fatty beef and pork, sausage, and bacon • dark-meat poultry with the skin on it • full-fat dairy products • coconut and palm oils
Trans Fats	• Trans fats are even worse for your heart than saturated fat. These fats raise your unhealthy LDL cholesterol levels and lower levels of healthy HDL cholesterol in your blood. Intake should be as low as possible, or no more than 1 gram a day on a low-calorie diet.	• Fried foods, such as French fries, fried chicken and fried fish, and doughnuts; • Many processed snack foods, such as crackers, cookies, and snack cakes
Monounsaturated Fats (You'll also see them referred to as MUFA.)	• Monounsaturated fats are known to help lower blood pressure and improve your cholesterol levels. Heart-healthy Mediterranean diets are known for their high levels of monounsaturated fats. Your intake should be about 10% to 20% of total calories, or 14 to 25 grams per day on a 1,200 calorie diet.	• Olive oil • Olives, • Peanut and canola oil • Avocados • Peanuts • Nuts
Polyunsaturated Fats (Sometimes they're called PUFA.)	• Healthy in moderate amounts. • Better choices than saturated fats • Aim to get about 10% of your total calories from polyunsaturated fats. That's about 14 grams per day on a 1,200-calorie diet.	• Nuts • Most vegetable oils, such as canola, sunflower, safflower, and soybean • Seeds • Peanuts; • Flaxseed oil
N-3 Fatty Acids (These are specific types of polyunsaturated fats that have important health benefits.)	• N-3 fatty acids are also called omega-three fatty acids • Lower your blood pressure • Lower your triglycerides, • Help control your blood sugar. • Get at least two servings of seafood per week to get enough n-3 fatty acids to improve your heart health • If you don't eat seafood, a fish oil supplement can get you to your recommended intake of n-3 fats. • The n-3s in vegetarian sources aren't quite as powerful, but they're still healthy.	• Fatty fish, such as salmon, herring, mackerel, and tuna • Shellfish, such as oysters, shrimp, crab, lobster, and mussels • Cod liver oil and fish oil supplements • Vegetarian sources, which includes flaxseed, flaxseed oil, walnuts, and canola oil

Table 35: Different types of fat & the general recommendations for healthy intake

Does Low-Fat Mean Low-Calorie?

No, not necessarily. With nine calories in each gram, fat is the nutrient with the most calories. A lot of low-fat and fat-free foods are lower in calories than their regular, full-fat versions. Non-fat and low-fat milk and cheese, for example, are lower in calories than full-fat milk and cheese. Lean ground beef is lower in calories per serving than regular ground beef, and the same is true for many reduced-fat salad dressings, although not all.

But, low-fat or fat-free does not always mean low-calorie. Fat adds flavor, takes up space (it adds volume to), and provides texture to many foods. When manufacturers take out the fat during their processing, they often add carbohydrates, such as sugars or starches, to replace the taste, volume, and texture that fat normally provides. The result can be a low-fat or fat-free product with just as many calories or more than the original one. These are some common examples of foods with similar amounts of calories in the reduced-fat and regular choices:

- Peanut butter
- Baked goods (e.g., cookies, cakes, pies, and pastries)
- Some condiments (but some reduced-fat versions are also reduced-calorie)
- Ramen noodles
- Canned tuna (i.e., oil-packed versus water-packed)
- Granola

This is quite a varied list, so how can you protect yourself? Read the nutrition facts panels on food labels. Place the regular, full-fat version of the food next to the reduced-fat option, and compare their calories per serving. Make sure you're looking at the same serving size so you don't get tricked!

Carbohydrates

Each gram of carbohydrates supplies four calories, and the only reason why you need carbohydrates from your diet is for energy. When you eat carbohydrates, your body breaks them down into small units of a simple sugar called glucose. The glucose goes into your bloodstream. Your brain depends on glucose for energy.[11] Other organs, such as your muscles, kidneys, and liver, also are good at using glucose when it is available. For most people, carbohydrates provide the most energy in your diet.

Tip

See Chapter 1 to read about how your body breaks down carbohydrates from foods. See Chapter 13, "Recovery and Your Post-Surgery Diet," for information on the nutritional differences between added sugars versus natural sugars.

315

Caloric Carbohydrates and Dietary Fiber

There are two main categories of carbohydrates: carbohydrates with calories and dietary fiber, which does not have calories. The kinds of carbohydrates with calories are divided into sugars and starches. Sugars are simple carbohydrates. They include added sugars that are used for sweetening foods and adding volume to food products and natural sugars, such as lactose in milk and fructose in fruit.

Food Sources of Caloric Carbohydrates

So what foods have caloric carbohydrates? This list contains some of the foods that provide sugars, starches, or both. Not all of them have *a lot* of carbohydrates, and some have fat and protein too. As you can see, foods with sugars can be healthy OR unhealthy, and foods with starches can be healthy OR unhealthy.

- *Grains:* (mainly starches) whole grain and white bread, cereal, pasta, rice, oatmeal, bulgur, barley, popcorn
- *Legumes:* (mainly starches) split peas, black-eyed peas, lentils, and all kinds of beans, such as black, pinto, and garbanzo
- *Fruit:* (mainly simple sugars) fresh, frozen, canned, dried, and juice
- *Nuts, seeds, soy nuts, and peanuts:* (mainly starches)
- *Dairy products:* (mainly simple sugars) milk, yogurt, cheese, frozen yogurt
- *Starchy vegetables:* (mainly starches) potatoes, sweet potatoes and yams, acorn and butternut squash, corn, beets
- *Non-starchy vegetables:* (small amounts of starch) green beans, broccoli, cauliflower, eggplant, lettuce, carrots
- *Sweets:* (mainly simple sugars) candy, ice cream, pudding, chocolate, fudge
- *Sugar-sweetened beverages:* (mainly simple sugars) soft drinks, coffee with sugar, energy drinks, smoothies
- *Baked goods:* (both starches and simple sugars) cakes, cookies, pies, pastries
- *Condiments:* (both starches and simple sugars) ketchup, salad dressing, sauces, gravies, jams and jellies
- *Mixed foods:* (both starches and simple sugars) battered fried chicken and fish, pizza, sandwiches

You might be wondering what *doesn't* have carbohydrates! Eggs, meats such as beef and pork, poultry, fish, and most shellfish are carbohydrate-free. Pure fats, such as butter and oil, are also carbohydrate-free. Just like the foods *with* carbohydrates, the foods *without* carbohydrates can be healthy or unhealthy, high or low in calories, and high or low in protein. What's the bottom line? Use your common sense to make good decisions about which carbohydrates to choose, and stick to your recommended portion sizes.

Dietary Fiber and Your Health

Dietary fiber is a different kind of carbohydrate. It's made up of the same small units as other carbohydrates, but fiber doesn't technically have calories. That's because your body can't break down the big pieces of fiber into small enough pieces to get energy. When you eat a food with fiber, your body breaks down the larger nutrients, such as the proteins, fats, and most carbohydrates. Then you absorb these and smaller nutrients, such as vitamins and minerals, into your body. The fiber stays behind in your gastrointestinal tract—and this fact surprisingly leads to a bunch of health benefits! These are some of them:[12]

- *Helps control your weight.* Dietary fiber ties in very well with the sleeve. Many high-fiber foods, such as fruits and vegetables, take a long time to chew, so they slow down your eating and help you eat less and lose weight. Slow chewing is exactly what you're already doing on your sleeve diet! Another reason why dietary fiber helps control your weight is that it makes food take longer to empty from your stomach.

- *Helps prevent constipation.* The undigested fiber helps add bulk and water to your stool so bowel movements are softer and more regular. Keep drinking water too, to prevent constipation.

- *Helps control blood sugar.* Since fiber slows absorption of carbohydrates, sugar is slower to enter your bloodstream as blood glucose. Your blood sugar doesn't spike as high after a meal, and it doesn't drop as quickly. That's great news if you have prediabetes or diabetes. It's also good because it helps prevent hunger that occurs when your blood sugar drops.

- *Lower your cholesterol levels.* Fiber lowers the amount of cholesterol that you absorb from food, so blood levels of unhealthy LDL cholesterol drop. That's good for your heart.

- *Lowers blood pressure and reduces inflammation.* Scientists aren't quite sure how fiber helps with these, but the evidence for these two heart-healthy benefits looks pretty clear.

Many nutritious, plant-based foods with carbohydrates are good sources of dietary fiber. These are some good sources:

- Whole-grain cereal: oatmeal, whole-wheat cereals, bran cereals
- Whole-grain breads and crackers
- Other whole grains: brown rice, whole-grain, multi-grain pasta
- Vegetables: *Fibrous* is not necessarily the same as *high-fiber.* While you may need to avoid very stringy vegetables like asparagus stalks and raw celery, there are plenty of high-fiber choices, such as butternut squash, onions, and carrots, which you can probably tolerate with the VSG. Vegetable juice does not contain much fiber.
- Fruit: fresh or frozen. Canned fruit has some fiber, and fruit juice is not a good source of fiber.
- Legumes: peas, beans and lentils, including dips and soups
- Nuts and peanuts: Of course, chew them very well and watch your portion sizes!

The recommended intake of fiber is based on the amount of calories that you eat. The general recommendation is to get at least 14 grams for every 1,000 calories that you eat. Don't worry—you don't have to start counting your fiber grams to make sure that you're getting enough. On the sleeve diet, you're probably not going to be counting calories, and you're almost certainly not going to be counting grams of fiber. You can be confident that you're getting enough fiber if you eat a balanced diet and make the healthy food choices that you know you're supposed to. That means choosing whole grains when you can and getting at least five servings of fruits and vegetables per day.

What's the Best Amount of Carbohydrates, Protein, and Fat in Your Diet?

If you follow the trends in weight loss diets, it's hard to avoid hearing about high-protein diets, low-fat diets, low-carb diets, and everything in between. Each of these diets has its die-hard fans and its critics, so how do you know what to believe? And where do calories fit into this?

For Your Health

A healthy diet is one that includes a variety of foods and comes as close as possible to meeting your nutrient needs. A balanced diet, with lean proteins, healthy fats, and nutrient-dense carbohydrate foods is probably best. That's what the sleeve diet emphasizes too. Your priorities include getting lean proteins; choosing vegetables, whole grains, and fruits for your carbohydrates; and eating healthy fats while limiting sweets, unhealthy fats, and refined grains.

For Weight Loss

It takes 3,500 calories to burn a pound regardless of where your calories come from. You can lose weight on high-protein, low-carb, or low-fat diets as long as your calorie intake is less than your calorie expenditure. As with any kind of diet, they work as long as you follow their rules for food choices and portion sizes. They don't work if you eat foods that aren't allowed or eat more than you're allowed.

How Does Your Diet Affect Weight Loss with the Sleeve?

The sleeve diet is based on healthy choices and portion control. As long as you meet your daily recommendations for protein, fluid, and other nutrients, you have a lot of flexibility with the sleeve diet. You can make a variety of menus that let you stick to the sleeve diet and continue to lose weight. One study found that a low-carbohydrate, high-fat diet was less effective for weight loss after the sleeve gastrectomy than a high-carbohydrate or moderate-carbohydrate diet. Based on this study and common sense, it appears that a balanced diet with sufficient protein is likely to be the best choice for your weight loss.

Source[13]

The Micronutrients: Vitamins and Minerals

Vitamins and minerals are known as the micronutrients because you only need small amounts of them compared to the macronutrients, which include carbohydrates, proteins, and fats. You might eat hundreds of grams per day of macronutrients, but you only need a gram, a milligram (one one-thousandth of a gram) or even just a few micrograms (one one-millionth of a gram) per day of micronutrients. Vitamins and minerals don't have calories, but they're just as important as the calorie-providing nutrients.

An Overview of the Micronutrients

There are *a lot* of vitamins and minerals. There are 13 vitamins and at least 15 minerals that are essential. Many of them are not worrisome to most Americans; you're not likely to be deficient in them if you eat a generally balanced and adequate diet. As a sleeve patient, though, you need to be a little more concerned about your vitamin and mineral intake. That's mainly because of your limited food intake.

Meeting Your Vitamin and Mineral Requirements

You can get enough of the micronutrients you need by:

- Eating a balanced diet.
- Taking your supplements as recommended.
- Getting tested regularly for deficiencies so you can be sure to catch them early, before they become serious.

All of the micronutrients are essential, but you're more likely to be deficient in certain vitamins and minerals than others. These include the following[14]

- Iron
- Calcium
- Vitamin D
- Zinc
- Vitamin E
- Vitamin K
- Folic acid
- Vitamin B12

Table 30 includes some of the most likely nutrients of concern. It includes their functions in your body—why you need them—as well as why you might be deficient and which foods you can get them from.

You definitely *do not* need to memorize this table! These are some of the main points to get:

Vitamin or Mineral and Requirement	Why You Need It and Other Background Information15	Reasons for Potential Deficiency	Food Sources
Iron (8 milligrams per day for men and postmenopausal women; 18 milligrams per day for menstruating women)	• Lets your red blood cells carry oxygen to the cells in your body. • Iron deficiency is the most common micronutrient deficiency in the world. • Iron deficiency is pretty widespread in the U.S. too especially among women and teenage girls. • Deficiency leads to anemia, with symptoms of fatigue and weakness.	• Lower intake of iron because of restricted diet (low-calorie diet) • Increased losses if you have bleeding from complications with the sleeve or during/after your surgery • Lower intake of vitamin C, which increases iron absorption from vegetarian foods • Intake of vitamin C not at the same time as intake of iron from plant-based foods • Having a heavy menstrual cycle; anemia is common in women with heavy blood losses.	• Red meat, including beef, liver, and pork • Seafood, such as oysters and tuna • Legumes, such as kidney beans and lentils • Fortified grains, such as bread, breakfast cereal, rice, and pasta • Potatoes, tofu, and nuts • Raisins and prunes
Calcium (1,000 to 1500 milligrams per day)	• Forms a major part of bone mineral • Necessary for strong bones • Prevents osteoporosis later in life • Losing bone mineral density is nearly irreversible.	• Rapid weight loss, as with the sleeve, increases calcium excretion (you lose more calcium from your body and bones). • Inadequate intake from diet, which is likely if you're having less than three servings per day of high-calcium dairy products on your sleeve diet • Decreased absorption from the diet after the sleeve	• Milk, cheese, and yogurt • Fortified breakfast cereals and breads; check the label to see if it has at least 10% of the daily value (DV) for calcium. • Canned fish, such as salmon and sardines, because it has bones in it. Of course, you'll only be able to eat canned fish with bones when you're well into Phase 4 of the sleeve diet, or the solid foods diet. • Fortified tofu, soymilk, and other soy products

Vitamin or Mineral and Requirement	Why You Need It and Other Background Information15	Reasons for Potential Deficiency	Food Sources
Vitamin D (400 to 4,000 International Units [IU] per day)	• Helps your body absorb calcium from food • Helps your body regulate calcium so you can have strong bones • Deficiency can lead to bone problems such as osteoporosis and osteomalacia. • Deficiency may increase your risk for heart disease.	• Low dietary intake, which is common because it's not in many foods • Reduced absorption due to very low-fat diet • Not enough exposure to high-intensity sun (common in northern climates and if you stay indoors) • Older adults • Dark-skinned individuals	• Vitamin D-fortified milk • Fish oil and fatty fish • Some fortified products (e.g., some breakfast cereals, orange juice, and yogurt [read the label])
Zinc (15 milligrams per day)	• Supports a healthy immune system • Needed for proper wound healing16	• Low dietary intake, especially if you don't have much red meat or shellfish • Low fat intake on the sleeve diet	• Shellfish (e.g., oysters and crab) • Dark-meat chicken and turkey • Beef and pork • Beans • Nuts • Milk and yogurt
Potassium (at least 4,700 milligrams per day)	• Needed to maintain a healthy (lower) blood pressure • Can prevent muscle cramps	• Diet low in fruits and vegetables, which can occur if you're not careful to eat them right after protein on the sleeve diet • Diet high in processed foods and sodium because that increases your need for potassium	• Potatoes • Beans, lentils • Winter squash • Most fruits, including bananas • Most vegetables • Meat and fish • Potassium supplements are rare.

Vitamin or Mineral and Requirement	Why You Need It and Other Background Information15	Reasons for Potential Deficiency	Food Sources
Vitamin E (15 milligrams, or 22.5 international units, per day)	• Has heart-healthy antioxidant functions • May reduce your risk of developing cataracts and macular degeneration • Severe deficiency is rare, but lower-than-optimal levels are common in the U.S. and sleeve patients.	• Low-fat diet, such as the sleeve diet, because of reduced vitamin E absorption • Low intake of vitamin E because it's mostly in high-fat foods and you're not eating many of those on the sleeve diet.	• Avocados • Nuts and peanut butter • Seeds (be sure you chew them well!) • Vegetable oils and salad dressings • Whole grains • Carrots • Spinach
Vitamin C (60 milligrams per day)	• Strong immune system • Antioxidant functions • Supports heart health • Necessary for proper wound healing • Increases your absorption of iron from plant-based foods • Deficiency is rare but higher intake can be healthy.	• Low intake of fresh fruits and vegetables • Diet high in processed foods	• Citrus fruits, such as oranges and tangerines—but be sure to wait until later in Phase 4 when you're used to eating solid foods • Vegetables, such as red peppers, tomatoes, broccoli, and kale • Many other fruits, such as papaya, pineapple, kiwis, cantaloupe, and berries • Potatoes
Vitamin A (900 micrograms, or 3,000 international units, per day for men; 700 micrograms, or 2,333 international units, per day for women)	• Antioxidant functions • Night vision and maintaining eye health • Deficiency can cause night blindness • Toxicity from supplements can lead to liver damage • A high amount of beta-carotene, the form of vitamin A in plant foods, is not dangerous.	• Very low intake on the sleeve diet can prevent absorption. • Low intake of fruits and vegetables • Toxicity can result from unnecessary vitamin A supplements.	• Orange vegetables, such as carrots, sweet potatoes, yams, and acorn squash • Orange fruit, such as cantaloupe and mangos (watch for strings) • Green leafy vegetables, such as spinach • Butter • Liver and cod liver oil

Vitamin or Mineral and Requirement	Why You Need It and Other Background Information15	Reasons for Potential Deficiency	Food Sources
Vitamin K (120 micrograms per day for men; 90 micrograms per day for women)	• Normal blood clotting • Supplements can interfere with blood-thinning medications (anti-coagulants, such as warfarin).	• Very low intake of dietary fat on the sleeve diet • Low dietary intake of vitamin K from restricted sleeve diet	• Leafy green vegetables • Other vegetables • Fruits • Vegetable oils
Folic Acid (vitamin B-9) (400 micrograms per day)	• Adequate intake is needed for preventing neural tube birth defects, such as spina bifida. • May be heart-healthy • May lower your risk for some cancers • Healthy red blood cells • Deficiency can cause anemia.	• Low intake of folate or folic acid from the diet • The sleeve diet emphasizes proteins, but meats and poultry don't have folate.	• Fortified grains—the same ones as for iron • Legumes, such as lima beans, garbanzo beans, and lentils • Orange juice • Leafy green vegetables, such as kale, and spinach • Asparagus
Vitamin B-12 (12 micrograms per day)	• Good nerve functioning; deficiency can cause permanent nerve damage. • Only naturally in animal-derived products • Healthy red blood cells • Deficiency can cause anemia.	• Plant-based diet; avoiding animal foods • Low intake from limited sleeve diet • Slightly decreased absorption because of a smaller stomach • Medications used to treat esophageal reflux17	• Seafood, such as clams, mussels, crab, salmon, and tuna • Meat and poultry, such as beef and chicken • Eggs and dairy products • Fortified foods, such as some breakfast cereals—read the label
Other B vitamins: Thiamin (B1), Riboflavin (B2), Niacin (B3), Pantothenic acid (B5), Vitamin (B6)	• Needed for energy production with many food sources; most Americans get plenty. You need these B vitamins for proper metabolism of nutrients.	• Low dietary intake from limited amount of food on a low-calorie sleeve diet • Vomiting can cause thiamin deficiency shortly after the VSG surgery.18	• Whole grains • Protein foods • Nuts and beans • Bread • Milk • Potatoes • Vegetables • Eggs

Table 36: Selected vitamins and minerals and their functions and food sources

- Eating a variety of foods will help you get the nutrients you need.
- Choosing healthy foods will help you get the nutrients you need. You already know that healthy, nutrient-dense foods include meat and poultry, seafood, legumes, vegetables, whole grains, dairy products, and fruit. These come up a lot on the table.
- The table doesn't include junk foods—they're not your best sources of nutrients.

When in doubt, choose healthy! Go for unprocessed foods instead of processed. Even without thinking about calories, saturated fat, and sugar, you can see that unprocessed foods are healthier—most of the good sources listed are foods that we think of as "healthy."

Don't Forget Your Supplements!

You can't overestimate the value of a balanced, nutritious diet. However, a well-planned assortment of dietary supplements can greatly reduce your risk of developing nutrient deficiencies when you're on the sleeve diet. A daily multivitamin is common. These specific supplements are also common:[19]

- Iron (likely with vitamin C to increase absorption)
- Vitamin B12
- Calcium
- Vitamin D
- Folic acid (most likely if you're a woman who may become pregnant)

Your surgeon and dietitian might also recommend taking supplements of one or more of these if they think you're at risk for developing deficiencies:

- Zinc
- Selenium
- Thiamin, or vitamin B1
- Vitamins A, E, or K

Anemia and the Sleeve

Anemia is a big problem among sleeve patients. One study found that 26% of sleeve patients had anemia within 6 to 12 months after their surgeries.[20] Anemia makes you feel tired and irritable and can interfere with concentration. More severe anemia can cause shortness of breath, brittle nails, and lightheadedness.[21]

The reason why you get these symptoms when you have anemia is because anemia is caused by lower-than-normal levels of healthy red blood cells. That can happen when you have one or more of the following problems:

- *Your red blood cells are not formed correctly / they are immature or deformed* – This can happen with a folic acid or vitamin B12 deficiency, since your body needs those vitamins for making red blood.

- *You don't have enough red blood cells / you lose a lot of blood* – This can happen during or after surgery.
- *Your red blood cells don't do a good job of carrying oxygen to the cells in your body, including your muscles and brain* – This can happen with iron deficiency because iron is what allows your red blood cells to carry oxygen.

Taking another look at the above table, you can see that nutritional anemia can result from a deficiency of folic acid, vitamin B12 or iron. You can be low in these nutrients because of low intake from your diet and low absorption. You're always at risk for anemia after you get the sleeve, so it's important to continue to follow your physician and dietitian's recommendations for nutritious foods, dietary supplements, and regular blood tests to monitor your status.

Long-Term Consequences of Nutrient Deficiencies

Nutrient deficiencies are a threat for as long as you're following the sleeve diet, so you're almost certain to need supplements for life.[22] Nutrient deficiencies are serious; they're not to be taken lightly. Some nutrient deficiency symptoms aren't permanent, and they go away when you get your nutrient levels back to normal. Other nutrient deficiency diseases, though, have irreversible symptoms, and unless you get tested regularly, you may not notice that you're deficient until it's too late. Osteoporosis, peripheral neuropathy, and heart disease are some of the potential long-term consequences of certain nutrient deficiencies.[23]

Osteoporosis

Osteoporosis is a condition with lower-than-normal bone mineral density and a higher-than-normal risk for fractures or broken bones. We tend to think of this as an old person's disease because that's when fractures are most likely to occur, but your bones might become increasingly thin and brittle for years before you break a bone and realize that you have osteoporosis. You're already at higher risk for osteoporosis after getting the gastric sleeve because of your rapid weight loss. Fast weight loss increases the rate at which you lose bone mineral density. Inadequate amounts of calcium and vitamin D also cause osteoporosis. You can reduce your risk for osteoporosis by:

- Getting enough calcium
- Getting enough vitamin D
- Participating in weight-bearing physical activities or exercises

There's no easy blood test to tell whether you're getting enough calcium. The best way to ensure that you are is to have at least three servings per day of high-calcium foods. Fortified foods, fatty fish, and plenty of sunshine help you get vitamin D. Also take any supplements recommended by your surgeon or dietitian.

Peripheral Neuropathy

Peripheral neuropathy is damage to one or more nerves that connect your brain to your spinal cord or your spinal cord to other parts of your body.[24] Peripheral neuropathy has many possible causes, and as a sleeve patient, you're at risk for peripheral neuropathy caused by deficiency of vitamin B12. Symptoms may become permanent, and they include the following: *numbness and tingling of the feet and hands, a sore tongue, loss of appetite, constipation, trouble walking, confusion and loss of memory*

- Following these steps can reduce your risk for peripheral neuropathy:
- Get plenty of protein from animal-based sources: meat, fish, poultry, dairy products, eggs.
- Choose breakfast cereals and other foods that are fortified with vitamin B12 (check the label).
- Get your levels of vitamin B12 tested regularly.
- Take dietary supplements if recommended by your surgeon and/or dietitian.

Fortified Foods: What Are They, and What's in Them?

We've already mentioned fortified foods several times because they're great ways to get certain nutrients. Fortification means that the manufacturer adds extra vitamins or minerals to food. Certain foods are required to have certain nutrients. For example, fortified milk in the United States always contains vitamin D and vitamin A. Fortified grains, including bread, flour, cereal, rice, and pasta, contain extra amounts of these nutrients:

- Vitamin B1 (thiamin)
- Vitamin B2 (riboflavin)
- Vitamin B3 (niacin)
- Folic acid
- Iron

Fortified foods may also contain additional nutrients. They're not required by law, though, so you need to check the label to see whether your food contains them. These are some examples of common nutrient–food combinations, but you need to read the label to make sure that these foods contain the nutrients you're looking for:

- Calcium and vitamin D in fortified breakfast cereals, orange juice, and soy milk
- Vitamin B12 in breakfast cereals and vegetarian meat substitutes
- Vitamin D in yogurt
- Calcium in pudding

Don't Let Vitamin and Mineral Supplements Turn into Too Much of a Good Thing

Overdoses and chronic toxicity from high levels of vitamins and minerals from supplements can be just as dangerous as deficiencies. For that reason, it's best not to automatically take supplements without first asking an expert. One study of bariatric surgery patients found that 48% had high blood levels of vitamin A, 31% were high in vitamin B1, and 30% were high vitamin in B6.[25] Consequences depend on which vitamins and minerals you're taking, how much extra you're taking, and how long you've been taking more than you need. They can include liver problems, an increased risk for heart disease, higher risk of kidney stones, and/or other nutrient deficiencies because of blocked absorption.[26]

Condiments, Water and Alcohol While on the Sleeve Diet

Sometimes we treat condiments as afterthoughts, but they're worth thinking about. They can throw off your weight loss if you're not careful. Condiments include the sauces, spreads, spices, dips, and garnishes that can make your food taste better or make your meal feel complete. Some condiments are pretty innocent, but others have enough calories to threaten your weight loss. Most of them are low in essential nutrients.

How Many Calories Can Condiments Contribute?

Take a look at the following table to get an idea of how many calories you can get from what seems like just a few condiments. The table shows a day on the sleeve diet with just one or two "extras" at each meal.

Table 37 is a sample day on the sleeve diet with a few condiments. Notice how quickly just a few small amounts of condiments can add up!

Meal or Snack	Foods with Condiments	Extra Calories from Condiments
Breakfast	Toast with 1 tablespoon jam (50 calories) and 1 teaspoon butter (30 calories)	80 calories
Snack 1	Tuna salad with 1 tablespoon mayonnaise (90 calories)	90 calories
Lunch	Deli turkey with 2 tablespoons cream cheese (100 calories); green beans with 1 teaspoon butter (30 calories)	130 calories
Snack 2	½ cup pasta with 2 tablespoons pesto sauce (110 calories)	110 calories
Dinner	Ground turkey burger with 2 tablespoons ketchup (30 calories) and 1 tablespoon sweet relish (20 calories)	50 calories
Snack 3	Fruit salad with 2 tablespoons sweetened whipped cream (30 calories)	30 calories
Beverages	Coffee with 1 container creamer (30 calories) and 2 sugar packets (30 calories)	60 calories
Total		550 calories

Table 37: Notice how quickly just a few small amounts of condiments can add up!

What's the Scoop on Sodium?

Sodium is an essential nutrient because it's necessary for life. Like potassium, sodium is a mineral and an electrolyte. Both help maintain water balance in your body. So why are you always hearing that you should lower your sodium intake? While potassium helps lower blood pressure by letting your body get rid of extra water, sodium is linked to high blood pressure because it encourages your body to hold onto water.

You already know that salt makes you retain water if you've ever felt bloated after eating a salty meal! Water retention doesn't just make you feel uncomfortable. It's actually unhealthy. The extra water that you retain gives you an extra high volume of blood, which raises your blood pressure and puts strain on your kidneys.

The average American gets 3,400 milligrams of sodium per day. That's more than the recommended maximum of 2,300 milligrams and far more than the amount you really need to survive, which is probably slightly over 500 milligrams per day. You can get about that much by having a cup of milk, an egg and two slices of bread. You can get to 500 milligrams just by eating three ounces of canned salmon, or a half-cup of canned soup! You're only going to be deficient if you have some sort of health problem, such as severe dehydration.

Another reason to keep your sodium intake in check is because excessive sodium makes your sleeve experience more difficult. A high-salt diet makes you thirstier so that you want to drink more, but drinking extra fluid can be a challenge when you're already struggling to hit your 1.5 liters of water per day on the sleeve diet. You can't drink within 30 minutes of eating solid food, so it's hard to increase your fluid intake when you're trying to make up for extra sodium consumption.

Most high-sodium food sources are prepared and processed foods because of their high amount of salt, which is very high in sodium. In fact, a single teaspoon of salt has more than 2,300 milligrams of sodium! These are some foods that are high in sodium:

- Canned soups; broth and bouillon powders and cubes; dry soup mixes
- Other canned foods, such as canned beans and other vegetables,
- Frozen meals and appetizers
- Bread – Surprisingly, bread is the single biggest source of sodium for Americans!
- Ready-to-eat foods, such as pasta dishes, pizza, and Chinese food
- Salty snack foods, such as peanuts, pretzels, popcorn, crackers, and potato chips
- Salty sauces and dressings, such as soy sauce, tomato sauce, and Italian salad dressing
- Cheese
- Cured foods, such as pickles, olives, and sauerkraut

A general guideline for when you're trying to limit your sodium intake is to choose less processed options. The more processing steps and the further the food is from its natural source, the more sodium it is likely to have. Yes, many kinds of foods naturally have a small amount of sodium. Meat, fish, celery, and tomatoes are examples. But, fresh meat is far lower in sodium than sausages or cold cuts; fresh fish is lower than canned, and celery and tomatoes are lower in sodium than vegetable juice.

You can also lower your sodium intake by choosing low-sodium or reduced-salt options, such as low-sodium canned vegetables and unsalted pretzels. Using herbs, spices, and low-sodium dressings can also help you reduce the amount of salt and salty seasonings you use while still enjoying flavorful foods.

Source[27]

As you can see, this sample day is pretty realistic. It has only one or two extras at each meal or snack. Those extras, though, add up to 550 calories! If you add an extra 550 calories per day to your sleeve diet without realizing it, your weight loss will slow by more than a pound a week. If you're trying to maintain your weight loss or you've hit a plateau, you might even gain weight because of extra condiments.

Tips to Keep Condiments in Check

So what can you do to maintain a tasty, satisfying diet while you prevent condiments from sabotaging your weight loss? These suggestions may help:

- Measure and record your condiments—don't just let them sneak into your diet.
- Limit your portion size. Using ½ tablespoon mayo instead of 1 tablespoon in your tuna salad saves you 50 calories, and you probably won't even notice the difference.
- Use fewer condiments at a time. Instead of butter *and* jam to make your toast less dry, try using butter *or* jam. Another benefit of using fewer condiments is that your toast will be a little bit drier. It'll help you eat slower because it will take longer to chew.
- Make better choices. Substitute more nutritious, lower-calorie choices for regular high-calorie options. In general, try to avoid high-fat, high-calorie, high-sugar condiments.

Condiment Substitutions to Try

Table 38 compares some poorer condiment choices with some substitutes that can be healthier or lower-calorie choices. Regularly choosing better options will eventually show up on the scale.

Instead of...	Consider...
1 tablespoon of butter on a baked potato or vegetables: 100 calories and high saturated fat	Melted low-fat cheese: 60 calories, including some protein and calcium
2 tablespoons full-fat salad dressing: 200 calories	2 tablespoons reduced-calorie dressing: 20 calories
1 tablespoon of regular mayonnaise: 90 calories	1 tablespoon of fat-free mayonnaise: 15 calories
2 tablespoons of ranch, French onion, and other regular dips: 120–200 calories, high-fat	2 tablespoons of hummus (garbanzo bean dip): 60 calories, high in protein 2 tablespoons salsa: 20 calories, fat-free
1 tablespoon flavored coffee creamer: 35 calories	1 tablespoon fat-free milk: 5 calories
1 tablespoon of fruit preserves, jam or jelly: 50 calories, high-sugar	½ cup applesauce or half mashed banana: 50 calories
1 ounce (2 tablespoons) pesto or alfredo sauce: 50 calories, high-fat	¼ cup tomato or pizza sauce: 50 calories
1 tablespoon of butter or margarine: 100 calories	1 tablespoon reduced-fat margarine: 50 calories
Salt and salty seasonings	Herbs and spices (e.g., oregano, thyme, rosemary, black pepper, marjoram, caraway, dill, garlic)
1 tablespoon of sugar or honey (50 calories)	½ tablespoon sugar or honey plus cinnamon and cloves (25 calories)

Table 38: Condiment Substitutions to Try

Good Condiment Choices Can Promote Success on the Sleeve Diet

Well-chosen condiments can encourage good choices on the sleeve diet. For example, you can use teriyaki sauce or fat-free marinade, such as a lemon-pepper or Italian herb marinade, to prevent dryness and persuade you to grill or bake chicken breast or fish instead of frying it. Soy sauce with some herbs and spices, such as garlic and ginger, can liven up your vegetables to encourage you to eat healthier.

Balance the benefits you get from the extra taste and change in texture from condiments with the possible disadvantages of the extra calories. You can still have great-tasting food on the sleeve diet. Just be mindful of your condiments the same way you are with all your other food

Water

Water is actually the sixth nutrient; the other five are protein, carbohydrates, fat, vitamins, and minerals. You need about 8–13 cups of fluid per day.[28] Watery foods such as soups, vegetables, and fruits count toward your fluid needs, and the recommendation for VSG patients is to aim for at least 1.5 liters, or 6 to 7 cups, of non-caloric beverages per day. Besides keeping you hydrated, water has the advantage of being a natural appetite suppressant—it helps you fill up without adding calories.

Alternatives to Plain Water

Some people don't like drinking water. That may just be because you're not used to it. With some practice, you might be able to train yourself to like water instead of sugar-sweetened soft drinks or other sugary options. There are still plenty of alternatives to plain water if you just can't bring yourself to drink enough. These are some suggestions for calorie-free or low-calorie beverages:

- Ice water. Ice-cold water can be more palatable than room-temperature.
- Water with a slice of lemon or lime or a sprig of fresh mint (you can find it in your grocery store's produce section with the other fresh herbs)
- Diet drinks. diet fruit drinks, diet iced tea (avoid carbonated beverages—they will increase your risk of stretching your sleeve and causing leaks)
- Calorie-free flavored waters (still water; not sparkling or carbonated)
- Hot or iced coffee, green tea, or black tea—without cream or sugar. You can use artificial sweeteners, such as saccharin in the pink packet, aspartame in the blue packet, or sucralose in the yellow packet. They have almost no calories. Be careful about the caffeine content, especially when you're still close to your surgery date.

Milk is high in protein, calcium, and vitamin D, but it does have calories. Your surgeon or dietitian might allow fat-free or 1 percent reduced-fat milk on the sleeve diet but only in moderation. Better choices for weight loss might be a calorie-free beverage for your fluid and fortified fat-free yogurt and reduced-fat cheese for getting your calcium and vitamin D.

Caffeine and the Sleeve

A lot of people worry that caffeine will dehydrate them. It's true that caffeine is a diuretic; it increases the amount of water that your body loses in urine. However, the effect is small enough so that caffeinated beverages such as coffee and tea still count toward your daily water requirements. Avoid caffeine if you notice that it keeps you up at night or gives you heartburn.

Plan Your Fluid Intake Carefully!

Your weight loss and health will be better if you take your hydration as seriously as you take your diet. These are a few reminders and tips to help you plan your fluid intake:

- Aim for 6 to 7 cups per day.
- Stick to water or other non-caloric (or low-calorie) beverages.
- Keep water handy so you remember to drink it. Have a water bottle in your car and desk and keep a pitcher of water in the fridge.
- Don't drink within 30 minutes before or after eating solid foods.

Alcohol and the Vertical Sleeve

What about alcohol? It's not an essential nutrient. Moderate consumption of red wine may have some benefits for your heart. It may raise your levels of healthy HDL cholesterol and help protect your blood vessels against damage.[29] Alcohol also helps you relax. However, drinking alcoholic beverages can throw off your weight loss and cause health problems.

Calories, Alcohol, and Your Weight

Alcoholic beverages are high in calories. Each gram of alcohol has seven calories, and that's not even counting the carbohydrates that are in some alcoholic beverages.

- A 5-ounce serving of wine has 130 calories; an 8-ounce cup has 200 calories, or about twice as many as a glass of juice.
- A 1.4-ounce shot of vodka has 103 calories, or nearly 600 calories in an 8-ounce cup.
- A 12-ounce can of beer contains 164 calories.

Drinking alcohol can cause you to take in more calories than you wanted to. Beyond the calories in the alcoholic beverage, the alcohol relaxes you so much that it makes you lose your inhibition. That means that you're less able to resist high-calorie foods and more likely to give in to temptations. You're also more likely to eat without planning for it or writing it down. Drinking alcohol may not be worth it after the sleeve because you don't want to work so hard to lose weight and then end up taking in way more calories than you wanted just because your judgment isn't good.

Other Concerns with Alcoholic Beverages

Alcohol, even in moderation, can cause problems in addition to interfering with weight loss:[30]

- It can make your blood sugar levels spike.
- It interferes with memory.
- It can increase blood pressure.
- It can damage your liver.

Alcohol Metabolism and the Sleeve

You may be more susceptible to the effects of alcohol after the sleeve gastrectomy than you were before it.[31] Your blood alcohol content may get to higher levels than before, and alcohol can stay in your system for longer than it did before the sleeve. Although not all studies have found that the sleeve changes your alcohol metabolism,[32] it is best, based on current knowledge, to avoid alcohol with the sleeve.

Pay attention to Food Labels & Make Healthy Choices

We're very lucky in the U.S. to have such strict standards for food labeling. If you've grown up in the U.S. and haven't left the country much, you probably take our food labels for granted. They're relatively complete and are fairly straightforward. Almost every food item that you can find has a label with these required components:

- The weight of the package
- The number of servings in the package
- A nutrition facts panel with nutrition information per serving
- A list of ingredients
- Any common allergens

The Nutrition Facts Panel: One of Your New Best Friends

The nutrition facts panel is tightly regulated, so it's easy to use. Federal regulations require that nutrition facts panels be standardized, so they all look very similar and have certain information.[33] Once you learn your way around one label, you'll be able to navigate your way around any food label.

The nutrition facts panel is required to contain information on the nutrients that are most likely to be of concern; that is, the nutrients which Americans eat too much or too little of on average. A typical nutrition facts panel looks like this. *Figure 3* is a picture of a standard nutrition label and some of its components.

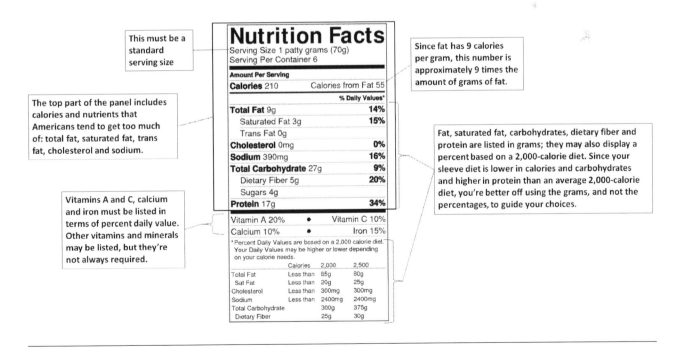

Figure 3: Standard Nutrition Label

It's relatively easy to use food labels to your advantage once you know how. Each food has a required set of information that must be listed, and in many cases, the information must be listed in a certain order so that it's easy for you to find. In this section, you'll learn your way around the food label so you know how to make the best choices.

The nutrition label can be a key to your success with the sleeve. The nutrition label provides a wealth of information. Nearly all packaged foods are required to have nutrition labels, and they have to have specific information on them. The required nutrients on the nutrition label are mandated because they're concerning to the general population—because most people get too much of them or too little of them.

Food Regulation in the U.S.

The Food, Drug and Cosmetic Act, or FDCA is the groundbreaking legislation that governs most food products in the U.S. The Food and Drug Administration, or FDA, and the U.S. Department of Agriculture, or USDA, are the two main federal agencies that carry out the FDCA and regulate food in the U.S. They're responsible for food safety and for helping consumers make informed decisions about the food they eat.

- The USDA regulates raw meat, poultry, and egg products. Some of the nutrition labeling requirements are the same as the FDA's, but some aren't. The USDA doesn't require small businesses to provide nutrition information about their products. The USDA also administers the National Organic Program (NOP). Foods that are USDA-certified organic are produced without synthetic pesticides, fertilizers, or other chemicals. They are all-natural.

- The FDA regulates most food products, including fish and mixed dishes containing meats and poultry, such as frozen dinners. Most of the food products and labels that you see in stores are regulated by the FDA. The nutrition label that we discussed above is the label required by the FDA on these products. If you're choosing unpackaged foods like raw fish, fruits, and vegetables, the nutrition information might be posted in the section of the grocery store right near the food product, but it's not yet required by law.

- The Bureau of Alcohol, Tobacco and Firearms regulates alcoholic beverages. That's why the information you see on bottles of beer, wine, and liquor is a little different than labels on foods and other beverages.

Source:[34, 35, 36, 37, 38, 39]

The List of Ingredients Is Full of Useful Information

The ingredients list is more than "the fine print" to skim over. It often provides extra information that you might not gather just from reading the nutrition label. The ingredients are listed in order of weight. That means that the first ingredients that are listed are the main ingredients, and the ones listed toward the end are only there in small amounts. This information can help you make healthier choices.

- A grain product whose first ingredient is a "whole" grain or flour has more whole grains than a product whose first ingredient is "enriched" or "refined."
- A product with sugar, corn syrup, honey, or another kind of sugar listed first has more sugar than any other ingredient and is probably not very healthy.

You can also use the list of ingredients to avoid certain ingredients. These are some examples of ingredients that you might want or need to avoid to protect the vertical sleeve and your health:

- Ingredients that you might be allergic to, such as soy or eggs
- Partially hydrogenated oils, which contain trans fat
- Additives that you're sensitive to, such as monosodium glutamate (MSG)
- Foods that aren't allowed on your current diet, such as nuts and raisins when you're still recovering from the VSG and you're not yet on a fully solid foods diet

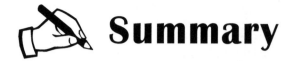

Summary

☞ By now you're not only an expert at the sleeve diet but you're also close to being an expert nutritionist. You know what it means to make nutritious choices that will promote weight loss and your health.

☞ This chapter has the information you need to select the healthiest foods and meet your nutrient needs. You now have the tools you need to create and follow a gastric sleeve diet:

  • Which foods to select

  • How much to eat

  • How to create a daily menu

  • Which nutrients to emphasize

  • Vitamin and mineral supplements to consider

  • How to stay hydrated

  • Pitfalls to avoid

☞ The book has covered the diet part of your sleeve lifestyle. Now it's time to take a look at another factor in your weight loss: exercise. It's not as scary or hard as you might think. The next chapter goes over the basics of starting an exercise program from the very beginning— even if you're not used to exercising at all.

Your Turn: Keeping a Detailed Diet Record

The diet record may become a key to your weight loss success with the vertical sleeve. It helps you stay truthful to yourself about your diet intake. This is some information that should go in a diet record—give it a try! Be very specific about quantities and condiments to make sure you don't forget anything.

Meal or Snack	What did you eat?	Describe the meal setting and how it affected you.	Record other notes here. How hungry were you before and after the meal or snack? Did you eat what you planned?
Sample	3 ounces lean ground turkey, 1 tablespoon ketchup, one-half whole-wheat English muffin, half-cup cooked carrots	Family dinner with the wife and kids. I focused on talking to them rather than wolfing my food.	Pleasant meal. Chewed everything well and felt satisfied (but could have eaten more) by the end. Ate exactly what I'd planned.
Breakfast			
Lunch			
Dinner			
Any snacks			

Table 39: Maintain a detailed diet record

A Glimpse into My Life with the Sleeve...Queen of Crop

Snapshot

59 years old

Starting Weight: 223 pounds

Current Weight: 151 pounds

Height: 5'3"

Wife and former Internet hotel salesperson

Loves traveling, dogs, interior design, gardening, and entertaining

First Things First: Why "Queen of Crop?"

Because for the last 10 years every photo I have had taken I have either "cropped" me out or cropped below my neck or cropped whatever I could get away with so I wouldn't have to see how big I was compared to others. As they say, photos are worth a thousand words. But they were words I didn't want to hear; so began my long descent into denial about my weight as I kept gaining year after year.

Not "Even" a Yo-Yo Dieter

I was never a yo-yo dieter—ever. I could never lose enough weight to gain it back. I basically kept gaining a few pounds every year. I got irritated when people would talk about how easy it was to lose weight, and that it was maintenance that was hard. I was mad because I never lost anything significant on any diet, so maintenance was never even a consideration for me. It isn't that I didn't try every diet out there; I did. And after a week or two or three or a month after what seemed like a lot of effort and feeling hungry and deprived, I had only lost one pound or maybe two if I stood a certain way on the scale and remembered to take my earrings off. So I would get very discouraged and bag whatever diet I was on—one more failed attempt.

It was so depressing because I never felt that I had an eating disorder: I wasn't a closet eater, I ate pretty healthily (not perfect, but I never ate huge portions or binged or ate late at night), and I didn't feel like I ate more than my husband who is 6' tall and usually weighs in the 150s. I'm 5'3" and went from 165 lbs to 223 lbs from 1991 to 2011. I was a fat baby, a fat kid, a fat cheerleader, and a fat bride, but at 165 pounds, I felt pretty good given I had been fat all my life. Now, as I was approaching my 60s and topped the scales at 223 pounds, I had almost lost hope that I would ever be a normal size.

Even though I didn't eat a lot of food, I gained. About three pounds a year doesn't sound like much. But over the course of 20 years that's almost 60 pounds on top of a starting weight that was already high. And as anyone knows who has struggled with their weight (or managed it as my husband always has), it's not hard to gain three pounds in a year. Most of us could do that in one meal!

So even though I never felt my eating was out of control, I didn't move. I barely exercised from 2003 to 2011. I've never been that physical to begin with, we were building a business, and

I just never made it a priority. Plus, as the weight piled on, it got harder. My husband, on the other hand, ran three miles every day, and if he gained three pounds, he focused on what he ate until those three pounds came off.

Diets Would Never Work, but Something Needed to Be Done

So bottom line, I was never successful at diets, and at some level, I think I knew I never would be.

Some people have "ah-ha" moments — they see a horrible photo of themselves, they bend over to pick something up and rip their pants, they sit down and the chair breaks — and decide they have had enough and opt for weight loss surgery. Mine was a little different. It went like this: My husband and I had retired, and we were traveling for a year. We had landed in Amsterdam and stayed for four months because we loved it. In Europe, especially Amsterdam, the women are tall, healthy, unbelievably gorgeous, and just amazing to look — okay, stare — at; even I couldn't take my eyes off these beauties. We also had lots of company, both European and American friends, who were all thin and elegant. We were basically dazzled by these women, and as my normally strong sense of self went down the toilet, my husband started wondering how he wound up with the fattest girl in the room. He loved me very much, but let's be honest, he was feeling pretty conflicted, understandably. And not just because he adores beautiful women (which was a big part of it) but also he could see my weight was killing me. I limped because my hip and knees and feet hurt, I had high cholesterol, and I was grumpy because I was the fattest, worst-dressed person around. He had lived with it for a long time and saw it getting progressively worse; it finally got to him, and he had a meltdown about it. It was really hard for him to get to this point, but it got us talking about the elephant (me) in the room.

Choosing the Sleeve over the Band

We decided it was time for surgery — which we knew little about — but we instinctively knew that another diet attempt was not the answer. We thought about coming back to the U.S. to have it done, but I was pretty sure our insurance wouldn't cover it, or if it did, because of my hip and knee problems, it would still be a very long, bureaucratic process, and we didn't want to go back to the U.S. just yet. So, we started looking at options in Europe, and we found a U.S.-based service called European Medical Tourist. They, in turn, found a hospital and doctor not far from Amsterdam, who specializes in WLS. In the meantime, I had started reading everything I could about the options, including a blog from a woman who had had the lap band procedure, and she was very successful with it. I found the blog inspiring, and it helped me make the decision to have a lap band myself.

When it came time to have my phone consultation with Dr. Rudolph Weiner, known as the "rock star" of weight loss surgery in Germany, I got a big shock. He basically told me in his no-nonsense way that he would NOT recommend the lap band but the vertical sleeve procedure. Now, I had never heard of VSG or done any research on it, but he was a bit intimidating on the phone, so I timidly said okay.

I immediately started doing research on this procedure, and of course, the first thing that stood out was that it was not reversible. After I had wrapped my head around that fact, I also learned that the lap band had many problems and the sleeve was the most effective outside of the bypass, which was really out of my comfort zone. My husband found the Vertical Sleeve Talk forum [now known as BariatricPal], and once I started reading and participating in that, I started getting excited about my new future.

Using the Forums and Preparing for Surgery

The European Medical Tourist (EMT) program organized my stay at the Krankenhaus Sachsenhausen hospital in Frankfurt, Germany. I was very pleased with the quick responses to our questions from the EMT group but not very happy that I received very little pre-surgery information, especially after reading in the posts on the forum all the details that people had to go through. And the entire process was fast: I decided on the vertical sleeve at the end of September 2011 and less than four weeks later was having the surgery. During that time, I was given very little information on how to prepare. The forum was a huge resource to me during this time. I have never had a dietician, nutritionist, support group, or psychologist — not before, during, or after — so the forum became the place for me to go with questions.

Checking into the hospital was a bit surreal. I think I was the smallest one in the waiting room. Most people were solemn, scared and quiet and had very little eye contact with anyone. It was sad; I think most people felt embarrassed that they had to resort to such drastic measures to become acceptable to society, and most probably thought it was their fault and that they were big fat failures. I felt a little of that, but mostly, I was excited and ready to get it over with.

I do remember going into several different rooms for paperwork or weighing in; I would go in one, then they would send me back out to the waiting room. Go in another, send me back out. They would call me again; and again, I would go back out to the waiting room. Then they called a fourth time, had me climb up on a gurney (fully clothed), asked me if I was allergic to anything — I said "no" — and then a nurse put something over my nose, the doctor waved and said "bye-bye," and I was out cold.

The next thing I knew, I was in a hospital room, still fully clothed and groggy. It turns out I had had my endoscopy done, and they had put me out — I sure wasn't expecting it to happen that way! I guess they do things differently in Europe. They then had me undress and put my hospital gown on. I put it on with the ties in front; I had never had any surgery before, so this was all new to me!

That night (Day 1) they gave me something to drink, and I had a wild poop fest. The next day I was wheeled into surgery and woke up in ICU, where I spent the night (Day 2). So, unlike U.S. hospitals where they get you in and get you out, I didn't even know what hit me until Day 3 when I woke up in my room; this is where I would spend the next five (yes, five) days. My entire hospital stay was supposed to be seven, but on Day 6 I got a serious bladder infection, so I stayed eight days. In those eight days, I had a liquid diet only, and I was just fine with that. I didn't feel hungry, my head was in a good space, my husband visited daily, and I had a series of roommates. The nurses were polite and spoke English, and Dr. Weiner came and visited me each day with his "entourage" of young groupie interns behind him, all with their requisite clipboards and all laughing and agreeing with every tidbit the professor would say. You could tell everyone adored him.

I always felt I was in good hands and well taken care of; looking back I am so grateful for the long stay in the hospital. When I hear about these overnight or two-day stays in the U.S. or Mexico, I personally can't imagine it. On the forum, some people talk about how they check into a hotel for a few days after surgery. I think I still had tubes in me on Day 4, including the self-administered pain reliever. They made sure I got up and walked and that I drank my liquids, and they brought me broth and took my vitals three or four times a day. When I got my bladder infection, they hooked me up to an antibiotic IV immediately. What would I have done if I were hours away from the hospital?

Blogging a Sleeve Success Story – Anonymously

Because I was inspired so much by another woman's blog, I decided to chronicle my story every Sunday for the first year on my own blog, www.queenofcrop.com. I think my first year was a little different than most people's first year because of my living situation. After the operation, my husband and I went back to Amsterdam for three weeks, then we traveled throughout Europe and the U.S. for the next three to four months, which created its own challenge as I navigated the world of "What can I eat today without having a kitchen?" I'm quite sure I was the only person who spent two weeks in Italy and had no wine, no pasta, and no pizza! I was tired during that time, but it all worked out fine.

I made the personal decision to tell only a close circle of friends, and this decision has been validated over and over for me. Everyone is different, but this was the right decision for me. From those closest to me — my sister, several of my best friends, and, most especially, my husband — I could not have asked for more support. For my husband and me, this has turned out to be "our" journey, not just mine. Once we started talking about my weight and how it affected our past and our future, the floodgates just opened up. We started talking about our history together, what we liked, what we loved, what pissed us off, and most importantly, what we wanted the rest of our life to look like. We cried a lot, laughed some, and talked, talked, talked. By the time I went into surgery, I think we both knew our relationship had taken a big step forward. Having this life-changing surgery and going through it together has made us closer than any diet ever would have. The main reason we can talk so easily about it now is that it has worked; had it not been effective, it would still be an emotional, difficult topic.

Expensive but Worth It!

Cost: At the Euro-to-USD conversion rate at the time (which was high), we estimated the cost to be about $18,000. It was worth every penny of it.

The surgery has been successful beyond my wildest dreams. The first few months were tricky (especially since we were traveling). I had some friends who were visiting bring me some saltine crackers (can't find those in Europe), and I savored the two I ate every day. They helped keep my stomach settled. I ate very little and threw up a lot in the beginning. I couldn't drink coffee and was so sad about that, because I love a good cup of coffee. It took a few months, but I got my taste back for it. I experimented here and there with what I could eat; pasta, cereal, rice, and bread didn't make the cut for a long, long time. I still don't eat most of those, but I also don't miss them much. And when I do, I think about the tradeoffs, and I'm fine.

Along the way, while figuring out what my new stomach could handle, the weight came off. Week by week, my body was changing, and it was thrilling. In many ways, my body started matching my brain. Until we got to Amsterdam (the land of the beautiful people), I always felt confident, capable, and certainly comfortable with any group of people. I might have been overweight all my life, but I never felt that it stopped me from doing what I wanted to do. Now, finally, my body was on the same page as my mind! In less than a year, I lost over 80 pounds and reached my goal.

I learned so much during that first year. I could list a hundred things that I love about being thinner. Topping the list is being more healthy, being able to exercise, looking better, and having a closer relationship with my husband, but there are so many little things: crossing my legs, getting dressed, having lots of seatbelt left over on an airplane, eating a cookie without feeling guilty, buying clothes, feeling more in control, and who doesn't love all the compliments?

But I also became convinced beyond all doubt that some people (and I was one of them) cannot lose weight on traditional diets. Even with the sleeve, eating less than 500 calories a day for the first four months, then about 1000 calories a day for the next four months, and eventually working up to about 1200 calories and faithfully exercising for an hour a day, I lost an average of less than 1.7 lbs a week in the first year; more in the beginning, and then it leveled off. Weight Watchers and Jenny Craig told me I could eat between 1600 and 1900 calories a day and lose two to three pounds a week, and those plans felt much more restrictive and cumbersome and made me cranky. No wonder I (and so many others) failed. It might work for some, but it never worked for me and only made me feel like more of a failure.

There is little I'm not happy with. I have some saggy skin on my arms and breasts and upper legs. If I want to, I could have some cosmetic surgery to correct it. I'm not against it, and sure, I'd love to be firm — and my husband wouldn't mind either — but I'll have to see about the costs and risks to figure out if it's right for me. Even with saggy skin, our sex life is better and so much more fun. I'm used to eating very little at this point, and when we go out and I see these huge portions (especially in America), it's unsettling. I can't say I love eating anymore, but there are things I like, and that's good enough. Even at almost a year out, I cannot judge portions; I think I can eat something I order and end up eating just a few bites. Doggie bags are a normal sight at the house of a sleever.

The best part of this decision has been waking up each day and feeling well. I feel good about myself, good about my marriage, and good that I have much to look forward to as I move into my 60s. I'm happy and humbled by those who read my blog and let me know that I am an inspiration to them as they start their own journey.

One of my girlfriends once asked her father what was the happiest time in his life (we were in our 30s at the time and having a blast). He replied that his 60s were the best time of his life. We were shocked. Now I know how he felt; at almost 60 years old, I feel pretty happy myself.

1   Critical Care Pediatrics. Basal energy expenditure: Harris-Benedict equation. Joan and Sanford I. Weill Medical College, Cornell University. Web site. http://www-users.med.cornell.edu/~spon/picu/calc/beecalc.htm. 2000, October 3. Accessed October 19, 2012.

2   U.S. Department of Health and Human Services and U.S. Department of Agriculture. Dietary guidelines for Americans, 2010. http://www.health.gov/dietaryguidelines/dga2010/DietaryGuidelines2010.pdf. 2011. Accessed October 19, 2012.

3   Gropper, S.S., & Smith, J.L. Advanced Nutrition and Human Metabolism (5th ed.). 2008;Wadsworth Publishing: Belmont, California.

4   U.S. Department of Health and Human Services and U.S. Department of Agriculture. Dietary guidelines for Americans, 2010. http://www.health.gov/dietaryguidelines/dga2010/DietaryGuidelines2010.pdf. 2011. Accessed October 19, 2012.

5   U.S. Department of Agriculture, Agricultural Research Service. (2010). What we eat in America, NHANES 2007-2008, individuals 2 years and older (excluding breast-fed children), day one dietary intake data (revised August 2010). http://www.ars.usda.gov/SP2UserFiles/Place/12355000/pdf/0708/tables_1-40_2007-2008.pdf. Accessed October 19, 2012.

6   Snyder-Marlow G, Tayle D, Lenhard MJ. Nutrition care for patients undergoing laparoscopic sleeve gastrectomy for weight loss. J Am Diet Ass. 2010;110(4):600-607

7   Andreu A, Moize V, Rodriguez L, Flores L, Vidal J. Protein intake, body composition and protein status following bariatric surgery. Obes Surg. 2010;20(11):1509-15.

8   Agricultural Research Service, National Agricultural Library. Nutrient Data Library Foods List. US Department of Agriculture. Web site. http://ndb.nal.usda.gov/ndb/foods/list. December, 2011. Accessed October 17, 2012.

9   Ziegler O, Sirveaux MA, Brunaud L, Reibel N, Quillot D. Medical follow-up after bariatric surgery: nutritional and drug issues. General recommendations for the prevention and treatment of nutritional deficiencies. Diabetes Metab. 2009;35(6 Pt 2):544-547.

10 Harvard School of Public Health. Fats and cholesterol: out with the bad, in with the good. The Nutrition Source. Web site. http://www.hsph.harvard.edu/nutritionsource/what-should-you-eat/fats-full-story/index.html. 2012. Accessed October 19, 2012.

11 Berg, J.M., Tymockzo, J.L., & Stryer, L. (2002). Biochemistry. 5th edition. New York, W.H. Freeman.

12 Mayo Clinic Staff. Dietary fiber: essential for a healthy diet. Mayo Clinic. Web site. http://www.mayoclinic.com/health/fiber/NU00033/METHOD=print. November 9, 2009. Accessed October 19, 2012.

13 Bielohuby M, Stemmer K, Berger J, Ramisch J, Smith K, Holland J, Parks K, Pfluger PT, Habegger KM, Tschop MH, Seeley RJ, Bidlingmaier M. Carbohydrate content of post-operative diet influences the effect of vertical sleeve gastrectomy on body weight reduction in obese rats. Obes Surg. 2012;22(1)140-51.

14 Aills L, Blankenship J, Buffington C, Furtado M, Parrott J. ASMBS Allied Health nutritional guidelines for the surgical weight loss patient. Surg Obes Relat Dis. 2008;4(5Suppl):S73-S108.

15 Gropper, S.S., & Smith, J.L. Advanced Nutrition and Human Metabolism (5th ed.). 2008;Wadsworth Publishing: Belmont, California.

16 Dietary supplement fact sheet: zinc. Office of Dietary Supplements, National Institutes of Health. Web site. http://ods.od.nih.gov/factsheets/Zinc-HealthProfessional/. Reviewed September 20, 2011. Accessed October 20, 2012.

17 Aills L, Blankenship J, Buffington C, Furtado M, Parrott J. ASMBS Allied Health nutritional guidelines for the surgical weight loss patient. Surg Obes Relat Dis. 2008;4(5Suppl):S73-S108.

18 Aills L, Blankenship J, Buffington C, Furtado M, Parrott J. ASMBS Allied Health nutritional guidelines for the surgical weight loss patient. Surg Obes Relat Dis. 2008;4(5Suppl):S73-S108.

19 Ziegler O, Sirveaux MA, Brunaud L, Reibel N, Quillot D. Medical follow-up after bariatric surgery: nutritional and drug issues. General recommendations for the prevention and treatment of nutritional deficiencies. Diabetes Metab. 2009;35(6 Pt 2):544-547.

20 Aarts EO, Janssen IM, Berends FJ. The gastric sleeve: losing weight as fast as micronutrients? Obes Surg. 2011;21(2):207-11.

21 Chen YB, Zieve D. Anemia. Medline Plus. Web site. http://www.nlm.nih.gov/medlineplus/ency/article/000560.htm. Updated 2012, February 7. Accessed October 20, 2012.

22 Ziegler O, Sirveaux MA, Brunaud L, Reibel N, Quillot D. Medical follow-up after bariatric surgery: nutritional and drug issues. General recommendations for the prevention and treatment of nutritional deficiencies. Diabetes Metab. 2009;35(6 Pt 2):544-547.

23 Ziegler O, Sirveaux MA, Brunaud L, Reibel N, Quillot D. Medical follow-up after bariatric surgery: nutritional and drug issues. General recommendations for the prevention and treatment of nutritional deficiencies. Diabetes Metab. 2009;35(6 Pt 2):544-547.

24 Zieve D, Eltz DR, Dugdale DC. Peripheral Neuropathy. Medline Plus, US National Library of Medicine and National Institutes of Health. Web site. http://www.nlm.nih.gov/medlineplus/ency/article/000593.htm. Updated 2011, April 26. Accessed October 22, 2012.

25 Aarts EO, Janssen IM, Berends FJ. The gastric sleeve: losing weight as fast as micronutrients? Obes Surg. 2011;21(2):207-11.

26 Dietary supplement fact sheet: calcium. Office of Dietary Supplements, National Institutes of Health. Web site. http://ods.od.nih.gov/factsheets/Calcium-HealthProfessional/. Reviewed August 1, 2012. Accessed October 20, 2012.

27 Agricultural Research Service, U.S. Department of Agriculture. USDA national nutrient database for standard reference, release 18: sodium, Na (mg) content of selected foods per common measure, sorted by nutrient content. http://www.nal.usda.gov/fnic/foodcomp/Data/SR18/nutrlist/sr18w307.pdf. 2011. Accessed October 20, 2012.

28 Myklebust M, Wunder J. Healing foods pyramid: water. University of Michigan Health System. Web site. http://www.med.umich.edu/umim/food-pyramid/water.htm. 2010. Accessed October 20, 2012.

29 Cordova, A.C., et al. The cardiovascular protective effect of red wine. Journal of the American College of Surgeons. 2005;200:428-438.

30 Beyond hangovers: understanding alcohol's impact on your health. National Institute on Alcohol Abuse and Alcoholism, National Institutes of Health. Web site. http://pubs.niaaa.nih.gov/publications/Hangovers/beyondHangovers.pdf. Accessed October 22, 2012.

31 Maluenda F, Csendes A, De Aretxabala X, Poniachik J, Salvo K, Delgado I, Rodriguez P. Alcohol absorption modification after a laparoscopic sleeve gastrectomy due to obesity. Obes Surg. 2010;20(6):744-8.

32 Changchien EM, Woodard GA, Hernandez-Boussard T, Morton JM. Normal alcohol metabolism after gastric banding and sleeve gastrectomy: a case cross-over trial. J Am Coll Surg. 2012;215(4):475-9.

33 Guidance for industry: a food labeling guide. Center for Food Safety and Applied Nutrition. Food and Drug Administration. Web site. http://www.fda.gov/Food/GuidanceComplianceRegulatoryInformation/GuidanceDocuments/FoodLabelingNutrition/FoodLabelingGuide/default.htm. Revised 2009, October. Accessed October 22, 2012.

34 U.S. Congress. (2010). Food, Drug and Cosmetic Act. U.S. Code of Federal Regulations. Government Printing Office, Washington, D.C

35 U.S. Congress. (2011). Title 21, U.S. Code of Federal Regulations. Government Printing Office, Washington, D.C

36 National Organic Program. US Department of Agriculture. Web site. http://www.ams.usda.gov/AMSv1.0/nop. 2012, June 6. Accessed October 22, 2012.

37 Nutrition information for raw fruits, vegetables and fish. U.S. Food and Drug Administration. Web site. http://www.fda.gov/Food/LabelingNutrition/FoodLabelingGuidanceRegulatoryInformation/InformationforRestaurantsRetailEstablishments/ucm063367.htm. 2009. Accessed October 22, 2012.

38 U.S. Congress. (2011). Title 9, U.S. Code of Federal Regulations. Government Printing Office, Washington, D.C.

39 Bureau of Alcohol, Tobacco and Firearms. Web site. http://www.fsis.usda.gov/PDF/Nutrition_labeling_Q&A_041312.pdf. 2012. Accessed October 22, 2012.

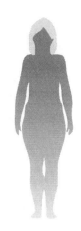

16

Getting and Staying in Shape with Exercise

The past few chapters covered recovery from the sleeve surgery. You know what to expect at the hospital and how to take care of yourself to minimize your risk of complications. The book covered the post-surgery sleeve diet progression from liquids to solid foods, and it detailed your everyday sleeve diet. You know what to eat and how much, and you know how to make meal plans that fit your needs.

The gastric sleeve isn't just about eating though. It's about an overall lifestyle change to improve your health. This chapter covers another part of your new lifestyle: physical activity, or exercise. You might have avoided exercise for years because it was uncomfortable, you felt self-conscious, it felt useless, or simply because you hated it. Maybe you didn't even know what to do!

This chapter can change all that by covering the following topics:

- Why exercise is good for your weight and health
- Recommended amounts of exercise
- How a complete beginner can safely and gradually start a physical activity program when you still have a lot of weight to lose
- How to make your program more advanced as you progress
- How to stick to your exercise program for the long term

Exercise and physical activity are used interchangeably in this chapter, so don't worry about which term is used. Now, let's get moving!

The Importance of Physical Activity

Exercise is good for you for almost unlimited reasons. Most people think of weight loss first when they think of exercise; next, you might think about heart health. Those are just the beginning of the list of physical and mental benefits of exercise. Of course, exercise makes you look pretty good too! At any weight, a firmer, more toned body always looks more attractive!

Physical Activity Burns Calories and Helps You Control Your Weight

Physical activity helps you control your weight because it burns calories. You burn calories while you're actually exercising, and physical activity boosts your metabolism so that you burn additional calories throughout the day. Plus, building muscles is good for your weight because muscles use more calories than your body fat whether you're exercising or resting.

In general, the more you exercise, the more calories you burn and the faster you lose weight. The National Weight Control Registry, which follows individuals who have lost weight and kept it off for at least a year, reports that more than 90 percent of its members included physical activity in their successful weight loss and weight maintenance programs.[1]

So how many calories does exercise burn? It depends on the specific type of exercise, how long you do it for, how hard you go, and how much you weigh.

Burn Calories and Control Weight Loss with Physical Activity

For pretty specific information on your calorie burn, you can always use an online calculator that will give you a good estimate of how many calories you burned through exercise. There are a lot available online, and the U.S. Department of Health and Human Services suggests one from the Calorie Control Council.[2]

For a quick reference, just so you can get an idea of how many calories different types of activities burn, *Table 40* is a table of calories burned doing different activities at different weights.[3] These numbers are for an hour of exercise.

Activity	Your Weight			
	160 pounds	200 pounds	250 pounds	300 pounds
aerobics, low-impact	364	455	568	682
basketball, shooting baskets	327	409	511	614
bicycling, stationary, easy effort	255	318	398	477
bicycling, stationary, vigorous effort	495	618	773	927
circuit training	313	391	489	586
dancing, average	291	364	455	545
elliptical trainer	436	545	682	818
frisbee or catch	218	273	341	409
golf, walking, carrying clubs	313	391	489	586
Pilates	218	273	341	409
run and walk combination	436	545	682	818
running/jogging, 6.0 mph (10 minutes per mile)	713	891	1114	1336
Stretching	167	209	261	314
Swimming	423	528	632	737
tennis, doubles	327	409	511	614
walking, slowly, 2.0 miles per hour (mph)	204	255	318	382
Walking, medium, 3.0 mph	255	318	398	477
walking, fast, 4.0 mph	364	455	568	682
walking, uphill at 3 percent grade, 3.5 mph	385	482	602	723
water aerobics	385	482	602	723
weight lifting, 8 to 12 repetitions per set	255	318	398	477
yoga, Hatha	182	227	284	341
yoga, power	291	364	455	545

Table 40: Calories burned doing different activities at different weights

Keeping Your Calorie Burn High

As you can see, you burn calories faster doing the same activity when you're heavier than when you're lighter. At first glance, that can seem kind of discouraging because, of course, you're just going to get lighter as you progress along your weight loss journey. The more weight you lose, the fewer calories you'll burn doing the same activity.

On the other hand, you're going to be in much better shape a few months down the road. You'll be able to exercise for longer and at a higher intensity. So, you can still keep your calorie burn up pretty high. As an

Tip

Chapter 2, "Weight Loss Options," talks about burning calories through exercise and the fact that exercise on its own isn't enough to get you to lose weight and keep it off. You also need to follow your sleeve diet.

example, you might walk slowly for 20 minutes when you weigh 300 pounds and burn about 182 calories.[4] Let's say that you keep your exercise program up for a while and lose a lot of weight. Let's say that you get down to 200 pounds. You'd only burn 85 calories if you walked slowly for 20 minutes. More likely, though, you'll be more comfortable working out longer and harder. You might be able to jog for 40 minutes and burn 242 calories without feeling as tired as you did when you were walking slowly at a weight of 300 pounds.

You lose a pound of body fat every time you burn off an extra 3,500 calories. You can see from these numbers that exercise helps, but it's just a small component of the lifestyle changes that you're making in order to lose weight as fast as you hoped. At 300 pounds, you'd have to burn 500 calories per day, which is the equivalent of walking for an hour a day, to lose an extra pound per week. Sticking to your sleeve diet, even if you're pretty active, is absolutely necessary to keep the pounds coming off.

Physical Activity Helps Prevent or Manage Obesity-Related Diseases

We've already talked about the numerous diseases that are related to obesity, and these conditions might have been a major factor in why you got the sleeve. You might already have been feeling the effects of obesity-related health conditions, or you might have been afraid of developing them. Losing weight can reduce your risk of developing many health conditions or make them less severe. Exercise not only helps you lose weight, but it also improves your physical health. Regular physical activity can prevent or lower your risk for a variety of obesity-related conditions.[5]

Exercise Improves Your Heart Health

Heart disease is the top killer of Americans. If you didn't already have heart disease because of your obesity, there's a good chance your obesity contributed to high blood cholesterol levels and blood pressure, which are risk factors for heart disease. Exercise has many positive effects on your heart health:[6]

- It lowers your risk of developing cardiovascular disease.

- It raises levels of your HDL cholesterol, which is the healthy kind.

- It lowers your blood pressure. That means that your heart doesn't have to work so hard, so you're less likely to get congestive heart failure. Also, you're at a lower risk for having a stroke.

- It lowers your LDL cholesterol, which is the bad kind of cholesterol.

- It lowers your levels of unhealthy triglycerides in your blood.

- It reduces your chances of developing atherosclerosis, or hardening of the arteries.

- It makes your lungs stronger, so your blood flow is more efficient and your heart doesn't have to work as hard.

Physical Activity May Lower Your Risk for Certain Cancers

Cancer is the second leading cause of death in the U.S., right behind heart disease. While scientists don't know everything about every kind of cancer, they are pretty sure that exercise can protect you against certain kinds. The American Cancer Society recommends regular physical activity to lower your risk for breast, colorectal, kidney, pancreatic, prostate, stomach, and lower esophageal cancers.[7] Of course, achieving a healthy weight helps too, and you're already trying to do that with the gastric sleeve.

> **Tip**
>
> Chapter I, "Obesity – A Costly Epidemic," describes the obesity-related diseases in more detail. It's a great review if you've forgotten about how chronic health conditions, such as cardiovascular disease, diabetes, cancer and osteoarthritis, are related to obesity.

Physical Activity May Improve Your Blood Sugar Control

Exercise helps your body regulate blood sugar to help prevent prediabetes or diabetes or to manage diabetes if you already have it.[8] Better blood sugar management is great news because it helps prevent complications such as heart disease, kidney disease, blindness, and amputations. Exercise helps your body regulate your blood sugar, or blood glucose, levels by increasing the blood flow to your working muscles so that they use fat and glucose for energy instead of letting the glucose sit in your blood. Another important way that physical activity helps is by increasing your body's sensitivity to insulin.[9] Remember, insulin resistance, or a decrease in insulin sensitivity, is the underlying cause of type 2 diabetes, which is the kind of diabetes that's related to obesity.

Physical Activity Often Helps Relieve Osteoarthritis

You may have osteoarthritis if you have pain in your knees, hips, and other joints that's chronic—it's there most days and isn't because of a recent injury. Chances are that obesity was responsible for keeping you in pain from arthritis each day before your gastrectomy. Osteoarthritis is the kind of arthritis that's from wear and tear on your joints—too much excess body weight really puts the pressure on. Sometimes all you want to do when you have osteoarthritis is sit or lie down, but exercising is more likely to help than doing nothing.

It's hard to believe, but almost any kind of gentle or moderate physical activity can actually reduce your pain and swelling. This may be because physical activity increases your blood flow to the injured joint, helping to heal it. Exercise may increase your flexibility and range of motion so that you can start to feel like you're *moving* your body instead of *straining* it. People with arthritis that exercise are more mobile and have better quality of life. Stick with exercises that don't cause pain, and ask a physical therapist or your doctor if you're not sure about what to do.

If you have osteoarthritis because of your obesity, you can probably start exercising sooner after your sleeve surgery than you think. You don't have to lose hundreds of pounds before you can exercise. In one study, bariatric surgery patients had significantly less pain and better mobility after only three months.[10]

Exercise Helps You Live Longer!

By the way, you're more likely to live longer if you exercise regularly than if you avoid physical activity. That's a pretty good reason to start exercising!

Exercise Supports Healthy Bones

Some kinds of exercise are good for your bones. That's an important benefit for everyone but especially crucial for you as a sleeve patient. Many bariatric surgery patients develop low bone mineral density, or osteoporosis, and a high risk for bone fractures.

- Your intake of bone nutrients, such as vitamin D and calcium, may be low because of your restricted diet.

- You can have lower absorption of bone nutrients.

- People who lose weight fast, as you do after bariatric surgery, can lose bone mineral density quickly. You can't get it back.

How Physical Activity Can Improve Bone Health

Physical activity can be a powerful weapon in your collection of tools to prevent osteoporosis. Your bones are constantly changing. Their bone mineral is always breaking down and building back up in a process called remodeling. When you're under 30 years old, the net effect is that you gain bone mineral density (BMD) faster than you lose it, so your bones are getting stronger.[11] You hit your peak bone mineral density around 30 years old; after that, your goal is to maintain as much bone mineral density as possible. You can slow down the loss of bone mineral density by eating plenty of calcium and vitamin D, as we talked about in earlier chapters, and by doing appropriate physical activity.

Here's how it works. Exercise stresses your bones so that they respond and compensate by growing stronger. It's a lot like how your muscles work; when you lift heavy weights, your muscles compensate by growing stronger.

Choosing the Best Exercises for Your Bones

The exercises that help your bones are known as *weight-bearing activities*. You can choose to do high-impact or low-impact weight-bearing activities to help your bones out.[12]

Low-impact activities: In low-impact activities, you never completely leave the ground—at least one foot is always on the ground. These are good ones to start with when you're not that experienced with exercise. They don't burn as many calories as high-impact activities, but they aren't as likely to cause injuries. Here are some examples:

- Strength or resistance training. You can lift weights, do exercises that use your own body weight, or use a resistance loop. We'll talk more about strength training later in the chapter.
- Using the elliptical machine at the gym. The elliptical machine is a great machine—it's a huge calorie-burner, it helps your bones, it works your arms and legs, and it's great for injury prevention.
- Dancing
- Walking
- Low-impact aerobics
- Stair or step machines
- Downhill skiing
- Light dancing

High-impact activities: These usually involve jumping and leaving the ground. A lot of them are high-intensity and a ton of fun, but you'll definitely not want to start an exercise program with high-impact activities. They're a little more challenging and can increase your risk for injuries if you're not truly ready for them. Save them for when you're in good shape and you've lost a good amount of weight.

These are some examples of high-impact activities that can help your bones:

- High-impact aerobics
- Jogging or running
- Dancing
- Basketball, soccer, and tennis
- Jumping rope
- Cross-country skiing
- Dancing with a lot of jumping

You'll notice that some activities are on both lists. A lot of activities, such as dancing and aerobics, can be modified to be high-impact or low-impact.

Exercises with Other Health Benefits That Don't Strengthen Your Bones

Swimming, water aerobics, rowing, and biking are examples of activities that are non-weight-bearing. These exercises provide many of the other great benefits of exercise, such as burning calories, helping with arthritis, reducing stress, and improving your cardiovascular fitness. But, they don't have much effect on your bones. You also need to regularly include weight-bearing activities in your exercise program if you want to protect your bones.

Staying active is just as important as *getting* active because you can lose bone density quickly when you stop exercising. This can happen within just a few weeks, and the effects can last for months. Here's the information:

- People who are confined to a few weeks of bed rest lose some bone mineral and continue to have lower bone density for more than five months after their hospital stays.[13]

- Being in outer space is a lot like skipping weight-bearing activity because of the lack of gravity that makes astronauts feel weightless. Astronauts can lose their bone mineral density 6 to 12 times as fast as the average adult on Earth.[14] What's the take-home message? Start an exercise program and stick with it—consistency really pays off!

The Psychosocial Benefits of Physical Activity

Physical activity isn't just good for your physical health. It's also great for your psychosocial health, or your mental and emotional health. These benefits are very well-documented, and many of them have biological explanations—so they're not just in your head!

Exercise Relieves Stress

Physical activity reduces stress.[15] Exercise might help you relax through a variety of possible ways:

- Repetitive motions, such as walking, can be calming. Taking a walk is a far healthier repetitive motion than emotional eating if you're trying to handle stress!

- The regularity of your exercise sessions can be comforting. You get to look forward to your exercise, and once you start, the familiar activities let you feel in control instead of anxious.

- Your mind gets a chance to wander. You can think through your day without interruptions or the pressure of coming to any conclusions immediately.

Exercise Improves Your Energy Levels

Morning exercisers find that they are sharper and more alert throughout the day. Some people find that they like exercising in the evening because it takes the fatigue away after a long day at work. And still others like to exercise on their lunch hour—because they say it prevents them from wanting to take a mid-afternoon nap. Find the time or times that you enjoy most—it's your choice!

Regular exercise is also good for your energy because it improves sleep. You'll sleep more deeply and wake up refreshed when you get into a regular exercise routine. Starting an exercise program can reduce insomnia, too.[16]

Exercise is Good for Your Brain

It sounds too good to be true, but exercise can make you smarter. Exercise increases your blood flow to your brain, so your brain gets more oxygen and nutrients. Physically fit adults have more active brains and better performances on cognitive tests[17] and are mentally sharper[18] than adults who don't exercise. Better yet, the effects don't stop when you're done exercising for the day. Adults who exercise have more white matter, which is the thinking part, in their brains.[19] So keep exercising and becoming smarter! Nobody will believe you when you tell them why you're suddenly being even sharper on the job!

Exercise Makes You Happier

Plenty of anecdotal and scientific evidence show that exercise improves your mood. One reason is related to what's known as the "runner's high." It's the release of chemicals, called opioids or endorphins, that activate different parts of your brain to make you happy.[20] Luckily, the "runner's high" isn't just for runners. Anyone who exercises can get the same effects!

Exercise Improves Your Confidence

The victories that you achieve during an exercise program increase your confidence in the rest of your life. Exercise provides so many opportunities for you to succeed. You can be proud of yourself for:

- Getting up early and going to the gym even though you didn't want to.
- Going a minute longer or 0.1 mph faster on the treadmill than you ever had before.
- Trying a new fitness class that you never would have dared to do before getting the sleeve.
- Finishing what's now "just a regular" workout—because in the old days, you wouldn't have even started.
- When you succeed at these challenges, you start to realize that you can succeed at challenges in your everyday life.

Exercise Can Improve Your Social Life

You have many opportunities to meet people through exercise:

- *At the gym:* Anyone who's at the gym has the same goals as you. You might be able to become someone's workout partner—you can encourage each other on the cardio equipment and help each other lift weights. Don't be afraid to be friendly—the worst that can happen if someone doesn't want to work out with you is that they'll let you know, and you can each go your separate ways.
- *In group fitness classes:* Strike up a conversation before or after class. You might want to schedule a workout together for the next day or even find that you hit it off and want to be friends for completely social reasons.

Help! I'm Afraid That People Are Making Fun of Me When I'm Exercising!

You walk into the fitness center. To the right, heavily muscled men are pumping iron. To the left, skinny women in tank tops are using treadmills, stationary bikes, and elliptical trainers. And in the group exercise room, there are about 20 highly fit and coordinated people following their aerobics instructor in perfect sync. The whole scene makes you want to turn around and run out of there as fast as you can before anyone sees your imperfect body and questionable fitness skills. But wait!

A huge concern for many obese people is that other people will look down on them. It can be such a strong fear that it can interfere with your fitness program. Yes, it's tough to walk into a gym full of strangers that look like they're confident and that are in great shape when you're not feeling so confident in yourself. They might even come off as snobbish or arrogant. But you know what? In most cases, it's all in your head.

Most of the people at the gym are just like you. They have careers and families too, and the gym is just one part of their busy lives. They have the same reasons for exercising that you do—they want to be healthy, control their weight, and relieve stress. They have their good workouts and bad workouts, just like you, and they have to drag themselves out of bed or away from the couch to get to the gym, just like you. They're focused on their own workouts and lives and may not even notice you. If they do, these regular exercisers are so much more likely to admire than disrespect you because they know what kind of effort you're putting in.

Remember we said that "in most cases, it's all in your head"? Well, we admit that, occasionally, you'll run into gym snobs, just like you run into snobs occasionally in the rest of your life. There are the clothing snobs who judge your lack of designer clothing, the car snobs who think your car isn't worth driving, the coffee snobs who wouldn't be caught dead drinking anything other than their favorite brand of coffee, and…well, you get the point. In every crowd, there's bound to be someone who tries to ruin it for everyone else, and it's true at the gym too. So, keep in mind that it's in their head, not yours, and let it be their problem if they don't like the way your biceps look. You have just as much right to the dumbbells as they do.

So what do people think about you when exercising? These are some likely possibilities:

"Who cares?" (They don't notice you enough to think much about you.)

Probably nothing. (They haven't even noticed you because they're wrapped up in their own workouts.)

"You're the best." (They recognize the challenges you're overcoming and are inspired by your dedication.)

"You're not good enough." (These are snobs who don't think anyone's good enough, so don't take it personally. In fact, take it as a compliment because, really, who would want the snob's approval?)

- *Online:* Use search engines to see if you can join up with individuals or groups in your area. Many groups are specifically started for obese adults who want to lose weight, and you can make unbelievable deep connections if you are able to exercise your way through your weight loss journey with someone who's in the same boat as you. Members who attend your sleeve or bariatric surgery support group meetings are great candidates because you know they live in your area.
- *In the park:* Tag along with walkers—you'll be surprised at how many of them are looking for company too.

Exercise doesn't just help you make new friends. You can take advantage of your new exercise program to strengthen your old relationships with friends and family. Getting through workouts together is one of the most supportive things you can do for each other.

Even if you prefer to exercise alone, your exercise program can improve your social life because of the way you carry yourself. Instead of being ashamed of yourself, you'll be proud of that body of yours that's capable of doing the physical activity that you've demanded of it. People will respond better to you when you are proud of yourself.

How Much Should You Exercise?

How much do you need to exercise to get the benefits? The ASMBS guideline for bariatric surgery patients is to aim for 30 minutes on most days.[21] Only one-quarter of patients tend to hit that amount though.[22] An average of 33.8% of sleeve patients who never had a bariatric procedure before exercise regularly, while about 16.7% of patients who got a revision from the laparoscopic adjustable gastric band are exercisers after getting sleeved.[23]

The 30 minutes-per-day recommendation is consistent with national guidelines from the Centers for Disease Control and Prevention, or CDC, for healthy adults to aim for at least 30 minutes on most days of the week.[24] Later in this section, we'll break down the types of exercise that you should include to get to your 30 minutes per day.

Don't Limit Yourself!

Extra exercise may have additional benefits. You'll still get a lot of the benefits of exercise if you hit your 30 minutes per day on most days of the week, and you'll be way ahead of the average American. In fact, only half of Americans meet CDC recommendations to exercise at least 30 minutes a day for five times a week at a moderate intensity or for at least 20 minutes three times a week at a vigorous intensity.[5]

But, you can get even more benefits if you increase your exercise beyond these goals. The Weight-Control Information Network, or WIN, is part of the National Institutes of Health. The organization states that aiming for about 60 minutes per day can help you lose weight.[26] And you've heard—and maybe even experienced for yourself in a previous yo-yo diet cycle— that keeping the weight off is even harder than losing it in the first place. The WIN suggests aiming for 60 to 90 minutes per day of exercise to maintain significant weight loss—like you'll have within a couple of years of getting the sleeve if you follow the sleeve diet.

Exercise Like the Weight Loss Pros: The National Weight Control Registry

The National Weight Control Registry, or NWCR, is a nationwide database, or even "club," of people who have successfully lost weight. It was started by doctors at Brown Medical School, in Rhode Island, and the University of Colorado. You can only sign up to join the registry after you've lost at least 30 pounds and kept it off for at least a year, and there are currently more than 10,000 members.

The goal of the NWCR is to help people figure out how to lose weight and maintain their weight loss. The NWCR conducts a lot of research through surveys and questionnaires, asking members about their diet, physical activity, and other health habits that may be related to their weight loss success.

Habits That Prevent Weight Regain

The NWCR has found a lot of interesting information! For example, just under half of participants lost their weight on their own; the other half used a program. And how do these role models keep their weight off? Well, two-thirds watch no more than ten hours of television per week, and about three-quarters of them eat breakfast every day and weigh themselves at least weekly. They follow a low-fat, low-calorie diet and tend to have a healthier diet than the average American—it's higher in calcium and is high in vitamin C and vitamin A too.

Exercise and Weight Maintenance

What is the role of exercise in preventing weight regain? It helps! According to the NWCR website, nine out of every ten NWCR members report exercising at least an hour per day. They average about 400 calories per day through a variety of activities, such as running, aerobics, bicycling, and weight lifting. This amount and intensity of exercise is a little more than the CDC's minimum recommendation to get at least 30 minutes per day on most days of the week, but it's doable. It's very motivational to know that your hard work can pay off, just like it does for members of the NWCR.

Source:[27, 28, 29, 30]

Types of Exercises

Aerobic Exercise: What It Is and How Much to Do

Aerobic exercise is often called cardio because of its effects on your cardiovascular system. Aerobic exercise is what a lot of us just think of as "exercise." It gets your heart rate up for a continuous period of time. You breathe a little deeper and faster to get more oxygen into your lungs and to your blood. Your heart pumps harder and faster so you can circulate more blood and get enough oxygen to your working muscles.

Recommendations for aerobic exercise depend on intensity. National recommendations for healthy adults are to get at least 150 minutes of moderate-intensity aerobic exercise per week, or at least 75 minutes of vigorous intensity aerobic exercise per week, or a combination of the two.[31] You can do any combination of moderate or vigorous activity. Here are some examples:

- 30 minutes of moderate intensity physical activity on five separate days
- 15 minutes of moderate intensity on five separate days
- 30 minutes of moderate intensity physical activity on two days and 15 minutes of vigorous intensity physical activity on three days
- An hour of moderate intensity physical activity on two days, and 15 minutes of vigorous intensity physical activity on one day
- 25 minutes of vigorous physical activity on three days

Moderate versus Vigorous Physical Activity

How do you know if you're doing moderate or vigorous physical activities? The National Heart Lung and Blood Institute provides several examples of common lists of activities and their intensities.[32]

Moderate physical activities:

- Walking
- Dancing
- Leisurely bicycling
- Water aerobics
- Mowing the lawn and other gardening activities
- Washing the windows
- Shooting hoops, non-competitively
- Using a rowing machine at the gym

Vigorous physical activities:

- Jogging or running
- Walking uphill
- Swimming laps quickly
- Playing full-court basketball, soccer, or an intense game of tennis
- High-impact step aerobics
- Elliptical machine at the gym

Moderate and vigorous physical activity can change depending on how fit you are and how much effort you put into it. At the beginning of your sleeve journey, you might sweat buckets and be huffing and puffing just by walking slowly around the block. That's vigorous physical activity. By the time you've lost some weight and you're getting to be in pretty good shape, slow walking might be moderate physical activity. To make walking count as vigorous, you might focus on going faster and swinging your arms more forcefully.

You Can Break Up Your Exercise Sessions

On some days it can be tough to set aside an entire 15- to 60-minute workout all at once. It's always okay to break up your exercise into smaller sessions. You might be able to squeeze in a quick 10-minute walk during your lunch period, another 10 minutes around the block before coming home from work for the day, and your final 10 minutes after dinner.

Breaking it up can make your exercise easier mentally too. If you're feeling tired after dinner, you might find it easier to get moving for 10 minutes. If you feel obligated to do 30 minutes, you might just stay on the couch and do nothing. Everything you do counts, so don't let an all-or-nothing attitude turn your exercise routine into "nothing." In general, when it comes to exercise, some is better than none, and more is better than less.

How Hard Should You Exercise?

Exactly how do you know if you're exercising at the right level for the maximum benefits when you're in the middle of a cardio workout? Your perceived exertion is the simplest method, and it's a pretty good one. Aerobic exercise should be tough enough to make you feel like you're working but not so hard that you think you're going to collapse. A general way to tell if you're in your aerobic zone is to do the talk test. You should be able to talk in short sentences but not have enough breath to sing a song.

You can also use your heart rate as a guide if you know your maximum heart rate. If you don't, you can use the standard formula of 220 minus your age to estimate your maximum heart rate, but keep in mind that individual maximum heart rates can vary a lot. Once you get your maximum heart rate, multiply it by 0.5 to get the target by getting the value of 50 percent of your maximum heart rate, which is the low end of an aerobic workout. Multiply your maximum by 0.8 to find out 80 percent of your maximum heart rate, which is about the high end of your aerobic workout zone.

Here's an example. Let's say you're 42 years old.

- Your estimated maximum heart rate is 220 minus 42, or 178 beats per minute.
- Your lower end goal is 0.5 times 178, or 89 beats per minute.
- Your upper end goal is 0.8 times 178, or 142 beats per minute.

- You want to keep your heart rate between 89 and 142 beats per minute. That's a pretty big range. It gives you plenty of room for easy days, hard days, and everything in between.

Here are a few tips for keeping it simple:

- Online calculators can save you trouble. Organizations like the American Council on Exercise, American Cancer Society, and National Institutes of Health, along with a bunch of other websites, have calculators that will tell you your goal heart rate. You can just put in your age and get the guidelines.

- You can use a heart rate monitor that consists of a chest strap and a wrist watch or just a wrist watch. Most sporting goods stores sell them, and a sales associate can help you out when you're choosing one.

- You can take your pulse by yourself if you don't want to buy or wear a heart rate monitor. Place your index and middle finger (not your thumb) on your carotid artery on either side of your Adam's apple in your neck. Count the beats for 6 seconds, multiply by ten, and that's your heart rate. So, if you count to 13 in 6 seconds, your heart rate is 130 beats per minute.

- It's not a precise science. It's okay if your workout ends up harder or easier than you had intended. Over time you'll figure out the zones that work best for you, and you won't even have to consciously think about staying in your aerobic zone.

- Give yourself a while to warm up before worrying about your heart rate. Your heart rate will take at least five minutes to increase from resting up to your aerobic zone.

Source: [33, 34]

Strength or Resistance Training: What It Is and How Much to Do

Strength training is also known as resistance training or weight training. This portion of your exercise program is good for your muscles and bones as well as your looks. Strength training isn't just for body builders and men. It's for anyone who's interested in a well-rounded exercise program, a tight and toned appearance, faster metabolism, and increased confidence from being stronger.

Aim for Two Sessions per Week for Each Major Muscle Group

Your major muscle groups are your hips, legs, shoulders, back, abdomen, and arms. Try to include exercises that target each of these groups at least twice per week.[35] You don't have to hit all the major muscle groups each time you do your strength training. You can break up your workouts however you want. These are some examples:

- You can do all of your muscles in one workout and do that twice per week.

- You can do your legs and hips two days a week and your back, shoulders, abdomen, and arms on two other days.
- You can do your hips and legs on two days, your core (back and abdomen) on two days, and your arms and shoulders on two days. That's a great schedule if you just want to get in a quick strength-training session after your cardio workouts but you don't want to set aside too long for your resistance training.

When you do your strength training, you should choose activities and weights that get you tired after 8 to 12 repetitions.[36] Those 8 to 12 repetitions count as one set, and you should be tired and want to rest after them. To count as a strength training session, you only have to do one set for each muscle! You can do two sets if you want though. Just rest for a little bit after the first set before you start your second set of 8 to 12 repetitions. If 8 to 12 repetitions becomes too easy, increase the weight until it becomes challenging again.

Ask for Help if You Need It

Proper form, or technique, reduces your risk for injuries from strength training, and it gives you better results. Resistance training isn't as natural as, say, walking, so it's a good idea to ask an expert to show you good form when you're first starting your resistance training program. A physical therapist can give you beginner modifications and watch to correct your form and technique. Trainers at the gym can help too. You can also look online for descriptions, photos, and videos of various exercises for more guidance.

You Have Many Different Options for Strength Training Equipment

Familiar weights, such as dumbbells and barbells, are just the start of your options for your strength training sessions. Below are some traditional and less traditional choices for improving your strength.

Traditional options:

- *Dumbbells* – These are great to have at home or to use at the gym. Just hold them in your hands and get your workout in.
- *Barbells* – These include a bar with weights in the shape of disks at the end. Barbells can be pretty heavy, so you probably won't be using them for a while.
- *Big resistance machines* – Weight benches and exercise-specific weight training machines at the gym are designed to target certain muscles. They work pretty well, but they may be uncomfortable for you to use when you're still very overweight.
- *Multi-Gyms* – These are available at most gyms, and they come in home-designed models in case you get very enthusiastic about your weight-training program. You can work out each major muscle group on a multi-gym.
- *Kettlebells* – These are round, steel balls that have a handle. A lot of workouts are designed using one kettlebell. Kettlebells are pretty fun to use and give you some

variety. Kettlebell workouts often double as cardio workouts because they can get your heart rate up in a hurry.

Less conventional options:

- *Body weight* – There are so many exercises you can do that don't require any equipment at all! You can do pushups (start on your knees, not your toes, when you're a beginner), sit-ups and crunches, arm raises, calf raises, squats, dips, and lunges without needing to hold any extra weight. Your own body weight is great resistance, especially when you're still carrying around so much extra weight shortly after your sleeve surgery.
- *Resistance band or loop* – These elastic bands come in different sizes and resistance levels so you can use them to work your whole body.
- *Stability ball* – These big balls look like giant beach balls. They're good for challenging your whole body because you have to work on balancing while you're using them for exercises.[37] You can use them for almost anything, such as crunches, push-ups, squats, and planks.
- *Medicine ball* – These are heavy balls that you can use to work your arms, shoulders, back, and abdominals. You can even use them to strengthen your legs if you hold one while doing lunges.
- *Soup cans* – Each one weighs about a pound, so soup cans are great for making the transition from no weights to heavier weights.

Strength Training Can Help You Lose Weight

Most strength training exercises burn fewer calories per minute than most aerobic exercises, but strength training can play an important role in your weight loss that aerobic exercise doesn't; strength training builds and maintains your muscle mass. Muscle tissue is *metabolically active*; that is, it burns a lot of calories at rest compared to fat. Strength training can keep you from losing muscle mass and having a slower metabolism as you get older. Even more important for sleeve patients is that your rapid weight loss can make you lose muscle as well as fat. You can't avoid losing a small amount of muscle mass when you lose weight, but strength training can greatly reduce the amount of muscle mass that you lose.

Strength training can do double duty as an aerobic workout. We just talked about aerobic exercise as being physical activity that keeps your heart rate up for a continuous period of time. You can turn strength training into an aerobic workout by moving without stopping. Here are a couple of ideas for getting your heart rate up while strength training.

- Progress to the next set of repetitions as soon as you finish one set. The first set will make your muscles tired, so the next set of repetitions should target a different muscle group. For example, if you just worked your arms, do some leg exercises for your next set of 8 to 12 repetitions. Then move on to your back and then back to your arms. Think about moving on to the next muscle group as soon as one becomes tired.

- Keep moving in between sets instead of sitting still to recover. Walking or marching in place can keep your heart rate up as your muscles recover for the next set of 8 to 12 repetitions.

When you turn your strength training into an aerobic workout, you burn more calories and don't have to spend as long on your exercise. This is how you can turn resistance training into an aerobic workout.

You'll know that you're getting a good cardio workout in if your heart rate is in your zone (that's 50 to 80 percent of your maximum heart rate), if your breathing is heavy, and if you can talk but not sing. You're getting a good resistance training workout if your muscles are burning at the end of each set of 8 to 12 repetitions.

Stretching, Flexibility, and Balance

There aren't firm guidelines for these parts of your exercise routine, but these components aren't just "extras." A good goal is to stretch at each workout, or at least three times per week. Stretching improves your flexibility, which makes you less likely to get injured. It lengthens your muscles and helps them recover better from your workouts so that you're feeling ready to go again by the next day or the next time you have a workout scheduled. Other potential benefits of stretching include reducing stress and improving your posture.[38]

When you stretch, think about working the same muscle groups that you do when you lift weights. That is, try to hit each of the major muscle groups. A physical therapist or staff member at a gym can get you started with effective stretches. Traditional stretching, yoga, and stretching with a rope can all help you improve your flexibility.

Beginners need to build up slowly to prevent injuries.

The above goals for the amount of exercise you should do are long-term goals for more experienced exercisers. Don't worry about hitting these goals for exercise when you're first starting your program. Instead, just focus on getting in the amount that's comfortable for you. That might be just one or two minutes at a time to start with. You have plenty of time to build up the time you spend exercising as your weight continues to come off and your physical fitness improves.

Everyone Needs Regular Rest Days

Rest is a crucial part of an exercise program for beginners and world-class athletes. It has the following benefits:

- It lets your body heal so you're less likely to get injured.
- It gives your muscles a chance to build back up so they're stronger than before.
- It gives you a mental break so you're eager to get back in the game the next day.

Just as you've been learning to listen to your body as you follow the sleeve diet, you need to learn to listen to your body when you're starting an exercise program. Learn to recognize the difference between being lazy and truly needing a day off. A general rule of thumb is that if you're not sure, you can get through your warm-up and start your workout. When you're five minutes in, try to decide – do you still feel tired? If you do, then you need a day off. Stop exercising now, or plan to take the next day off. However, if you feel good after warming up, you probably don't need a day off.

Restrictions after the VSG

Such a life-changing experience as getting the sleeve naturally can make you wonder whether you need to avoid certain activities. As long as your sleeve is fully healed and you start new activities only slowly and gradually, the sleeve shouldn't interfere with your workout routine. Just be sure to get your physician's approval before starting any new activity. Sleeve patients can successfully participate in a range of activities, such as the following:

- Water activities, such as swimming, water jogging, and water aerobics
- Weight-lifting, as long as you don't strain yourself
- Walking, running, and hiking
- Dancing and aerobics
- Sports such as basketball and tennis

The main precaution that you can take is to warm up well before exercising, which is what everyone should do anyway. Warming up helps prevent you from straining your abdominal muscles and taking the risk of splitting your gastric sleeve's seam. Your surgeon can advise you on any restricted activities, but there won't be many of them.

Everything Counts!

As you develop your exercise program and count your minutes of exercise, try to keep your ultimate goals in mind: You want to lose weight and get healthy. Each bit of movement that you do takes you a step closer to achieving your goals in the following ways:

- *It helps you develop new lifestyle habits as part of a new lifestyle*. Making a conscious effort to walk an extra minute or two to cool down after your workout, park farther away from the store, and take the stairs at work can become habitual.
- *A few extra minutes of exercise can translate into measurable calories and noticeable weight loss*. Every bit helps you lose weight and improve your health, even if you're not counting it as part of your exercise for the day.
- *It keeps you motivated*. It's easy to get discouraged if you think that you have to do a lengthy workout just to benefit from exercise. Instead, you can be confident that walking to the corner after dinner and doing knee bends during commercial breaks are absolutely worth the effort.

Everything counts, so keep moving!

Starting and Developing Your Exercise Routine

The first part of the chapter covered why exercise is beneficial and how much you should eventually aim for. You know the *what, why,* and *when*. Now, it's time to get down to the nitty-gritty—the *how* of exercise. You're geared up and ready to go, so you need to know exactly what to do. Starting an exercise program can be almost overwhelming if you've never exercised before or if it's been a while, but this section will walk you through it step by step.

Getting Active after Your Sleeve Gastrectomy

You can't jump into a full-blown exercise program the second you get home from the hospital after your VSG. Your body just isn't ready. It will take a few weeks until you're able to do a full range of activities. By that time you'll be into the solid foods diet phase and getting comfortable with the gastric sleeve, so it's a great time to develop a regular exercise routine.

Activity after the Sleeve Surgery

Even though you can't do vigorous exercise right after you get the sleeve, you can start some light activities. Light exercise will make the transition easier as you shift to more intense exercises later. It also might speed your recovery from surgery. Any gentle, painless movements you make increase blood flow and can help your wounds heal faster.

Small movements around the house can give you the benefits of exercise. You'll be surprised about how much activity you can easily add to your daily life once you start trying. Here are a few possibilities:

- Walking around the house
- Folding the laundry (being careful not to carry a heavy, full laundry basket!)
- Standing up instead of sitting
- Cooking, setting the table, and washing the dishes
- Playing with children (without lifting them up, if you're still close to surgery)
- Light housecleaning, such as making the beds and washing the windows (but avoid carrying or pushing a heavy vacuum cleaner or scrubbing the floors if you're still close to surgery)
- Playing golf

> **Tip**
>
> Chapter 11, "Recovering from Surgery," talks about the slow return to activity after the sleeve surgery. The chapter talks about avoiding heavy weights and water activities until you've healed a little bit and also about the benefits of keeping your body moving even during your recovery period.

You can start these activities as soon as you feel comfortable after getting home from the hospital. They're not formal parts of a specific exercise program, but they help you prepare for your planned exercise that will start about six weeks after surgery. Until then, slow walking is probably a safe option until you get your surgeon's go-ahead to add in aerobics or other, more intense activities.

Getting Medical Support and Clearance

People should check with their doctors before starting exercise programs if they have certain conditions. These include being overweight or obese, having heart disease, diabetes, arthritis, or asthma or other respiratory problems and if you haven't exercised regularly for a while.[39] Sound familiar? Well, yeah. As a gastric sleeve patient, you definitely need medical clearance before starting your program because you're starting off at an obese weight, and you might have other medical conditions that you need to be careful of. Plus, you want to be absolutely certain that you're fully healed from your surgery so that you don't reopen wounds and risk infections or leakage. Your surgeon or your primary care physician can give you the go-ahead for an exercise program.

Take Advantage of Expert Help

We recommend taking advantage of any physical therapy services that you are entitled to through your insurance plan or as part of the aftercare package that your sleeve surgeon provides. Physical therapists and physical therapist assistants are trained to diagnose your physical abilities and limitations and design an appropriate exercise program for you.[40]

In our experience, physical therapists and physical therapist assistants are phenomenal. Their goals are the same as yours: to improve your daily function, to let you enjoy exercise while it makes you healthier, and to improve your overall quality of life. They seem like magicians because they can come up with exercises that are interesting and pain-free. They can get you started in a program and work with you until you're comfortable taking charge of your own physical activity.

Even if you don't have a physical therapist, you can get help designing a safe and effective exercise program that meets your needs. Here are a few ideas:

- *A personal trainer at a local gym.* You might not want to pay the fees for a personal trainer, but many gyms and fitness centers provide free services to help you plan a program.

- *Your own friends, family members, and coworkers, if they know a bit about exercise.* Most regular exercisers are rightfully proud of their routines and are happy to share the knowledge they've gained.

- *A coach at a local high school or community college.* Some will be too busy to help you, but many will be glad to play a role in improving your health and helping you lose weight.

- *Online resources.* The American Council on Exercise has an assortment of articles for beginning exercisers on goal-setting and performing various exercises.[41] There are also links to other resources.

- *This book.* We'll guide you through a basic program starting at the beginning.

Online communities are great for advice too. BariatricPal.com, for example, is an online community whose members include thousands of gastric sleeve patients. They can share their own experiences with you so you have some ideas of what kind of exercises and progressions work for other sleeve patients. The forum is encouraging and has a zero tolerance for rudeness, and new members are always welcome and warmly greeted.

	Monday	Tuesday	Wednesday	Thursday	Friday	Saturday	Sunday
Week 1	5 minute warm up 5 minute cool down	5 minute warm up 5 minute cool down	Day off	5 minute warm up 5 minutes medium-speed walking 5 minute cool down	5 minute warm up 5 minute cool down	5 minute warm up 5 minutes medium-speed walking 5 minute cool down	Day off
Week 2	5 minute warm up 10 minutes medium-speed walking 5 minute cool down	5 minute warm up 5 minutes medium-speed walking 5 minute cool down	Day off	5 minute warm up 10 minutes medium-speed walking 5 minute cool down	5 minute warm up 5 minutes medium-speed walking 5 minute cool down	5 minute warm up 5 minutes brisk walking 5 minute cool down	Day off
Week 3	5 minute warm up 15 minutes medium-speed walking 5 minute cool down	5 minute warm up 5 minutes brisk walking 5 minute cool down	Day off	5 minute warm up 15 minutes medium-speed walking 5 minute cool down	5 minute warm up 5 minutes medium-speed walking 5 minute cool down	5 minute warm up 10 minutes brisk walking 5 minute cool down	Day off
Week 4	5 minute warm up 20 minutes medium-speed walking 5 minute cool down	5 minute warm up 10 minutes medium-speed walking 5 minute cool down	Day off	5 minute warm up 20 minutes medium-speed walking 5 minute cool down	5 minute warm up 10 minutes medium-speed walking 5 minute cool down	5 minute warm up 15 minutes brisk walking 5 minute cool down	Day off
Week 5	5 minute warm up 20 minutes medium-speed walking—can add in 15 seconds of jogging if you feel good—can do this up to 5 times during the 20 minutes and walk in between each one 5 minute cool down	5 minute warm up 10 minutes medium-speed walking 5 minute cool down	Day off	5 minute warm up Same as Monday—jogging is optional 5 minute cool down	5 minute warm up 15 minutes medium-speed walking 5 minute cool down	5 minute warm up 15 minutes brisk walking—can run up to 5 times but only if you feel great! 5 minute cool down	Day off

	Monday	Tuesday	Wednesday	Thursday	Friday	Saturday	Sunday
Week 6	5 minute warm up 25 minutes of brisk walking alternating with up to 6 short jogs 5 minute cool down	5 minute warm up 15 minutes of medium-speed walking 5 minute cool down	Day off	5 minute warm up 20 minutes of brisk walking with up to 6 short jogs 5 minute cool down	5 minute warm up 20 minutes of medium-speed walking 5 minute cool down	5 minute warm up Same as last Friday—You can jog up to 5 times if you feel good. 5 minute cool down	Day off
Week 7	5 minute warm up 25 minutes of brisk walking with as many as 10 short jogs 5 minute cool down	5 minute warm up 15 minutes of medium-speed walking 5 minute cool down	Day off	5 minute warm up 15 minutes of brisk walking with up to 5 jogs 5 minute cool down	5 minute warm up 20 minutes of medium-speed walking 5 minute cool down	5 minute warm up 20 minutes of brisk walking with up to 6 jogs 5 minute cool down	Day off
Week 8	5 minute warm up 30 minutes of brisk walking with jogs as you feel like it! 5 minute cool down	5 minute warm up 20 minutes of medium speed walking 5 minute cool down	Day off	5 minute warm up 20 minutes of brisk walking with short jogs 5 minute cool down	5 minute warm up 25 minutes of medium-speed walking 5 minute cool down	5 minute warm up 20 minutes of brisk walking and/or jogging 5 minute cool down	Day off
	Saturday	Sunday	Monday	Tuesday	Wednesday	Thursday	Friday

Table 41: Sample Plan for Starting a Workout Plan

367

A medical professional should approve any new exercise that you plan to try. It's safest to inform your doctor or surgeon about your plans before you try anything new just to be sure you're ready.

Start Slowly after You Get Medical Clearance

Medical clearance to start your exercise program is permission to start slowly, not to jump into an intense Olympic training schedule. Starting out conservatively has a few benefits:

- It gives you a chance to find out how exercising with the sleeve feels.
- It reduces your risk of injuries.
- It prevents burn-out, or mental fatigue, from feeling obligated to do too much.
- It increases your motivation because you're more likely to achieve conservative goals than unrealistic ones.

Sample Plan for Starting a Workout Plan

Table 41 is an example of how you can get from being sedentary—doing almost no regular physical activity—to becoming a regular walker–jogger. It's closer to your grasp than you probably think! This chart provides an example of an eight-week progression that is gradual and safe to follow with the supervision of your physician. Don't forget to include your warm up, your cool down, and some stretching!

Of course, feel free to "start" your week on any day that works for you—you don't have to start on Mondays and take your days off on Wednesdays and Sundays. You could, as you see on the bottom row of the chart, "start" your weeks on Saturdays and take days off on Mondays and Fridays.

Don't ever be afraid to repeat a week or two; for example, if you get through Week 3 and feel like it was a struggle, go back to Week 2 again and then try Week 3 again. This strategy is similar to the strategy you used during your post-surgery dietary progression from liquid foods to solid foods. When a new food was too much for you to handle, you had to step back a bit to the liquid, pureed, or soft foods diet that you were already comfortable with. Then, when you felt better, you could try the new food again. That's how it is with exercise too. When a week makes you especially tired or sore, just go back a week and repeat it until you feel better. Try the new week again when you're ready. There's no need to hurry—you're trying to develop an exercise program for life, not rush through a specific exercise plan that ends after a few weeks.

All about an Exercise "Workout"

We've mentioned "workout" a few times. A "workout" is a single exercise session. It goes from the time you get off the couch (or step into the gym) to the time you take off your sneakers. A workout includes your main cardio and/or strength-training components as well as additional components. In this section, you'll learn exactly how to get started and get through an entire workout so that you get the most out of your workout.

Components of a Workout

A standard workout includes these components in this order:

- Warm-up
- Stretching (here and/or after cool-down)
- Main physical activity session: cardio and/or resistance training
- Cool-down
- Stretching (here and/or after warm up)

Start off Right with a Good Warm Up

Before you start exercising, your body is at rest, whether you're a morning exerciser who's just getting out of bed or an afternoon exerciser who's been sitting at a desk all day. The warm up is your bridge between resting and getting into the full swing of your exercise. It slowly raises your heart rate, gets you breathing a little faster and deeper, and may even have you breaking a sweat by the end. Your warm up should be some light aerobic activity, such as one of the following:

- Slow walking, gradually speeding up to brisk walking by the end
- Deep knee bends and lunges
- Swinging and lifting your arms
- Kicking your legs forward and to the sides, one leg at a time
- You can use almost any light aerobic physical activity as a warm up. Just go slower and easier than you would during the middle of a hard workout. Slow cycling before a hilly ride, walking in the pool before lap swimming, and shooting free throws or easy lay ups before a basketball game are some examples.

Your warm up should be 5 to 10 minutes. Start slowly and comfortably and gradually pick up the intensity so that, by the end, you're about ready to get into the main activity for the day. Warming up properly not only makes it mentally easier to start your workout, but it also lowers your risk of injuries.[42] In addition, a good warm up can reduce the amount of soreness that you feel over the next day or two.[43]

A Good Cool Down Can End Your Workout on a Strong Note

The cool-down is almost a mirror image of your warm up. It takes you from a high-intensity exercise to a resting state—but gradually. If you skip your cool down, you can get blood pooling in your legs and risk feeling lightheaded or dizzy. Any activity that you did for a warm up can also serve as a cool down.

The cool down should be about 5 to 10 minutes. It gradually goes from the intensity of your main physical activity down to a very light effort. You know when you've cooled down enough when your heart isn't pounding any more, your breathing feels relaxed and normal, and your face is no longer beet red.

Stretch When Your Body Is Warm

There's no single best time to stretch.[44] The key to remember is that it's very important to only stretch after your muscles are warmed up. You can stretch after your warm up or after your cool down, but don't try to stretch before you're warmed up. Stretching cold muscles is a lot like trying to stretch an old rubber band that's no longer very elastic. The rubber band can break if you force it—and your cold muscles can be pulled or strained if you force them.

How do you stretch? Here are a few tips:

- Be sure to hit each major muscle group. You'll get your calves (back of your lower legs), hamstrings (back of your thighs), quadriceps (front of your thighs), shoulders and neck, biceps (front of upper arms), triceps (back of upper arms), groin, hip flexors (front of hips), and outside of your hips.
- Ease into each stretch and hold it for at least 15 to 30 seconds. Don't bounce; instead, stay still or gradually go deeper into the stretch.
- Stretching should never be painful. Deepen each stretch until you feel gentle pressure but no pain.
- Everyone's at a different level of flexibility. Ask your physical therapist or look online for beginners' modifications if you need them.
- Continue to breathe as you stretch. Don't hold your breath.

As long as you're warmed up, it's really up to you to decide when you want to stretch—as long as you make sure that you *do* stretch! Stretching after your warm up and before the main part of your workout gives you a chance to get revved up for your upcoming workout.[45] Stretching after your workout and cool down lets you focus on your accomplishment and reduce the tightness in your muscles. Some people like to stretch after the warm up *and* before the cool down.

Cross Training Should Be a Regular Choice

Cross training just means doing something different. Hard-core runners might cross train by swimming; tennis players might cross train with running; triathletes, who swim, bike, and run, might cross train by lifting weights; and you might cross train by including at least two or three different types of activities in your regular schedule. Cross training has many mental and physical benefits.[46]

Injury Prevention

Cross training reduces your risk for injuries, such as overuse injuries. These injuries get their name from their causes—they come from overuse, or repeatedly doing the same motions over and over again. Tendinitis, muscle strains, and joint pain are common overuse injuries. Even your bones can get overuse injuries in the form of stress fractures. Cross training provides a break from the same motions.

Preventing Muscle Imbalances

If you always bicycle but never lift weights, you'll have strong legs but not strong arms. If you're a right-hander who's always playing tennis, you might get a very strong right arm but not a strong left arm. A balanced strength-training program in addition to playing tennis will make you stronger in both arms and give you extra strength in your legs, hips, back, and core to improve your game. Similarly, cross training promotes balanced muscles to not only look more proportioned, but it also prevents injuries.

Improved Fitness

Cross training improves your overall fitness. If you always work on cardio, you'll have a strong heart and lungs but might not have the strong muscles and bones that you can get from including strength training. If you regularly walk, adding some dancing to your schedule can improve your balance and agility. Often, increasing the variety of activities that you do can lower your resting heart rate and increase your metabolism.

It Gives You a Mental Break

Once or twice a week you get to look forward to a new activity. It gives you a break from your regular physical activities so they don't get boring.

How to Cross Train

Just include a couple of different activities in your schedule in a typical week. These are some examples of fitting in some cross training:

- If you normally walk five days a week, consider cutting back to three days, bicycling on one day, and swimming one day.
- Join a weekly sports league.
- Take a new group fitness class, such as Latin dancing, aerobics, or yoga.
- Try circuits at the gym. Pick 10 to 15 different exercises, such as squats, bicep curls, lunges, and treadmill walking. Do each exercise for about 30 to 60 seconds. When you're done, you can repeat the circuit. This counts as cross training because you're doing so many different activities. Try to vary your circuits regularly so that you don't get stale.

As you work on your schedule and include cross training, check to make sure that you are including aerobic activities, resistance training, and flexibility exercises in your regular schedule.[47]

Goal-Setting

Goal-setting is an important part of planning an exercise program. Goals give you a sense of purpose. They let you know where you're going, and they help you recognize the progress you've made.

Examples of Possible Goals

You can have several goals at once. You might have some goals related to types of activities to try, how often you want to exercise, or specific achievements. They can be short-term or long-term. These are some examples:

- To start with, your plan can be as simple as having a short-term goal of walking up and down the driveway twice, with a medium-term goal of walking to the end of the block and back. Your long-term goal might be to jog around the block.

- Your goal might be to do one strength-training exercise and one aerobic activity in the first week. You might plan to increase your amount most weeks until you reach your final goal of three strength-training days and five aerobic activity days each week (yes, you can do strength-training and aerobic activity on the same day if you want!).

- Your immediate goal might be to stay on the treadmill for five minutes at a slow walking pace at 0% incline. You might work up to 30 minutes at an incline of 3% within a month.

- Your goal might be to do two sessions of cardiovascular, strength training, and stretching exercises every week for the next four months so that when you get to Hawaii for your vacation, you'll be ready for whatever your surfing instructor throws at you.

Be Accountable and Stick to An Exercise Program

Specific goals are better than general goals. That way, you can know whether you've achieved them or not. That keeps you accountable to yourself so that you work harder, and it makes you feel prouder when you accomplish them. Having interim goals, such as walking to the end of the block in between going up and down the driveway and jogging around the block, guides you and lets you know that your goal is attainable. These interim goals keep you motivated because you see progress. Recording your workouts is a great way to track your progress toward your goals. It's a lot like recording your food intake because you hold yourself accountable.

Sticking to the Exercise Program

You are gung-ho at the beginning. You're right on time for each exercise session. The time flies by, and you nail each workout. Then your exercise program doesn't seem as fun. You cut a few workouts short because you're bored, and you sleep through a few workouts because you don't want to work out. Pretty soon you're feeling more like your old sedentary self than the fit person you want to be. You've gone down the exercise-quitting road before, and you're afraid you're going to do that again.

This Time Is Different

This time you're going to stick to your program. Why? This time you're committed. You invested in the sleeve, after all. That's a permanent commitment to your diet, weight loss, and health. Your exercise program can be just as successful as your weight loss journey. The same persistence and dedication that you use for your diet can carry through to your exercise program.

So how can you keep your exercise program on track? It's all about figuring out what's wrong and fixing it. We'll work through some of the common troubles in this section so that you can put the motivation back into your exercise program.

Problem: Disliking Your Exercise

If you don't like calculus, don't major in math; if you don't like reading, don't become an English major. If you don't like swimming, don't base your program in the pool. It's far harder to stick to an exercise program that you don't like. Exercise should not be a chore; rather, it should—and can!—be fun. You're more likely to stick to your program when you look forward to your daily workout instead of dreading it.

Choose Activities That Match Your Personality

People have different likes and dislikes for foods, clothing, and hobbies—so why not for exercise too? Choose the wrong activities, and you'll be bored out of your mind. Choose the right ones, and you won't be able to stop working out! And, just like in other areas of your life, your physical activity preferences probably include a range of options.

Since you're just beginning an exercise program, you may not already know your exercise personality. It can take a while to figure out your preferences, but these questions can help you get started. You'll almost certainly have multiple answers to each of these questions—and that's good. You can try new things and develop a range of interests.

- Do you want to work out alone, with one partner, with a group of friends, on a team, or with a group of strangers?
- Do you want to be indoors, in an air-conditioned and clean building, or outdoors, in the fresh air and changing scenery?
- Do you want to do a competitive sport, non-competitive activity, or something in between? You can find leagues and teams of all skill levels and time commitments to match whatever you prefer.

Don't Count Yourself Out!

Give all activities a try, even if you didn't like something the last time you tried it. For example, your last experience with weight lifting might have been 30 years ago in your physical education class during your freshman year of high school. Maybe it was the most miserable thing you've ever done if the football jocks teased you about your weight and ridiculed you for being weaker than them. Now, though, you might discover that lifting weight makes you feel strong and powerful, and you don't have to take showers in a locker room with 100 of your closest 14-year-old enemies.

Keep It Interesting!

Boredom is about the quickest and most preventable reason for wanting to quit an exercise program. If you aren't feeling motivated any more, take a step back and ask yourself whether you're simply bored. These are a just a few ways you can keep individual workouts and your entire exercise program more interesting and motivating:

- *Vary your workouts.* Try doing two or three different aerobic activities one to three times a week each. You might walk with your spouse on Mondays and Saturdays, go to an aerobics class on Tuesdays, and play tennis with your friends on Sundays. That way, you always get to look forward to something fun and different.

- *Try a circuit.* If you tend to get bored quickly, break up your workout by doing a circuit workout at the gym. Divide your workout into short segments of about three to five minutes each. Do one activity per segment, then move quickly to the next activity for the next segment. If you're just working on cardio, you can get in a quick twenty-five minutes by doing the treadmill, stair climber, stationary bike, elliptical trainer, and rowing machine for five minutes each. Another option is to alternate segments of cardio with segments of weight training. Your heart rate will stay up, and you'll get in a great resistance training session. The time flies by on these kinds of workouts because you don't have a chance to get bored before it's time to go to the next exercise.

- *Take a class.* Group fitness classes help prevent boredom because no two classes are the same, even if you have the same instructor teaching the same kind of class each week. There'll be minor changes mixed with the familiarity of the class. Group fitness classes give you the chance to challenge yourself even while you are getting more comfortable with the moves.

- *Vary the intensity.* Alternate fast cycling with slow cycling, uphill walking on the treadmill with level walking, and swimming laps with water calisthenics in the pool. Varying the intensity makes the time fly by because you're focusing on your hard and easy intervals. This type of training can get your heart rate up and burn more calories than a steady intensity workout.

- *Go social.* Surrounding yourself with fun people can prevent boredom. You never know exactly how the workout's going to go or what you'll get to talk about during it.

Challenge Yourself with New Activities

New activities give you more options for your exercise. The more new activities you try, the more options you have for enjoyable activities. Set a goal to regularly try a new activity. You might resolve to try one new exercise each month, or you can even tie your new activities to weight loss with the sleeve. Here is a sample progression of adding new activities when you hit certain weight loss goals:

- You might start your exercise program with walking.
- At 50 pounds, your next goal might be to go to a yoga class at the gym.
- At 100 pounds of weight loss, you might decide to add some running to your walking routine.
- At 150 pounds, you might start training to surf.
- At 200 pounds, you might take your dream trip to Hawaii and be ready for whatever your surf teacher throws at you.

Keep Trying

Whatever you do, don't give up. You may start to wonder if you're ever going to find the exercise that works for you. Walking is too boring, you're not coordinated enough to enjoy dance classes, aerobics is too old-school, you live in an apartment so you can't garden outside, you don't like team sports…and then a last-ditch effort leads you to meet up with a hiking group, and you fall in love with the scenery and your new best friends! Or maybe you feel as though you've tried and disliked everything…until you pick up your son after school and realize that you don't want to leave because you love being a referee for the children. There are so many different scenarios that can lead to finding the exercise or exercises to keep you healthy and losing weight. Don't give up until you find them!

Give It a Second Chance

A good rule of thumb is to always try something twice or more before deciding you don't like it. There's a good chance that you'll find the dance moves easier to follow, that you'll be able to build the mental strength to prevent boredom on a treadmill, and that you'll feel like a strong fish instead of a drowning landlubber.

Problem: Running Out of Time

This is probably the most common excuse that people give for not exercising. You probably are extremely busy and may even believe that this excuse is the truth, but it is just an excuse. You can get the physical activity you need if you try hard enough.

First, take a good hard look at your schedule. Make sure that you're truly short on time—and not that you're finding ways to fill your time so that you don't *have* to exercise. If that's what you're doing, it's time to find some activities that you genuinely enjoy and look forward to. That's what the above section is about.

Where There's a Will, There's a Way

Making time is possible if you want to badly enough. We're all busy. Ask anyone who's exercising at your local gym or park, and they'll tell you that they're busy too. You may be shocked at how busy some of the regular exercisers that you see are. Okay. Now that we've established that everyone's busy, it's time to think about *how*, not *whether*, you're planning to fit in your exercise.

You're Worth It

Some sleeve patients feel guilty because they think that their exercise commitments are taking away from the family. That's just not true. You're losing weight and following a healthy lifestyle so that you can be a better family member. You're gaining more energy and on the path to being a better contributor to the family. Compared to the 30 daily minutes you're dedicating to exercise, your family is going to get a ton more benefits from your health and happiness—and the possibility that you'll live longer. You need to remember every second of every day that *you are worth it*. You are on this sleeve journey because you chose to get healthy, so take advantage of every second of it.

A Few Way to Make Time

These are a few more ideas for making time in your schedule for exercise:

- Include your family—instead of having family time in front of the television, ask your kids about their school days while you're shooting hoops in the driveway. Walk them to school instead of driving them.
- Walk around the field instead of sitting in the stands while your children are at soccer practice. You'll still get to watch the action as you burn calories.
- Write down your exercise plans in your planner—you'll be amazed that treating it like a firm appointment will allow you to leave time available.
- Exercise on your lunch break. Invite a coworker to walk or go to the gym with you and you might make a new work friend as you get fit.
- Bike to work. You'd be surprised at how many workplaces support employees biking to work. You might be able to shower and store your clothes at work. If not, another option is to join a gym close to your workplace and shower there.
- Save time by keeping your exercise gear handy and ready to use so that you can grab it whenever you have a few minutes to work out.

Each Small Change Helps

Some days you won't be able to fit in a full, uninterrupted workout, but small changes in your lifestyle can add up to extra calories burned and better fitness without taking too much time. These are a few ideas that can get you moving without eating into your time. They're good not only for busy days but also for your daily routine.

- Park a few blocks away or at the far end of the parking lot instead of within feet of building entrances—and when parking lots are crowded, this can actually save time because you won't have to drive in endless circles looking for a parking spot.

- Take the stairs to get from floor to floor instead of using the elevator. This one is sometimes a time-saver too when elevators are slow or crowded.

- Stand up periodically when you're working at your desk. Stretch and do a few arm swings, deep knee bends, and lunges.

- Pace back and forth while talking on your cell phone instead of sitting down. If you're on a landline, buy a cordless phone so you can walk around the house or office.

- Walk to the other side of your workplace to talk to your colleagues instead of sending an email or phoning them. They will probably appreciate seeing you anyway.

- Do knee lifts while you're waiting for the microwave to go off, calf raises while you're washing the dishes after dinner, and squats during television commercials (of course, you can always skip the television program altogether and head off for a full exercise session…).

Problem: Self-Consciousness

Many new exercisers, especially obese ones, worry what others think of them. As mentioned earlier in this chapter, you have nothing to worry about as long as you know deep down that you're doing the best you can for your health. But, if you're so worried about what people think of you that you just can't face the thought of exercising in public, then don't. You have other options. Exercise in the privacy of your own home using your own equipment. Or, what some people do to avoid fearing the stares of others is to exercise in the dark. Depending on where you live, you might have several months a year when it's easy to exercise before sunrise or after sunset without getting up too early or staying out too late. You might even make the eventual change from being a shy, dark-only exerciser to an outgoing, anytime exerciser! If you choose to exercise in the dark, stay in well-lit areas, wear reflective clothing, and stay aware of your surroundings.

Problem: The Weather Won't Cooperate

You plan an outdoors workout, but it's too hot, cold, windy, wet, humid, or icy. Maybe you don't want to go outside in the snow during winter or face the heat of summer. What do you do when the weather's not on your side?

Get Used to It

Your body is a lot tougher than you might think. If you never tried walking in the drizzle or cross-country skiing, you might not have realized that you can. Tons of people just brave the elements and continue with their planned workouts. Another option is to change your workout time. So if you normally work out at lunchtime, try getting up super early in the summer to beat the heat. Or, if you know that the roads will be cleared of snow later in the day, postpone your workout until after work. Don't ever try to exercise in dangerous conditions, such as thunderstorms, freezing rain, heavy snowfall, or an excessive heat warning.

Modify Your Workout

If you just can't beat the weather, don't let it beat you. Change your workout so it's appropriate. Swim or go to an air-conditioned gym or recreation center in the summer; go to the gym or use an exercise DVD at home during the winter.

How Should I Change My Diet When I Start a Physical Activity Program?

Your exercise program burns calories and builds muscle. You need the right nutrition to support your activity, but your diet doesn't need to change much from your prescribed sleeve diet. That's especially true when you're near the beginning of your sleeve journey. At that time, you're already losing weight quickly, and one of your primary goals is to keep up your calorie deficit. That is, you want to keep a big difference between the calories you eat and the calories you burn. Exercise increases the deficit and supports weight loss.

In the beginning, the sleeve diet is also appropriate for your physical activity program for these reasons:

- It's nutritious. The protein and other nutrients that you emphasize on the sleeve diet are the same ones you need to support physical activity.
- You're not exercising too intensely at the beginning. You don't need a lot of extra calories to support intense exercise.
- You eat frequently. The small, frequent meals and snacks on the sleeve diet keep your energy levels up so you can be ready for exercise and recover from each workout

Water is the biggest concern with exercise, especially if you're a heavy sweater or are exercising in hot conditions. In addition to your regular 6 to 8 cups of water throughout the day, drink about 16 extra ounces of water about an hour before you work out. Then, drink another 16 ounces afterward. During exercise, drink water when you are thirsty. You almost certainly do not need a sports drink during exercise.

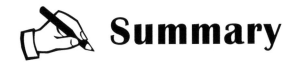 **Summary**

- ☞ This chapter has the information you need to go from being a sedentary person to an active, fit one.

- ☞ First, get your doctor's approval.

- ☞ Then, start with easy activities in short exercise sessions. Only gradually increase the intensity and length of your workouts. Most of all, enjoy your new freedom to find activities that you love and that will make you healthier and happier at the same time!

Your Turn: Keeping Your Exercise Log

An exercise log helps you plan and record your physical activity. Some people like to keep a weekly calendar; others prefer a monthly calendar. Keeping an exercise log can motivate you to keep going because you get to fill it in each day and watch it fill up. Include what you did, how long you did it for, how you felt, whether other people were involved, and any other details, such as hitting a goal or extreme weather conditions.

Table 42 is a four-week log for you to start. You can photocopy the blank one and use it again once you fill up the first one.

	Sunday	Monday	Tuesday	Wednesday	Thursday	Friday	Saturday
Sample	30 minutes hiking with Betty. Hard but so fun! Sunny—we took water bottles.	Planned day off. Needed it badly; sore from weekend.	Normal gym day. 20 minutes on treadmill, 15 minutes weight lifting. Nothing exciting.	Boot camp in the park! First class. I was nervous, but people were nice. They're something for me to strive for!	Sore everywhere from yesterday! Aqua aerobics at the gym for 50 minutes. Good workout.	Walked 20 minutes moderate with Bill, then 10 minutes at home with dumbbells. Tired, not into it. Glad to finish.	Off. Needed rest after yesterday and want to be ready for tomorrow's hike with Betty!
Week 1							
Week 2							
Week 3							
Week 4							

Table 42: Four-week exercise log

1   NWCR Facts. The National Weight Control Registry. Web site. Accessed http://www.nwcr.ws/Research/default.htm. Accessed October 31, 2012.

2   National Health Information Center. Get moving calculator: exercise and calories burned. U.S. Department of Health and Human Services. Web site. Retrieved from http://www.healthfinder.gov/docs/doc12322.htm. 2012, July 2. Accessed October 31, 2012.

3   Ainsworth BE, Haskell WL, Herrmann SD, Meckes N. Bassett Jr. DR, Tudor-Locke C, Greer JL, Vezina J, Whitt-Glover MC, Leon AS. Compendium of Physical Activities: a second update of codes and MET values. Medicine and Science in Sports and Exercise. 2011;43:1575-1581.

4   Calorie Control Council. Get moving calculator. Web site. Retrieved from http://www.caloriescount.com/getMoving.aspx. 2012. Accessed October 31, 2012.

5   Physical activity for everyone: physical activity and health. Centers for Disease Control and Prevention Web site. Retrieved from http://www.cdc.gov/physicalactivity/everyone/health/index.html 2011. Updated February 16. Accessed November 1, 2012.

6   Physical activity for everyone: physical activity and health. Centers for Disease Control and Prevention Web site. Retrieved from http://www.cdc.gov/physicalactivity/everyone/health/index.html 2011. Updated February 16. Accessed November 1, 2012.

7   American Cancer Society: Kushi LH, Doyle C, McCullough M, Rock C, Demark-Wahnefried W, Bandera EV, … Gansler T. American Cancer Society guidelines on nutrition and physical activity for cancer prevention. Cancer: A Cancer Journal for Clinicians. 2012;62:30-67.

8   Centers for Disease Control and Prevention, National Institutes of Health, U.S. Department of Health and Human Services. Chapter 4: the effects of physical activity on health and disease. In Physical activity and health: a report of the surgeon general. 1996;Washington, D.C.

9   American Cancer Society: Kushi LH, Doyle C, McCullough M, Rock C, Demark-Wahnefried W, Bandera EV, … Gansler T. American Cancer Society guidelines on nutrition and physical activity for cancer prevention. Cancer: A Cancer Journal for Clinicians. 2012;62:30-67.

10 Vincent, H.K., Ben-David, K., Conrad, B.P., Lamb, K.M., Seay, A.N., & Vincent, K.R. (2012).Rapid changes in gait, musculoskeletal pain and quality of life after bariatric surgery. Surgery for Obesity and Related Diseases, 8(3):346-354.

11 Weak in the knees – the quest for a cure. Exploration Systems Mission Directorate Education Outreach, National Aeronautics and Space Administration . Web site. http://weboflife.nasa.gov/currentResearch/currentResearchGeneralArchives/weakKnees.htm. 2012. Accessed November 2, 2012.

12 About osteoporosis: exercise for healthy bones. National Osteoporosis Foundation. web site. Retrieved from http://www.nof.org/aboutosteoporosis/prevention/exercise. 2011. Accessed November 2, 2012.

13 Belavy, D.L., Bansmann, P.M., Bohnne, G., Frings-Meuthen, P., Heer, M., Rittweger, J., Zange, J., Felsenberg, D. (2011). Changes in intervertebral disc morphology persist five months after 21-day bed rest. Journal of Applied Physiology, 111:1304-1314.

14 Human research program: areas of study: bone health. National Aeronautic and Space Administration. Web site. http://www.nasa.gov/exploration/humanresearch/areas_study/physiology/physiology_bone.html. 2012. Accessed November 2, 2012.

15 Kemper KJ. Complementary and alternative medicine therapies to promote healthy moods. Pediatric Clinics of North America. 2007;54:901.

16 Kline CE, Sui X, et all. Dose-response effects of exercise training on the subjective sleep quality of postmenopausal women: exploratory analyses of a randomized controlled trial. BMJ Open. 2012;2(4).

17 Rosano, C., Venkatraman, V.K., Guralnik, J., Newman, A.B., Glynn, N.W., Launer, L., Taylor, C.A., Williamson, J., Studenski, S., Pahor, M., & Aizenstein, H. (2010). Psychomotor speed and functional brain MRI 2 years after completing a physical activity treatment. The Journals of Gerontology. Series A, Biological Sciences and Medical Sciences, 65: 639-47.

18 Kemper KJ. Complementary and alternative medicine therapies to promote healthy moods. Pediatric Clinics of North America. 2007;54:901.

19 Colcombe, S.J., Erickson, K.I., Scalf, P.E., Kim, J.S., Prakash, R., McAuley, E., Elavsky, S., Marquez, D.X., Hu, L., & Kramer, A.F. (2006). Aerobic exercise training increases brain volume in aging humans. The Journals of Gerontology. Series A, Biological Sciences and Medical Sciences, 61:166-1170.

20 Boecker, H., Sprenger, T., Spilker, M.E., Henriksen, G., Koppenhoefer, M., Wagner, K.J., Valet, M., Berthele, A., & Tolle, T.R. (2008). The runner's high: opiodergic mechanisms in the human brain. Cerebral Cortex, 18, 2523-31.

21 Mechanick JI, Kushner RF, Sugerman HJ, Gonzalez-Campoy M, Collazo-Clavell ML, … Dixon J. American Association of Clinical Endocrinologists, The Obesity Society and American Society for Metabolic and Bariatric Surgery medical guidelines for clinical practice for the perioperative nutritional, metabolic and nonsurgical support of the bariatric surgery patient. Obesity. 2009;17:S1-S70.

22 McVay MA, Friedman KE. The benefits of cognitive behavioral groups for bariatric surgery patients. Bariatric Times. 2012;9(9):22-28.

23 Kafrik N, Valfer R, Nativ O, Shiloni E, Hazzan D. Behavioral outcomes following laparoscopic sleeve gastrectomy after failed laparoscopic adjustable gastric banding. Obes Surg. 2012.

24 Centers for Disease Control and Prevention. (2011, December 1). Physical activity for everyone: how much physical activity do adults need? Retrieved from http://www.cdc.gov/physicalactivity/everyone/guidelines/adults.html

25 Kaiser Family Foundation. (n.d.) Percent of adults who participated in moderate or vigorous physical activities, 2009. Retrieved from http://statehealthfacts.org/comparemaptable.jsp?ind=92&cat=2

26 Weight-Control Information Network, National Institute of Diabetes and Digestive and Kidney Diseases (NIDDK). (2006, November). Physical activity and weight control. Retrieved from http://www.win.niddk.nih.gov/publications/physical.htm

27 McGuire, M.T., Wing, R.R., Klem, M.L., Seagle, H.M. & Hill, J.O. (1998). Long-term maintenance of weight loss: Do people who lose weight through various weight loss methods use different behaviors to maintain their weight? International Journal of Obesity, 22:572-577.

28 Wing, R.R., & Phelan, S. (2005). Long-term weight loss maintenance. American Journal of Clinical Nutrition, 82:222S-225S.

29 National Weight Control Registry. (n.d.). NWCR facts. Retrieved from http://www.nwcr.ws/Research/default.htm

30 Shick, S.M., Wing, R.R., Klem, M.L., McGuire, M.T., Hill, J.O. & Seagle, H.M. (1998). Persons successful at long-term weight loss and maintenance continue to consume a low calorie, low fat diet. Journal of the American Dietetic Association,98:408-413

31 U.S. Department of Health and Human Services & U.S. Department of Agriculture. (2010). Dietary Guidelines for Americans. (7th edition). U.S. Government Printing Office, Washington, D.C.

32 National Heart, Lung and Blood Institute. (n.d.). Moderate-level physical activities. Retrieved from http://www.nhlbi.nih.gov/hbp/prevent/p_active/m_l_phys.htm

33 Heart rate zone calculator. American Council on Exercise. Web site. http://www.acefitness.org/calculators/heart-rate-zone-calculator.aspx. Accessed November 3, 2012.

34 Monitoring exercise intensity using heart rate. American Council on Exercise. Web site. http://www.acefitness.org/fitfacts/fitfacts_display.aspx?itemid=38. Accessed November 3, 2012.

35 Physical activity: how much physical activity do adults need? Centers for Disease Control and Prevention. Web site. http://www.cdc.gov/physicalactivity/everyone/guidelines/adults.html. Updated 2011, December 16. Accessed November 3, 2012.

36 Get fit facts: strength Training 101. American Council on Exercise. Web site. http://www.acefitness.org/fitfacts/fitfacts_display.aspx?itemid=2661. Accessed November 3, 2012.

37 American Council on Exercise. (n.d.). Get fit facts: strengthen your abdominals with stability balls. Retrieved from http://www.acefitness.org/fitfacts/fitfacts_display.aspx?itemid=2662&category=11

38 American Council on Exercise. (n.d.). Get fit facts: ACE's top ten reasons to stretch. Retrieved from http://www.acefitness.org/updateable/update_display.aspx?CMP=HET_0807&pageID=520

39 Mayo Clinic Staff. (2010, December 18). Exercise: when to check with your doctor first. Mayo Clinic. Retrieved from http://www.mayoclinic.com/health/exercise/SM00059/METHOD=print

40 PT careers: role of a physical therapist. American Physical Therapy Association. Web site. Retrieved from http://www.apta.org/PTCareers/RoleofaPT/. 2011, January 15. Accessed November 4, 2012.

41 American Council on Exercise (n.d.). Get fit facts: before you start an exercise program. Retrieved from http://www.acefitness.org/fitfacts/fitfacts_display.aspx?itemid=2612

42 Woods, K., Bishop, P., & Jones, E. (2007). Warm-up and stretching in the prevention of muscular injury. Sports Medicine, 37:1089-99. Retrieved from http://www.ncbi.nlm.nih.gov/pubmed/18027995

43 Law, R.Y.W., & Herbert, R.D. (2003). Warm-up reduces delayed-onset muscle soreness but cool-down does not: a randomized controlled trial. Australian Journal of Physiotherapy, 53:91-95.

44 Shrier, I. (2012). Should people stretch before exercise? The Western Journal of Medicine, 174:282-283.

45 American Council on Exercise. (n.d.). Get fit facts: flexible benefits. Retrieved from http://www.acefitness.org/fitfacts/fitfacts_display.aspx?itemid=2610

46 American Council on Exercise. (n.d.). Get fit facts: cross-training for fun and fitness. Retrieved from http://www.acefitness.org/fitfacts/fitfacts_display.aspx?itemid=2547

47 American Academy of Orthopaedic Surgeons. (2011, October). Cross training. Retrieved from http://www.orthoinfo.aaos.org/topic.cfm?topic=A00339

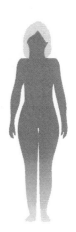

17

What to Expect in the First Year after VSG

So far this book has covered the gastric sleeve starting from the beginning of your journey. You know the strengths and weaknesses of the surgery, how to choose a surgeon, how to get prepared for and recover from your surgery, and how to plan and follow a nourishing sleeve diet that'll help you lose weight and prevent side effects from the gastric sleeve. Those are the parts of the sleeve experience that you might think of first when you think of the gastrectomy, but the journey continues beyond this.

The gastric sleeve experience affects all parts of your life. The changes that happen go far beyond the number on the scale. In this chapter, we'll cover some of the things you can expect during the first year after getting the sleeve. Things are easier when you know what to expect because you can prepare for them. Here's what the chapter will cover:

- Physical and emotional changes in the first year
- Common cosmetic surgeries that bariatric surgery patients get after losing a lot of weight
- More changes to expect with the sleeve

Of course, this chapter can't predict everything that will happen over this exciting year, but knowing even a little bit can be helpful. Something else that will help you get through this year is the knowledge that you're not alone.

The First Year Is Filled with Changes

The VSG is a life-changing experience. Along with your weight going down, you can experience plenty of other changes, both physical and otherwise. Your entire world may change — and mostly in great ways!

Physical Changes – Weight Loss and Other Effects

The first physical change is pretty obvious. You might lose 100 pounds or more in the first year after the sleeve. Your appearance is going to change pretty quickly. How quickly depends on your body type, your starting weight, and how quickly you lose weight.

Changes in Weight

- **People Won't All Notice Your Weight Loss at the Same Time -** The people who are closest to you, such as your family and close friends, may notice your weight loss soonest. Some people see you frequently but aren't too close to you. They may include coworkers and neighbors, and they might not notice your weight loss until you've lost quite a bit of weight. They're not ignoring your efforts or being intentionally unobservant; they're just not as familiar with your appearance.
- **Reacting Positively when People Notice Your Weight Loss -** You spent so long fighting obesity and defending your weight from other people that you might naturally get defensive when people comment on your weight loss after the VSG. This is especially likely if you're shy or if the comment comes from someone who you don't like or who

doesn't know about your surgery. People who don't often see you will be especially shocked by your weight loss. Try to take each comment as a compliment. Learn to enjoy each time you get to surprise someone with the new, more attractive you! You've certainly earned it.

- **You'll Re-Discover Body Parts That You'd Forgotten You Had -** This is meant in the best possible way, of course. As your fat comes off, you'll see new curves and even a few angles that you hadn't seen or dared to hope think about for years. Your knees and elbows might start to look like joints instead of cushions, and your jaw line— supporting only a single, not triple, chin!—will eventually emerge! Eventually, as you lose more weight and work out a little bit, your muscles will make their appearances. A huge milestone for many sleeve patients is the day they can see their feet while standing up straight. You'll start to enjoy looking at yourself instead of turning your head away from the mirror and avoiding the camera.

Other Physical Effects

- **You Might Lose Some of Your Hair[1] -** When you're losing weight so quickly, your body is doing everything it can to conserve energy and nutrients. Hair loss, also known as alopecia, is common in weight loss surgery patients because of your rapid weight loss. Low levels of selenium are linked to a higher risk for alopecia, so you might want to ask your doctor or dietitian about how to get enough of this essential mineral.[2]

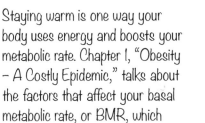

Tip

Staying warm is one way your body uses energy and boosts your metabolic rate. Chapter 1, "Obesity – A Costly Epidemic," talks about the factors that affect your basal metabolic rate, or BMR, which describes how fast you burn calories throughout the day and night.

Alopecia itself is not dangerous, but thinning hair can make you feel self-conscious. Luckily, it's probably more noticeable to you than to anyone else. In addition, the condition is temporary, and your hair will grow back to normal when you're at your maintenance weight and you're eating enough calories to sustain your weight and support hair growth.

- **You Might Feel Cold -** Feeling cold is another result of your body's effort to lose weight, and you might feel cold as you quickly lose weight during this first year of your sleeve journey. That's a sign that your body is conserving energy, or calories, as you reduce your intake. Remember, your body uses calories as part of your basal metabolic rate. Part of that energy expenditure goes towards "burning" calories to keep you warm. When you cut back on your calorie intake to lose weight, you may feel a little cooler than usual.

Emotional and Social Changes

Your weight loss journey isn't just about the number on the scale. It's not even just about your physical health and appearance. Getting the sleeve is also about personal emotional growth and improving your interpersonal relationships to improve your life. During this first year of your life-changing experience, it's natural to notice not only physical changes but also emotional ones. Your personal outlook and social relationships can change, and a positive attitude increases the likelihood that these changes will be positive.

Self-Confidence over Self-Doubt

You will probably gain more self-confidence as you lose weight. You get to take credit for the decreasing numbers on the scale week after week, and you will become confident that you can do—and are doing—everything what you need to do to lose weight with the sleeve. Your self-confidence in taking charge of your weight can translate into self-confidence in other parts of your life as well.

You'll have the occasional moment of self-doubt. It might come when you encounter someone who snubs your hard work, when you hit a weight loss plateau, or when you feel excessively hungry and give in to your craving even though you know you shouldn't. The important thing is that you keep it to a moment of self-doubt and don't let it turn into a rut. And once you get used to changing your self-doubt into self-confidence, you'll gain even more confidence that—yes!—you *can* do this!

Changes in Your Social Life

Most of the changes will be good. As you lose weight and gain confidence in yourself, you'll probably have a more positive attitude and more energy, and you will be more fun to be around. You'll probably have more fun with your friends and family and likely find it easier to meet people.

Some people might treat you differently than before.

- Some people who looked down on you because of your obesity might start to treat you with a bit of respect.
- Others might reject the idea of the bariatric surgery. They might treat you like a cheater or act as though you don't deserve to be happy and healthy.
- The people who you care about and who love you will treat you as you deserve: just as warmly as before the sleeve but with additional respect for your hard work to lose the weight and get healthy.

An important point to consider is that, in general, people react to the news of your sleeve based on how you present it. If you're embarrassed about it, they'll be embarrassed to talk about it, or they'll judge you for getting it. If you're proud and open, they will be far more likely to be interested and accepting.

Changes in Your Quality of Life

Your quality of life, or QOL, basically refers to how good life is for you. Most bariatric surgery patients who lose the amount of weight they had hoped for experience a higher quality of life.[3] This is because of:

- Improved health.
- Fewer physical limitations.
- More self-confidence.
- Better relationships with other people.
- Better mood.

Changes in Your Relationship with Food

Your relationship with food may change. Many obese patients spend years struggling with food, and you might start to overcome some of these challenges after the sleeve gastrectomy.

- **Less hunger.** Before surgery, you might have been hungry all the time, leading you to overeat and continue to gain weight. After surgery, you might not be as hungry before meals, and you might get full sooner when you eat.
- **Preference for healthy foods.** Before surgery, you might have craved salty, sugary, and fatty foods — think fast food, sweets, and fried foods. After surgery, as you eat the sleeve diet, your tastes might change. Your cravings for these high-calorie foods might decrease, and you might start to prefer more nutritious options, such as lean protein, vegetables, and whole grains.
- **Changes in how you use food.** Some obese patients use food as an emotional outlet or as a way to escape their feelings. After the VSG, you might stop turning to junk food to hide your feelings and instead use healthy foods in a healthier way: to provide essential nutrients.
- **Better self-control.** You got obese in the first place because you ate too much, and one of the biggest reasons for that might have been because you didn't have self-control. Taking a second helping, finishing the entire package instead of stopping at one serving, and sneaking a bite or two in the kitchen were probably regular occurrences that showed up on the scale. Self-control with your portions is essential with the sleeve to lose weight and prevent complications.

Changes in Your Health

You know that a lot of your health conditions were related to your obesity. Things like high blood pressure, high cholesterol, and type 2 diabetes are just a few of the examples that you've heard over and over again. What you might not have realized, though, is that you don't have to wait for years after the sleeve surgery to get good news about your health. Your health will be measurably better long before you reach your goal weight. That's right; by the time you lose about 5 to 10 percent of your initial body weight—that's about 15 to 30 pounds if you started at 300 pounds—you'll probably already have improvements in your health.[4]

Improvements in Chronic Conditions

Chronic conditions or risk factors for them may improve if you follow all of your surgeon's instructions. Some of these changes can occur regarding your heart health and diabetes, prediabetes, or risk for diabetes:

- Lower blood pressure
- Lower total cholesterol and lower "bad" LDL cholesterol levels
- Higher "good" HDL cholesterol (The biggest influence on your HDL cholesterol levels is exercise. So if you start a physical activity program during this time, your HDL cholesterol will go up, and your risk of heart disease will go down.)
- Lower blood sugar levels[5]

If you were on medications for high blood pressure to lower your cholesterol levels or to control your blood sugar, you may get to lower your dosage. Eventually, when you get closer to your goal weight, you may get to stop taking some or all of your medications altogether! That would let you avoid any side effects, let you stop worrying about remembering to take them, and save you money. Of course, don't ever stop taking your prescription medications without telling your doctor.

More Energy and Feeling Better

Losing weight from the sleeve gastrectomy can reduce or even get rid of your sleep apnea.[6]

- You won't have to worry about your breathing stopping while you sleep.
- You'll get higher-quality sleep and have way more energy during the day. That's the result of not waking up during the night.
- You might not have to sleep with a continuous positive airway pressure, or CPAP, machine.

You'll also have more energy during the day when your blood sugar levels are better controlled because they won't be going up and then crashing, leaving you exhausted. Finally, you'll have a lot more energy because, simply, it's easier to move. The more weight you lose, the less weight you have to carry around every single time you want to move.

Side Effects from the Sleeve

You'll almost certainly have side effects from the sleeve. They won't necessarily be serious, but they can be unpleasant. Before you got the sleeve, you could, and often did, eat more than you should have without any immediate serious side effects. After getting the sleeve, there are immediate consequences to eating the wrong foods or eating too much. You'll notice these most in the first few months after surgery, but their threats can stick around for years at times when your diet slips.

Gastrointestinal Side Effects Are Likely

- **Productive burps.** This is a polite term for having regurgitation—a tiny amount of vomit—slip back up from your sleeve through the esophagus into the back of your mouth after you eat. Regurgitation and heartburn are more likely when you eat too much or too fast. They can be a little embarrassing, especially when you get them in public while you're trying to eat.
- **Vomiting and nausea.** Vomiting and nausea can be more serious results from the same causes of productive burps: eating too much, eating too fast, or eating something you shouldn't have.
- **Diarrhea.** Diarrhea can result from eating too much, eating too fast, or eating high-fat or high-sugar foods that aren't on your plan.

First, be sure that the symptoms aren't serious. You might need to call your surgeon. Then, the best thing to do for these gastrointestinal symptoms is usually to go back to a liquid or pureed food diet until the symptoms stop. If you can pin down the food or eating behavior that triggered the symptoms, avoid it; only try it again in the future, in very small quantities, when you're over this particular episode of difficulty. Think about whether you've been chewing your food slowly enough, taken only the portions you're supposed to take, and have been careful to stop eating when you're full.

Avoiding Side Effects Can Motivate You to Stick to the Sleeve Diet

The best way to look at these unpleasant side effects is as a blessing in disguise. Although these symptoms are uncomfortable, they're often avoidable and predictable, making them ideal motivation for sticking to the sleeve diet. The chapter covers additional complications from the VSG. For all of them, continuing to follow your sleeve diet and surgeon's instructions is the best way to prevent them.

You Might Need or Choose Additional Surgical Procedures

One surgery, the sleeve gastrectomy, is enough of an experience! However, you might need or want additional surgeries. These are some of the possibilities:

- Surgery to correct a serious sleeve complication, such as leaking
- Conversion to the biliopancreatic diversion with duodenal switch (BPD-DS)
- Revisional surgery to another type of bariatric surgery, such as the adjustable gastric band or gastric bypass. This can happen in about 5% of patients.[7]
- Plastic surgery, also known as body contouring or cosmetic surgery

Serious complications requiring additional surgeries and the BPD-DS as the follow-up procedure to the VSG are covered earlier in this book. This chapter will discuss elective surgeries—the ones you choose—to improve your appearance. This type of surgery was probably far from your mind when you started looking into weight loss surgery, but you might find that you need or want other surgeries to get your body looking the way you'd imagined it from the beginning. Your impressive amount of weight loss can make you feel dissatisfied with your body, and it can also lead to health risks. Body contouring surgery is relatively common after successful weight loss following bariatric surgery; one study found that one-third of bariatric surgery patients had had at least one procedure.[8]

Surgeries to Remove Excess Skin

You're going to be losing a lot of weight, and your body will be changing *a lot*. That's great in almost every way, but with such dramatic weight loss, you'll develop folds of skin that aren't necessary any more. They can be uncomfortable and make you feel unattractive. They can even cause medical problems, such as the following:

- Back pain from the weight of your abdominal skin hanging down in front.
- Inability to keep yourself clean in the bath or shower because of so much extra skin. For women, excess skin between the legs can lead to frequent yeast infections.
- Risk of regaining the weight because you're too uncomfortable to exercise. When you try, the loose skin flaps and bumps, and you feel very heavy, so you quit.
- Interference with a normal life. Some extra skin, such as around your abdomen, under your arms, or between your legs may be so heavy and bulky that it makes you feel tired, and you can't even get through your normal daily routine in comfort.
- Rashes from constant rubbing of skin against skin. These can be painful and itchy and lead to infections because there is broken skin.

Common Types of Body Contouring or Plastic Surgery after Large Scale Weight Loss

You'll be losing weight from all over your body, and there are a ton of different procedures that might be beneficial for you depending on how much weight you lose. These are a few of the more common skin removal or body contouring procedures for bariatric surgery patients who've lost a lot of weight. In general, bariatric surgery patients who've lost a ton of weight are most likely to complain about excess skin around the waist and abdomen compared to other areas of the body and are most likely to be satisfied with surgery in those areas.[9]

Panniculectomy or Abdominoplasty

You can call it your evil twin, you can call it "Fred," you can call it whatever you want… but the fact remains that your abdominal skin often feels like you're dragging around a second person—who's not on your side! *Panniculectomy* is the term for removing the excess skin and fat of your belly; an *abdominoplasty*, also known as a "tummy tuck," involves removing the excess skin and fat while also tightening up your stomach muscles.

Brachioplasty

Come on, let's be serious. *Brachioplasty*? We all know it better as removal of the bat wings. Yes, you'll have scars under your arm. But at least your arms will be light enough so that you can actually lift them up to see the scars! After a brachioplasty, your arms will be closer to the tight and toned arms you might have dreamed of.

Breast Reduction and Breast Reshaping

Some women would kill to have bigger breasts. But you? If you've lost a lot of weight after getting the sleeve, you may be going through life with heavy, aching breasts, sore shoulders from your bra straps cutting in, and constant back pain from heavy breasts. Daily life can be painful and embarrassing, and don't even mention exercise—just the thought of unnecessary bouncing is painful! *Breast reduction* may be for you. *Breast reshaping,* or *mastoplexy*, is cosmetic and probably won't be covered by insurance, but you might choose to get mastoplexy if you're getting breast reduction anyway.

Lower Body Procedures

Walking is nice, but it's a little (okay, a lot) less pleasant when your thighs are going *swish, swish, swish* with every step. Losing so much fat will leave you with a lot of excess skin in your inner thighs and groin area. A *belt lipectomy*, or *lower body lift*, can take care of that so you're not constantly experiencing rubbing, burning, and chafing between your legs. Lower body procedures can also remove extra skin and fat from your buttocks.

The Logistics of Plastic Surgery

How do you go about getting your elective surgery done? You have to find a surgeon and figure out how you'll pay for the procedure. In fact, the whole process is similar to getting the gastric sleeve—but it's a lot simpler!

Many Plastic Surgeons Are Qualified

Choose a certified plastic surgeon whose qualifications and credentials inspire your confidence. The American Society of Plastic Surgeons is a private organization that aims to improve plastic surgery care. It includes surgeons from the American Board of Plastic Surgeons and its Canadian counterpart, the Royal College of Physicians and Surgeons of Canada.[10] You can use the Society's search engine to find a certified surgeon in your area. The advanced search function on the Society's website allows you to specify the procedure(s) that you're interested in.[11]

Another option is to go to the American Board of Plastic Surgeons' website and use its search function to find a certified surgeon.[12] The site also has a phone number that you can call to check whether a particular surgeon is certified.

Health Insurance May Cover Plastic Surgery for Medical Reasons

You won't get reimbursed for cosmetic surgery if it's for purely aesthetic reasons, but some health insurance policies cover plastic surgery procedures if you are getting them for health reasons. You and your physician may be able to persuade your health insurance company that your excess skin is a health hazard for which plastic surgery is the best treatment.[13] You'll need documentation of your health problems, and the American Society of Plastic Surgeons provides a sample letter, along with medical insurance coding, to assist you in persuading insurance companies to decide in your favor.[14]

Possible Side Effects of Extra Surgeries

Any surgery leads to risks. There's always a risk of complications whenever you go into surgery. Luckily, many of the risks are lower now than they were when you first got the gastric sleeve. That's because you lost a lot of weight and have been taking good care of yourself for a while. As you know, these are some of the general risks of surgeries:

- Infections
- Blood clots
- Excessive bleeding
- Long recovery times with overwhelming nausea and fatigue

Plastic Surgery Has Its Own Risks

In addition to the general risks of surgery, these are some of the risks that are more specific to cosmetic and reconstructive procedures. Your risks of severe complications are lower when your BMI is lower.[15]

- Seromas, or fluid, building up near the surgery site under your skin. You'll need your surgeon to drain it for you with a needle.
- Numbness at the site that your surgeon cuts. Your surgeon may cut a few nerves, so you'll feel tingling or numbness. It's usually temporary.
- Large scars at the site where the excess skin is removed and your remaining skin is stitched together. Many patients don't mind these, and they're often not in obvious places—they may be hidden by your clothes in most cases. But, you should be aware that your skin may not look perfectly smooth.
- Dehiscence, or splitting, of the scar site where the stitches are. Basically, this is a reopening of the wound from poor stitching techniques or too much stress on the wound. It can lead to bleeding, infections, or even another surgery. You can lower your risk by choosing a good surgeon and by avoiding stretching the wound too much before it is fully healed. Another potential cause of dehiscence is if you regain your weight—yet another reason to treat your sleeve diet as a new lifestyle and not as a temporary fix.

- Disappointment due to unrealistic expectations. If you didn't look like a Hollywood star before excess skin removal, you're not going to look like one after it.

Keep Your Expectations Realistic

Before you get your surgery or multiple procedures done, think carefully about your expectations in the short term and long term. You want to be able to enjoy your new body and feel pride in your hard work. Don't start criticizing your body for smaller and smaller details. Some bariatric surgery patients fall into the trap of wanting more procedures done, after they get the first, in pursuit of perfection.[16] Plastic surgery isn't a solution to your self-image problems,[17] but it can help you enjoy your new looks and your healthier body.

Celebrate Triumphs & Milestones

This can be a thrilling year! Do you remember all those times over the past 5, 10, 20 years, or your entire life, when you felt a sense of failure, disappointment, or shame that was related, in some way, to your weight? As you lose the weight, you're going to relive the *opposites* of those moments—and they'll come within the short period of a year or two. Every day or week that you stick to your diet and exercise plan will bring you pride and unforgettable moments on the scale and off the scale. Our advice is to appreciate each one of your personal triumphs.

Milestones

These are what will stand out in your mind when you think about your weight loss. The milestones on the scale come at numbers that are important. These might be some of your milestones:

- The day you break 300 pounds and get back into the 200s and the day you break 200 pounds and get into the 100s
- Getting below your pre-pregnancy weight, weighing what you did on your wedding day, or getting back to your weight on the day that you graduated from high school
- Losing a round number of pounds, such as 100 pounds or 200 pounds
- Hitting your goal weight

These might not all come in the first year after surgery, but you'll be well on your way to hitting them if you're dedicated to the sleeve lifestyle.

Non-Scale Victories

A non-scale victory or NSV is exactly what it sounds like. It's a triumph that comes during your weight loss journey, but it's not a specific number on the scale. You'll have tons of non-scale victories during your sleeve journey, and the NSVs are as important as your scale victories in making your gastric sleeve experience worthwhile.

Better Control over Food Can Be an NSV

In the past, food was in control over you. Many obese patients report having thoughts of food all day: when the next meal is, how soon can they go back for seconds and thirds, whether they can squeeze in trips through the drive-through on the way to and from work, and so on. After you get the sleeve, you might find that food doesn't control your mind. Instead, you might think about food less frequently or be able to control your thoughts rather than giving in to them.

A food-related NSV might come when you go to a party and don't overeat as you did in the old, pre-sleeve days. At that moment, you'll realize that *you* are in control. Just as good is when you realize that you had fun mingling and socializing instead of sneaking over to refill your plate over and over to avoid talking to people as in the old days.

Clothes Shopping Will Be Easier

Almost every lady dreams of fitting into her "skinny jeans," and quite a few gentlemen have their own dream belts, waist sizes, and other goals for fitting into clothes. The sleeve journey provides plenty of opportunities for clothes-related NSVs! These are some examples:

- Ordering a 4X dress online and finding that it's too big. You exchange it for a 2X, and by the time it comes…it's already too big because you're down to the 1X size!

- Having fun shopping with your friends because *you* get to shop too. In the pre-surgery days, you were probably good at pretending you were interested in their clothes but didn't want anything for yourself, but in reality, there was nothing in the store that fit. Even if there was, you wouldn't have wanted to try it on in public. The NSV comes when you get to browse and have your friends wait for *you* to try things on!

- Clearing out your closet because none of those ridiculously oversized clothes will ever fit you again.

- And for fun? It's an NSV when you drag your old jeans out of the closet and step into them—with both legs in one pant leg!

Life Will Become More Natural

This is an NSV to be truly thankful for. Until you gain freedom, you probably didn't even realize how much your obesity was holding you back. Sure, you knew that your knees hurt, you got out of breath easily, you felt self-conscious, and you didn't fit comfortably into regular chairs and cars. But until your obesity stops being such an obstacle, you might not realize *quite* how hard it was keep up with your grandchildren or friends, how much you avoided eating meals in public, and how often you had to make excuses so that people didn't feel bad leaving you behind while you sat and rested. You might not realize the changes all at once, but there may be a few NSVs that will be *ah-ha* moments, as in *"Ah-ha…This is what the sleeve journey is all about."*

- Your friends will invite you to the movies, and you'll say "yes" without worrying whether you'll fit into the car with them.
- You'll book a flight to your family reunion and choose the cheapest flight instead of scrambling to find the least full flight so that you can use two seats.
- Your daughter will ask you if she can take her tricycle out, and you'll go with her on your own bicycle without having to get the car out to accompany her down the block.
- You and your spouse will go to a work party, and you'll be able to focus on the people and the scene instead of wondering whether people are staring at you.

The list goes on—all of these new activities will become natural as you lose weight. You'll be able to focus on life, not on your weight.

Practice Watching for NSVs

Some will be obvious—who *wouldn't* be delighted with the ability to put her wedding ring on again for the first time in 30 years, for example? And others—you'll have to look for them. Not every VSG patient will automatically notice the first time that he was able to let his toddler sit on his lap when his lap appeared from under his belly. With practice, you'll be seeing NSVs everywhere and using them as motivation to keep up the good work.

What to Expect: Overcoming Challenges

You'll be facing tons of challenges during this year, but the difference now is that you have the sleeve to help you overcome them. You, like many obese individuals, might have gone through life giving in or giving up easily. You might have turned away from challenges and turned to food. Now, you're going to confront and overcome your challenges because you're a stronger person and have committed to success with the sleeve. Success breeds success, and better self-confidence goes hand in hand with more weight loss.[18]

Challenges that you can encounter include:

- Trouble sticking to your diet
- Disappointment in your rate of weight loss
- Feeling stress over changes in some of your relationships

It's important to be honest with yourself. Learn to recognize behaviors that contribute to weight regain and confront them instead of ignoring them. Some of these behaviors might be going back to drinking beverages with calories, snacking without recording your food, or going to drive-throughs. Another risky behavior is having an all-or-nothing attitude. A sure way to stop losing weight is to convince yourself that a small mistake is a sign of failure, so there's no point in trying any more. A better approach is to recognize a slip-up, think about why it happened and what you can do to prevent something like it in the future, and go on with your good habits.

Conquer Plateaus, Depression & Struggles with Food

Unfortunately, plateaus are to be expected in the first year and beyond. A plateau is when weight loss slows for a while. It might be a couple of weeks or even a month. Plateaus can come on suddenly—you might lose two pounds per week like clockwork for the first four months after surgery and then one week—bam. Nothing. The next week—nothing. You're still following the same diet plan, and your exercise has been consistent. What's going on? It's the dreaded…plateau.

Don't Let Plateaus Derail Your Diet

Everyone experiences plateaus while trying to lose weight. Plateaus are frustrating, and they can drive many dieters off of their diets. Some people throw in the towel, saying there's no point to trying so hard to lose weight if it's not working. Don't be one of those people! Instead, you can be one of the sleeve patients that perseveres through plateaus and emerges from them successfully.

Weight loss is all about the calories in and the calories out. If you keep up your VSG diet, you'll eventually break out of the plateau. It may take a couple of weeks, and it may take a couple of months. These are two sure things about plateaus:

1. It *will* end if you continue to follow your sleeve diet and burn off more calories than you eat.

2. It *won't* end if you give up and eat too much.

Sticking closely enough to your sleeve diet to be able to break through a plateau is something to be proud of. It's another challenge that you've faced successfully, and it's another reason to be confident in yourself.

Only Count Your Weekly Weigh-Ins

Your weight won't go down every day. If you weigh yourself every day, the number will often be the same as the day before. Sometimes, it may even go up. These small fluctuations in your weight are normal, and they're not a sign that you're gaining body fat. They're usually just from small changes in the amount of water in your body, and there's nothing you can do to prevent them.

That's why it's best to make a deal with yourself to only officially "count" a weekly weigh-in that you'll record as part of your weight loss journey. Choose a day of the week to be your weigh-in day, and be consistent with your official weigh-in.

- Weigh yourself in at the same time of day. The early morning, right after you go to the bathroom for the first time, is a good time because you haven't eaten anything yet so you don't have the extra weight of food or drink inside of you.

- Weigh yourself naked or wearing just your underwear. Light clothing is okay, but be sure not to wear shoes.

Daily Weighing for Accountability

Although daily weigh-ins shouldn't be taken as seriously as weekly ones, they can still be important in your weight loss plan. Knowing that you have to face the scale helps you stay accountable. Weighing yourself regularly will likely continue to be a part of your life for years to come. In fact, the National Weight Control Registry, or NWCR, reports that more than three out of every four people who lose at least 30 pounds and keep it off for at least a year weigh themselves regularly.[19]

Depression

Depression isn't likely, but it is a real possibility. Depression can be a normal response to the rapid changes in your life. After getting the sleeve, your whole world may seem upside-down. For the first time in years, possibly for the first time in your life, you're losing weight, you're in control of yourself, you're getting compliments about your appearance, and your self-esteem is increasing. Some of your personal relationships may improve while others may fall apart. These changes can be stressful because they're such big, important changes and because they affect all aspects of your life.

These changes can be overwhelming at times and make you thoughtful or moody. Everyone feels a little less energetic sometimes, but these periods should be short and infrequent. You may have mild depression if your feelings of hopelessness or lack of self-worth interfere with your regular activities or your symptoms last for more than two weeks.[20]

The risk for depression is one reason why keeping up your regular appointments with a mental health professional is so important as part of your aftercare plan. If you don't have regularly scheduled appointments, you should at least know how to contact a mental health professional in case you need to. An expert can determine whether your symptoms are normal and you should just wait them out or whether you should get treated for depression. The sooner you catch depressive disorder, the easier it is to treat.

Depression isn't ubiquitous. In fact, losing a lot of weight after your surgery is more likely to improve your mood than make you depressed. This is especially true if you were mildly depressed before surgery because of your obesity and health issues related to your obesity that prevented you from living the life you wanted.[21]

Continued Struggles with Food

The gastric sleeve is a powerful tool for weight loss, but it's just a tool. It doesn't instantly erase years of bad habits, get rid of all hunger, or eliminate food cravings. However, some bariatric patients report less hunger and lower cravings for sweets and fast foods.[22]

Unfortunately, not everyone finds the weight loss journey to be so easy. Some patients feel as though they're starving, especially at the beginning on the liquid diet. As you progress to pureed, soft, and finally, solid foods, the VSG diet will still be pretty tough because you're not used to eating such small portions and ending the meal when you're full.

Cravings Can Still Hit Hard

It seems unfair, but even post-surgery patients whose cravings decrease still tend to have stronger cravings than normal-weight patients.[23] Sometimes you'll want something that's not on your diet, like a slice of pizza (or, as in the old days, a half of a pizza!) or some fried chicken. When cravings strike, you have a few good options:

- *Ignore it until it goes away.* Distract yourself however you can, whether by talking on the phone or going for a walk, until the moment has passed. By the time you're finished with the phone conversation or walk, it'll be close to time for your next drink or meal or snack, so you can focus on a healthy food or beverage. Stalling tactics usually work, but sometimes you can't stop thinking of that food for weeks on end.

- *Reason with yourself.* Weigh the benefits against the disadvantages. A benefit of eating a small amount of the food might be preventing an eventual binge if you try to ignore your craving. A disadvantage might be having something that's unhealthy or likely to make you feel sick.

- *Have a very small amount.* Measure out a small portion, record it in your food journal and enjoy your serving at your next meal. Be sure to chew it slowly and savor it.

- *Have a healthier substitute.* For example, instead of regular meat-lover's pizza, try an English muffin pizza. Take half of a whole-wheat English muffin and spread it with a quarter-cup of tomato or pizza sauce. Add an ounce of low-fat shredded mozzarella and some diced onions, black olives, and mushrooms. Turkey or vegetarian pepperoni and sausage are good substitutes for pepperoni if you can't imagine a slice of pizza without pepperoni.

As long as you stay focused on making good decisions, you can get over your craving without doing much damage to your diet or your sleeve. The most important thing to remember is that there's always another chance, and there's never any need to slip into a rut. There's no giving up. Whenever you feel like you've gone off of your diet, pick yourself up and get right back to work.

Cravings	
Instead of...	Try...
Apple pie	Baked apple with cinnamon
Buffalo wings	Chicken breast with barbecue sauce
Fried chicken	Baked chicken breast with high fiber cereal or whole-grain bread breading
Banana split	Half of a banana on a stick dipped in dark chocolate with sweetener; freeze
Brownie or chocolate cake	1 square (1/2 ounce) dark chocolate; 1 cup sugar-free hot cocoa mix

Cravings	
Instead of...	**Try...**
Ice cream	Sugar-free frozen pudding cup; let thaw for 30 minutes
French fries	Oven-baked squash fries/sticks

Table 43: Cravings

Working Hard to Develop New Eating Habits

You will be breaking old habits and developing new ones after surgery. This requires persistence and hard work because old habits are hard to break, and new ones take a while to form. Your old habits might have been going on for years before your VSG. Examples of habits that you'll need to break include:

- Constantly snacking
- Eating while doing other tasks
- Nibbling while preparing your next meal or snack
- Going to drive-through restaurants
- Choosing food based on taste rather than nutrition
- Wolfing down your first portion to be sure there was time for a second helping

> **Tip**
>
> Chapter 13, "Recovery and Your Post-Surgery Diet," lists the foods that should and should not be regular parts of your sleeve diet. The following chapter goes into more detail about healthy choices.

Good habits to form include:

- Measuring and recording everything you eat and drink
- Focusing on your food and not on other tasks while you're eating
- Eating only at the table
- Choosing the most nutritious foods
- Stopping to decide whether you're full before considering another portion

You might have spent several pre-surgery years practicing the unhealthy eating behaviors, and teaching yourself better habits will take some time and effort. It'll be a while before you naturally weigh out each portion of food, choose proteins and vegetables instead of macaroni and cheese, walk to the store to buy bananas instead of drive to your nearest burger drive-through, and slow down your eating enough to enjoy your food. How long will it take? It depends on the person, but your new actions will start to become habits within weeks if you're consistent. Every time you consciously make a good decision instead of a poor one, your new healthy habits will become easier and more natural, and the old bad habits will seem less tempting.

Side Effects or Complications

You're still at risk for experiencing side effects or developing complications even after you're fully recovered from surgery.[24] [25] You could experience the following:[26]

- Gastric fistula
- Vomiting
- Leakage
- Staple line hemorrhage

You can nearly always prevent or reduce these complications by following the sleeve diet precisely. Try to figure out the cause of your symptoms. Ask yourself whether your diet changed, whether you chewed your food too fast, or whether you ate too much in one meal. These are common causes of the above side effects.

Remember to call your surgeon if you ever have a situation in which you can't swallow or drink for more than a few hours or if you're ever concerned for any other reason that your health is in serious danger. It's always better to be safe than sorry.

Tip

See Chapter 5, "VSG: Risks and Considerations," describes common side effects and complications of the sleeve. Chapter 13, "Recovery and Your Post-Surgery Diet," and Chapter 15, "The Sleeve Diet, Weight Loss," and Your Health, have advice on how to choose safe foods that aren't likely to cause problems plus what to do if you start to experience irritation or other symptoms caused by your diet.

Smoking

Question: What's the only lifestyle choice that kills more Americans each year than obesity, a poor diet, and not enough exercise?

Answer: Tobacco use

The Centers for Disease Control and Prevention state that smoking kills one out of every five Americans.[27] Smoking leads to coronary heart disease and peripheral vascular disease; lung cancer; esophageal, throat, pancreatic, and kidney cancer; high blood pressure and stroke; emphysema; chronic obstructive lung disease; and osteoporosis. In fact, smoking harms every organ in your body. What else does smoking do:

- It hurts the people around you because of your second-hand smoke.
- It makes your clothes and breath smell.
- It's expensive. At $5 per pack, a pack a day costs you more than $1,500 per year.
- It makes your teeth yellow.
- It makes your hands shake.
- It's inconvenient. You can't enjoy anything because all you can think about is getting out for your next smoke and making sure you have another pack handy.

Time to Quit

So where does smoking fit into your post-surgery plans? Hopefully you're not a smoker, but if you are, this post-surgery period is an ideal opportunity to quit for several reasons:

- *You're going to lose weight anyway.* A lot of people hesitate to quit smoking because they think it will make them gain weight, but that doesn't have to be true. If you follow your sleeve diet as prescribed, you'll still lose weight quickly even if you stop smoking. Because your diet is so low-calorie, the sleeve surgery is a golden opportunity to stop smoking without noticing the effects of a slower metabolism, so take advantage of it!

- *You're taking control of your life.* The next few months of your life are going to be all about you. You need to focus on yourself and your weight loss goals if you want to succeed with the sleeve. Now is a good time to take the attention that you're putting on yourself and apply the energy to quitting smoking too. Your post-surgery care program will require you to work closely with your medical team and attend group support meetings anyway; why don't you use this time to commit wholeheartedly to your health and go to the extra support groups or doctor's appointments that will help you quit smoking?

- *You're going to test your willpower anyway.* You will need to be strong-minded to be able to consistently make the diet and exercise changes necessary for success with the sleeve. As you're breaking old eating habits and forming new ones, you might as well break the smoking habit and live a smoke-free life.

- *It's time for a new you.* You've already decided that your body is going to be at the goal weight you've been dreaming of. Why don't you make it a healthy, smoke-free body?

Some Surgeons Require You to Quit Smoking

Some surgeons might ask you to stop smoking during the weeks leading up to your surgery as a way to prove that you have enough self-discipline. When you schedule the date of your VSG, you might have to sign a contract stating that you won't smoke until the surgery. Your surgeon can give you frequent drug tests to make sure that you are sticking to your end of the bargain leading up to surgery. By the time you have your surgery, you probably won't even be craving cigarettes anymore.

Replacement Addictions

Replacement addictions, also known as crossover addictions or substitute addictions, are a threat to a small proportion of bariatric patients. Some obese individuals were literally physically or psychologically addicted to food; you may have actually *felt a need* to use junk food to get you through the day. Your eating habits change drastically after you get sleeved as you focus on small portions of nutritious foods.

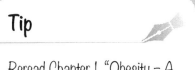

Tip

Reread Chapter I, "Obesity – A Costly Epidemic," for information on food, especially high-calorie, high-sugar, high-sodium foods, as an addiction.

Replacement Addictions Can Result from Physiological Reasons

Breaking your food addiction helps you lose weight for sure, but some people might actually develop addictions to replace the food addiction. Alcohol is among the most likely addictions to develop because there are actually biological mechanisms that are similar to those of high-sugar foods. Alcohol and sugar are both used to stimulate dopamine, which is a neurotransmitter, or chemical, that your brain produces that gives you a sense of pleasure. When you stop "abusing" sugar as a drug, you might end up replacing your sugar abuse with alcohol abuse.[28]

Replacement Addictions Can Result from Psychological Reasons

Even if you weren't chemically addicted to food, you might have been emotionally or psychologically addicted. That's true if you used to eat for comfort or out of boredom or habit. Smoking is an example of a dangerous replacement addiction that might develop if you start to smoke on your lunch hour and short breaks and when you want to take a moment to step outside. In the old days, you might have gone to the break room or stayed at your desk to eat; a replacement addiction could develop if you choose to smoke instead.

Choose Healthy Alternatives to Food or Replacement Addictions

If you're concerned that you're developing a crossover addiction, try to figure out why. What role did overeating fill in your life that you're now trying to fill with another unhealthy habit? Then, find a healthy alternative to junk food or replacement addictions:

- Your social support system can help if you're lonely or bored—phone a friend, write some emails, or hop onto BariatricPal.com.
- Find a new hobby to fill the gaps between meals, relieve stress, or keep your hands occupied—blogging, sewing, and gardening are examples.
- Crossword puzzles and other mind games can help you distract yourself.
- Go for a short walk or do a few stretches to relieve stress in a healthy way and let the craving pass.

✏️ Summary

☛ Losing significant amounts of weight after your surgery will lead to far greater changes than just the number on the scale. You'll look different and feel better. Your whole world can change after the VSG.

☛ This chapter covered some of these possible changes to help you prepare. We suggest greeting the changes with confidence, preparing for them as much as possible, and staying aware that you're facing the same challenges and situations as other sleeve patients.

Your Turn: Looking ahead to the First Year

List three things that you are most looking forward to in your first year after surgery.

Example: I can't wait to go biking with my son for the first time!

1. ....
....
....

2. ....
....
....

3. ....
....
....

List three challenges you expect to have and how you plan to overcome them.

Example: It'll be tough to go to parties and social events and stay on my diet. People are used to me pigging out, and I'm used to me pigging out. I plan to avoid any diet problems by focusing on enjoying the people, not the food, when I go to social events. Also, when it's appropriate, I will bring something healthy to eat so I won't be starving.

1. ....
....
....

2. ....
....
....

3. ....
....
....

1   Faria SL, Faria OP, Lins RD, de Gouvea, HR. Hair loss among bariatric surgery patients. Bariatric Times. 2010;7(11):18-20.

2   E, Riffo A, Papapietro K, Csendes A, Ruz M. Alopecia in women with severe and morbid obesity who undergo bariatric surgery. Nutr Hosp. 2011;26(4)

3   D'Hondt M, Vanneste S, Pottel H, Devriendt D, Van Rooy F, Vasteenkiste F. Laparoscopic sleeve gastrectomy as a single-stage procedure for the treatment of morbid obesity and the resulting quality of life, resolution of comorbidities, food intolerance and 6-year weight loss. 2011. Surg Endosc. 25(8):2498-504.

4   Losing weight: What is healthy weight loss? Centers for Disease Control and Prevention. Web site. http://www.cdc.gov/healthyweight/losing_weight/index.html. Updated 2011, August 17. Accessed November 24, 2012.

5   Gill RS, Birch DW, Shi X, Sharma AM, Karmali S. Sleeve gastrectomy and type 2 diabetes mellitus: a systematic review. Surg Obes Relat Dis. 2010;6(6):707-713.

6   Leonetti F, Capoccio D, Coccia F, Casella G, Baglio G, Paradiso F, Abbatini F, Iossa A, Soricelli E, Basso N. Obesity, type 2 diabetes mellitus, and other comorbidities: a prospective cohort study of laparoscopic sleeve gastrectomy vs. medical treatment. Arch Surg. 2012;147(8):694-700.

7   van Rutte PW, Smulders JF, de Zoete JP, Nienhuijs SW. Indications and short-term outcomes of revisional surgery after failed or complicated sleeve gastrectomy. Obes Surg. 2012.

8   Mitchell JE, Crosby RD, Ertelt TW, Marino JW, Sarwer DB, Thompson JK, Lancaster KL, Simonich H, Howell LM. The desire for body contouring surgery after bariatric surgery. Obesity Surgery. 2008;18:1308-12.

9   Steffen KJ, Sarwer DB, Thompson JK, Mueller A, Baker AW, Mitchell JE. Predictors of satisfaction with excess skin and desire for body contouring following bariatric surgery. Surgery for Obesity and Related Diseases. 2012;8:92-7.

10 American Society of Plastic Surgeons. Active membership process (United States and Canada). Retrieved from http://www.plasticsurgery.org/For-Medical-Professionals/Surgeon-Community/Join-ASPS/Active-Membership-Process.html. 2012. Accessed November 24, 2012.

11 Find a surgeon. American Society of Plastic Surgeons. Web site. http://www1.plasticsurgery.org/find_a_surgeon/. 2012. Accessed November 24, 2012.

12 American Board of Plastic Surgeons. Web site. https://www.abplsurg.org/moddefault.aspx. 2012. Accessed November 24, 2012.

13 Gurunguoglu R. Insurance coverage criteria for panniculectomy and redundant skin surgery after bariatric surgery: why and when to discuss. Obesity Surgery. 2012;517-520.

14 American Society of Plastic Surgeons. ASPS recommended insurance coverage criteria for third-party payers: surgical treatment of skin redundancy for obese and massive weight loss patients. Web site. http://www.plasticsurgery.org/Documents/medical-professionals/health-policy/insurance/Surgical-Treatment-of-Skin-Redundancy-Following.pdf. 2007, January. Accessed November 24, 2012.

15 Langer V, Singh A, Aly AS, Cram AE. Body contouring following massive weight loss. Indian Journal of Plastic Surgery. 2011;44:14-20.

16 Song AY, Rubin JP, Thomas V, Dudas JR, Marra KG, Fernstrom MH. Body image and quality of life in post massive weight loss body contouring patients. Obesity (Silver Spring). 2006;14:1626-1636.

17 Singh D, Zahiri HR, Janes LE, Sabino J, Matthews JA, Bell RL, Thomson JG. Mental and physical impact of body contouring procedures on post-bariatric surgery patients. Eplasty. 2012;12:e47.

18 Batsis JA, Clark MM, Grothe K, Lopez-Jimenez F, Collazo-Clavell ML, Somers VK, Sarr MG. Self-efficacy after bariatric surgery for obesity: a population-based cohort study. Appetite. 2009; 52:637-45.

19 NWCR facts. National Weight Control Registry. Web site. http://www.nwcr.ws/Research/default.htm. Accessed November 24, 2012.

20 Depression. National Institutes of Mental Health. Web site. http://www.nimh.nih.gov/health/publications/depression/complete-index.shtml.Revised 2011. Accessed November 24, 2012.

21 Rutledge T, Braden AL, Woods G, Herbst KL, Groesz LM, Savu M. Five-year changes in psychiatric treatment status and weight-related comorbidities following bariatric surgery in a veteran population. Obes Surg. 2012;22(11):1734-41.

22 Leahey TM, Bond DS, Raynor H, Roye D, Vithiananthian S, Ryder BA, Sax SC, Wing RR. Effects of bariatric surgery on food cravings: do food cravings and the consumption of craved foods "normalize" after surgery? Surg Obes Relat Dis. 2012;8(1):84-91.

23 Leahey TM, Bond DS, Raynor H, Roye D, Vithiananthian S, Ryder BA, Sax SC, Wing RR. Effects of bariatric surgery on food cravings: do food cravings and the consumption of craved foods "normalize" after surgery? Surg Obes Relat Dis. 2012;8(1):84-91.

24 Hamdan K, Somers S, Chand M. Management of late postoperative complications of bariatric surgery. Br J Surg. 2011;98(10):1345-1355.

25 Richardson WS, Plaisance AM, Periou L, Buquoi RN, Tillery D. Long-term management of patients after weight loss surgery. Ochsner Journal, 2009; 9:154-159.

26 Iannelli A, Dainese R, Piche T, Facchiano E, Gugenheim J. Laparoscopic sleeve gastrectomy for morbid obesity. World J Gastroenterol. 2008;14(6):821-827

27 Health effects of cigarette smoking. Centers for Disease Control and Prevention. Web site. http://www.cdc.gov/tobacco/data_statistics/fact_sheets/health_effects/effects_cig_smoking/. 2012. Accessed November 24, 2012.

28 Common mechanisms of drug abuse and obesity. National Association of Drug Abuse. Web site. http://www.drugabuse.gov/news-events/news-releases/2010/03/common-mechanisms-drug-abuse-obesity. 2012, March 28. Accessed November 24, 2012.

18

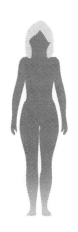

Build a Strong Support System

The last chapter discussed some of the changes to expect after your vertical sleeve gastrectomy. With so many changes, you'll need a lot of support. This chapter will talk about building a fail proof support system. This chapter will talk about the sources of support that may be available to you. These include:

- Yourself
- Your family and friends
- Members of your medical team
- Other bariatric surgery patients from your support group meetings and online communities.

A Strong Support System is Crucial

Your support system will be one of the most important factors in your sleeve success story.[1] You can't prevent the down times and struggles, but you can deal with them better. A solid support system can let you rise to the challenge. It encourages you to keep on track and helps you prevent depression.

A Strong Support System Is Like a Multi-Level Insurance Policy

Failure is nearly impossible when your support system is solid. A support system is a complex organization of people that will hold you up in any situation that you come across. It has many different aspects and people from all parts of your life and in all possible settings. When your support system is in place, you should have encouragement and advice coming from all directions. No matter what happens, someone in a strong support system can get help over the bump in the road.

The Center of Your Support System: Yourself

This may sound corny, but it's quite true. You are the center of your support system for these reasons:

- *You are your own biggest fan.* Nobody wants you to succeed as much as you do.
- *You're always there for yourself.* There's no denying that fact, so you might as well be a source of support for yourself!
- *You are in charge.* That means that you have the power to do the right thing.

How You Can Support Yourself

With a bit of effort, you can become a stronger source of support for yourself. These are a few tips:

- *Make yourself proud.* Follow your sleeve diet and your exercise routine.

- *Compliment yourself.* Make a conscious effort to recognize your accomplishments. Tell yourself that you're proud, just as you would tell your best friends when you're proud of them.

- *Believe in yourself.* You're much more likely to achieve your goals when you're confident that you can. If you let doubts creep in, they can prevent you from trying and succeeding. If you don't succeed the first time, try again. True failure comes when you give up.

- *Prepare to give yourself pep talks.* Sure, you'll slip up sometimes. You're only human. But you can prepare for it so that if you go off your diet or exercise program, you can pick yourself right back up. Pick yourself up and dust yourself off. Going right back to your original plans should become automatic.

- *Be your own best motivator.* Make a list of reasons why you're losing the weight, and post it where you can see it every day, possibly on the refrigerator or on the wall behind your desk.

- *Make a back-up plan.* When you're feeling down, you might not be thinking as clearly as you normally do. Have a list of your closest support allies with you so that you can easily decide whom to call when you need help.

Track Progress

Your role as part of your support system includes holding yourself accountable. You can do this by tracking your progress. These are some ways to do this:

- *Track your weight.* Write down the numbers or record them on the computer so you can see how well you're doing and be motivated to continue working hard.

- *Maintain a food diary.* Bariatric surgery patients who keep journals are more likely to lose more weight.[2]

- *Keep an exercise log.* The chapter on starting and continuing an exercise program has a sample log and some suggestions for keeping one.

- *Record body measurements.* Your waist and thigh circumference (distance around your upper thighs) will shrink as you lose weight. Recording these changes is motivating.

Family and Friends for Support

Some of us are closer to certain members of our family, while others are closer to our friends. Family and friends go in the same category because nearly all of us are in the same situation. Some of our family members and friends will be supportive, and others will not be. Often, you won't know which are which until you've told them that you're getting the sleeve or you've already undergone surgery. Each of your friends and family members will fall into one of these categories.

Automatic Supporters

Just like they love you unconditionally, they'll automatically support you in anything that you believe is best for yourself without demanding explanations. Of course, these are the people who are most likely to be open to explanations and interested in learning all about your journey and what they can do to help.

Dealing with Disapproval & Rejection

Many people are in this category. Their instinctive reaction to your surgery is that it's weird, cheating, or unhealthy, but they are likely to genuinely listen to your explanation of what the surgery is and what you have to do to make it work. When you explain your reasoning and they see you losing weight, eating healthier, and being happier, they'll start to understand your decision and support you. Even if they don't agree, most people in this category probably won't judge you as a person based on your surgery.

Flat-Out Rejection

Some people might be negative about the sleeve and bariatric surgery in general, and they might never change their minds. It might because they struggle with their own weight and are envious of the choice you've made and the commitment you're demonstrating. Others might decide that you're lazy or that weight loss surgery is bad—even if they never bothered to learn the first thing about it. Still others may be basing their judgment on a bad experience that a friend of a friend of a coworker's relative had with weight loss surgery. People like this can be frustrating and demeaning, but don't let them get to you. People who are so closed-minded are not worth getting upset over. Just ignore them while you keep losing weight and doing your best for yourself.

You'll find out soon enough who's going to support you, who's going to be neutral, and who's just there to bring you down. Don't waste your time and energy worrying about negative people.

Recruit Allies

Directly ask several of your friends and family members if they will be part of your official support system. Make a list of the ones who are willing to help you. Different friends and family members each have their own best roles. You can figure out how each of them can help you the best way they can. Here are some examples:

- You might need to ask your spouse to avoid eating chocolate chip cookies in front of you, if that's your weak spot.
- You might ask your sister to call you each day on your cell phone at 8:00 p.m. so that you can take your walk while talking to her.
- Your best friend might be your conscience and responsible for asking (politely and with genuine concern) if you're doing okay when he sees that you're down or notices

that you haven't been telling him proudly about weight loss recently.

- You might ask your children to help you make dinner so that you're not tempted to nibble on food while you're preparing it. Younger children will revel at being the food police and stopping their mom or dad from sneaking forbidden bites.

Here are a few more tips for making the best use of your friend and family member support system:

- Your spouse, friends, children, siblings, and parents all have different roles in other parts of your life. The same is true for your sleeve journey.
- Be specific about what you need them to do. They don't know unless you tell them.
- Understand and clarify the differences between being a shoulder to cry on, someone who gives advice, and someone who's there to give you some tough love or a kick in the pants. Some friends and family members will always be best at one of these. Others can fill multiple roles depending on the situation, but they may need you to tell them what you need in any given moment.
- Don't be afraid to be the weak one. Sometimes you hold your family and friends up; sometimes they hold you up. That's how life works. If you need help in your sleeve journey, ask for it.

A Supportive Work Environment

The average middle-aged working adult spends an average of nearly nine hours per day at work on a typical working day.[3] That's a lot of time. If you work, a healthy work environment can play an important role in your success with the sleeve. An unhealthy environment can make every step a struggle. You can make your work environment more supportive by recruiting coworkers to help you and by making your own workspace healthier.

People at Work

Everyone's employment situation is different, but what is likely to be common if you work outside the home is that you spend a *lot* of time with your coworkers. You may not know them all very well or like all of them, but your weight loss journey will be so much easier if you can find one or two supporters. Here are some potential sources of support at work. Your own personal work situation is unique, so just use the following as ideas as you search for your own effective source of encouragement.

A Friend

If you're lucky enough to have one or more close friends at work, by all means take advantage of them! Let them know about your sleeve journey and how they can help, if they're willing. Each friend you have at work can help keep you on track and listen to your problems.

How Can I Prevent Sabotage?

Other people can sabotage your diet if you let them. The sabotage often seems—and may be—intentional. These sneaky people are often the ones who make you feel bad for using the sleeve as a tool for weight loss, for following a diet and exercise plan, or for taking steps to become healthy. Their sabotage may include:

- Keeping certain foods in the house that you've specifically asked them not to have around. These might be foods such as fried chicken, ice cream, potato chips, or anything else you can't control yourself around.

- Inviting you to dinners without serving anything you can eat or pressuring you to eat more than you want.

- Making rude comments or staring at you to make you feel uncomfortable or doubt yourself.

What can you do about these people? Here are a few options:

- Avoid them. It's a sure-fire way to prevent them from getting to you, but it's not always possible.

- Prepare for them. Psych yourself up: Think ahead to what might go wrong when you encounter your saboteur, and prepare to react. What will you say and do? Also, give yourself a pep talk. Remind yourself what a wonderful person you are, how hard you're working to achieve your goals, and how much you deserve your success.

- Phone a friend or family member—before and after. When I know that I'm going to have an unpleasant encounter with someone who's about to make me feel bad, I ask my sister to be ready with her phone so that I can call her right afterward, and she can make me feel better.

- Be patient. Believe it or not, some saboteurs actually have the potential to become your friends and allies. Try to be kind, informative, and courteous. Over time and with persistence, you might be able to figure out why they're mean to you and how you can solve the problem. It's possible they're jealous of you or unsure of themselves and need a helping hand that you can provide.

- Be prepared. Bring a healthy dish to share if you're going over for dinner; decide ahead of time exactly how many bites you'll eat; and remember to take three deep breaths before even considering taking offense. You may be taking a lot of deep breaths, but the deep breathing practice will serve you well in the future too.

Everyone faces intentional or unintentional sabotage at some point. You can prevent it from delaying your weight loss as long as you stay cool, collected, and in control of yourself.

Your Boss

Not everyone has a sympathetic boss or a good personal relationship, but if you do, your journey can be easier. You need to decide for yourself exactly what and how much you want to tell your boss, since you always want to appear strong and professional in front of your boss. You may not feel comfortable divulging personal information. But, if you're pretty sure that your boss will be supportive, go ahead and tell about your weight loss surgery. Having a boss who's in your corner will make it easier to attend surgeon or other appointments in your post-surgery care program. It'll also help at those times, especially when surgery is still pretty recent, when you want to go home a little early or take it easy at work because you don't feel well.

A Colleague Who's Also Losing Weight

You're not likely to find someone in your workplace who also got weight loss surgery around the same time as you, but you might find a coworker who's making a serious effort to lose weight. You two can help each other stay on track and exchange tips and encouragement.

A Colleague Who's Working toward a Different Goal

A little creativity can go a long way when you're looking for support at work. Support can come from someone who's not trying to lose weight but who's trying to achieve a different life-changing goal. For example, someone who's trying to quit smoking can be a great source of support and inspiration for you. The two of you can go for walks together at lunch so that you can burn calories and your coworker has a distraction from smoking. Inside the office, you can confide in each other with your struggles and remind each other that you're rooting for each other.

If you work a 40-hour work week, you're spending one-third of your weekday life in your work environment. The more support you can get at work, the better off you'll be.

Your Workspace

You can design your workspace to be more encouraging to weight loss. Keep your food environment healthy by following many of the same guidelines as you do at home. These include:

- Keeping healthy snacks on hand so you never get too hungry
- Planning ahead so you know what you'll have for each meal and snack for the entire work day
- Keeping unhealthy foods out of your office and your space in the worksite's refrigerator
- Keeping water available on or near your desk at all times

These are some additional ways that you can promote weight loss at work:

- Keep some sneakers and workout clothes available. You can use them for lunchtime walks or for going to the gym.

Do I Have to Tell People That I Got the Sleeve?

The gastric sleeve is a new and permanent part of you. It's your tool for helping you lose weight and keep it off for good. The sleeve can change your life, and everyone who knows you can see the differences between the old you and the new you. Does that mean you have to tell people about the VSG? Absolutely not! You can decide whether you want to tell.

Keeping your weight loss surgery a secret is completely normal. If you're a shy, private person, your natural inclination is to say nothing, lose weight quietly, and smile and thank people when they point out your weight loss. Even if you're outgoing, you might not feel like telling many people about the sleeve simply because you don't feel that they need to know. On the other hand, if you love to share everything about your life and are super proud of your weight loss and success with the sleeve, you'll find yourself telling pretty much everyone.

To tell or not to tell? That seems to be the question…but the answer can lie somewhere in between! These are some of the decisions we've seen from a variety of weight loss surgery patients:

- Telling everyone because they're proud of their hard work and success.
- Telling close friends and family but not saying anything to more casual acquaintances—after all, weight loss can be a personal thing.
- Telling people who may be able to benefit from hearing about your experience with the vertical sleeve gastrectomy. It's a bit like using an NTK, or need to know, basis.
- Telling people who care. Some people are genuinely interested in you and your life; others are going through the motions. If they ask and sincerely seem interested in the answer, you might want to tell them.
- Telling almost nobody. They've heard some nasty, often uninformed, comments about the sleeve or weight loss surgery in general and don't feel like opening a can of worms.

By the way, your decision isn't necessarily related to your chances of being successful with the sleeve. Each of the above examples came from people who were losing weight at the rate they'd hoped or who had hit their goal weight and were maintaining their weight.

- Reduce the temptation of workplace foods, such as chocolates or doughnuts, by trying not to walk by where they're being offered.
- Remind yourself about your goals and motivating reminders.

Support from Your Healthcare Team

Your healthcare team's main goal is for you to succeed, and team members can play a large role in your success by being part of your post-surgery support system. You can take advantage of this support by participating fully in your aftercare program. Weight loss surgery patients who complete their aftercare programs and follow through with their one-year check-in after surgery are more likely to lose the weight they'd hoped for by the end of that year than patients who don't take aftercare seriously.[4]

Medical Support

A comprehensive support system includes having support for when you have a medical emergency or just a question. You should have the direct number to your surgeon or someone at the clinic or hospital where you got the sleeve so that you can get answers to urgent questions. You can call these numbers when you need to know whether the symptoms you're experiencing require medical attention or whether you can treat them at home.

Psychological Support

Your psychologist or mental health professional should be available for more routine support. Many VSG patients actually have regular appointments with their mental health professionals or maintain regular contact when the psychologist leads support group meetings. Psychologists are great for suggesting coping strategies for your situation and ways to stay positive during the tough times. Staying in touch with your psychologist lets you be monitored for signs of depression, which can occur with bariatric surgery patients because of the quick changes in your life. Post-surgery psychological support is recommended for sleeve patients.[5]

Dietitian or Nutritionist

Dietitians aren't officially responsible for keeping you emotionally grounded, but they can certainly help! Your dietitian is your trusted source for nutrition advice and meal plans. Beyond that, dietitians can be lifesavers, or at least diet-savers, when you're craving something that's not on your diet. Most dietitians understand your situation and are sympathetic; most are willing to accept your calls (or text messages or emails) and offer suggestions when you need help. For example, when you're craving a banana split and you're just about to give in, you can contact your dietitian, who might

> **Tip**
>
> Chapter 7, "Tips when Planning for the Sleeve," discusses the process of assembling a strong healthcare team and the role of each member in your success. Chapter 12, "Post-op Care," talks about taking full advantage of the follow-up appointments with your surgeon and other team members.

encourage you instead to stick with a half of a pureed banana mixed with some Cool Whip to save hundreds of calories and worlds of guilt. Knowing that your dietitian is there for you no matter what adds an extra layer of support to your system.

Support Group Meetings

Before agreeing to do the vertical sleeve gastrectomy, your surgeon is likely to have you promise to attend support group meetings for at least a year. It's an important part of your post-surgery care program. Support group meetings can help teach you better eating habits, ways to develop better habits, and strategies for getting through the tough times.[6]

In-Person Support Group Meetings

Research clearly shows that you're more likely to have better weight loss when you attend support group meetings.[7] In one study that followed bariatric surgery patients for a year, the patients that went to their recommended support group meetings lost an average of 42 percent of their original BMI. The patients that did not attend support group meetings lost only 32 percent of their original BMI, even though they had the same surgeon and other aftercare services as the group that attended support group meetings.

Online Support

Support group meetings are great when they fit into your schedule. You learn a lot and meet great people. But, online support groups can fill in huge gaps — the gaps in between your weekly or monthly support group meetings. Online support groups also have an advantage over your own friends and family. Like online friends, your family and friends are there for you every day. The difference is that most of them aren't vertical sleeve patients, so they don't know exactly what you're going through.

Online support resources are always there for you at every minute of every day, and you can get encouragement; advice about how to deal with sleeve issues; and information on diet and exercise just to name a few. Online support forums are composed of members who are gastric sleeve patients. There will be people who've been there and done that, and they can offer advice for any problem that you're experiencing or question that you have. There will also be people who are at the same point of their weight loss journey as you; you can form amazing bonds with these members as you support each other.

> **Tip**
>
> See Chapter 19, "Online Support & BariatricPal.com," for information on joining and using BariatricPal.com. The chapter covers the unique features of the site and some of the benefits of membership, which is free for everyone.

There are many weight loss surgery and gastric sleeve support groups online. Many are free to join, and they welcome everyone. BariatricPal.com is the largest such group, and it is an independently-run, non-biased board. It is not run by a healthcare company, a bariatric surgeon, or a hospital.

Summary

- You'll encounter plenty of challenges with the VSG, and you'll have a head start at overcoming them if you have a strong support system. You're at the center of your system.

- Also supporting you will be some of your friends and family members and, hopefully, a few people at your workplace. Your surgeon, psychologist, and dietitian will also be ready to give you a helping hand as you lose weight after surgery. You can get support from other bariatric patients from your support group meetings and online groups too.

- The Internet is likely to play a large role in your success with the sleeve, and the next chapter focuses on BariatricPal.com, an online community that's welcoming, free for everyone, and a potentially important component of your social support system.

Your Turn: Your Support System

List five sources of social support that you are going to recruit and maintain.

Example: I've already signed up for membership on BariatricPal.com, and I've gotten into some cool conversations with some of the members. I hope they'll continue to be sources of support for me!

1. ....

....

....

2. ....

....

....

3. ....

....

....

4. ....

....

....

5. ....

....

....

1   Positive relationships. Realize. Web site. http://www.realize.com/weight-loss-lifestyle-support.htm. Accessed November 24, 2012.

2   Butryn ML, Phelan S, Hill JO, Wing, RR. Consistent self-monitoring of weight: a key component of successful weight loss maintenance. Obesity (Silver Spring). 2007;15:3091-3096.

3   Bureau of Labor Statistics. Charts from the American Time Use Survey. Department of Labor. Web site. http://www.bls.gov/tus/charts/. Modified 2012, November 16. Accessed November 23, 2012.

4   Harper J, Madan AK, Ternovitis CA, Tichansky DS What happens to patients who do not follow-up after bariatric surgery? The American Surgeon. 2007;73:181-4.

5   Breznikar B, Divneski D. Bariatric surgery for morbid obesity: pre-operative assessment, surgical techniques and post-operative monitoring. J Int Med Res. 2009;37(5):1632-1645.

6   McVay MA, Friedman KE. The benefits of cognitive behavioral groups for bariatric surgery patients. Bariatric Times. 2012;9(9):22-28.

7   Orth WS, Madan AK, Taddecci RJ, Coday M, Tichansky DS. Support group meeting attendance is associated with better weight loss. Obesity Surgery. 2008;18:391-4.

19

Online Support &
BariatricPal.com

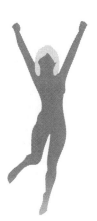

Congratulations on making it this far in the book! The previous chapters explained each step of your journey, including:

- Learning about the sleeve.
- Making the decision about the VSG.
- Choosing a surgeon and planning for the procedure.
- Getting the gastric sleeve and recovering from surgery.
- Your post-surgery diet progression and long-term sleeve diet.
- Exercise as part of your new lifestyle.
- What to expect in the first year after surgery.

Your knowledge practically qualifies you as an expert on the vertical sleeve, but there's so much to know that a single book can't possibly tell you everything you need to know for your entire weight loss journey. That's especially true for a new procedure, such as the gastric sleeve, because new information is always coming out. You also need additional resources for when you have sleeve-specific questions about your diet, a sleeve side effect, or anything else sleeve-related.

The Internet can be invaluable on your journey. It's not only an infinite source of information but also an increasingly popular option for social support. This chapter is dedicated to online resources. It begins with some general advice on using the Internet, and the main focus of the chapter is on BariatricPal.com. This social network has already been mentioned throughout the book, and this chapter will discuss BariatricPal.com in more detail so that you know what it offers and how to use it.

Online Resources Can Be Indispensible

The Internet is increasingly central to daily life. We use it for staying in touch, finding locations, researching products and services, and keeping up with the news. Connectivity is available at home and on mobile devices. With the emphasis on technology, information, and communication, counting on the Internet to help you through your sleeve journey makes perfect sense. This section suggests ways to use the Internet more effectively.

Online Social Communities & Informational Resources

You already know that your support system is fundamental to your success with losing weight with the sleeve. Your system likely includes your family, friends, and medical team, and virtual buddies can fulfill important, complementary roles. Social networking is a great resource for you on your sleeve journey because you can meet far more sleevers online than you'd ever be able to meet in person.

Some sites, such as Facebook and Twitter, let you find sleevers and communicate with them without ever meeting in real life if you don't want to. If you're looking for some in-person friends, you can try sites such as meetup.com to find bariatric patients in your area.

Discussion forums, such as BariatricPal.com, are where you're most likely to spend the majority of your online social time because they're filled with people just like you.

Online Informational Resources

Online resources are unlimited sources of information, and they're always available. You don't have to wait until business hours to get answers to your questions answered, and you can connect with friends around the world in different time zones when you have questions that just can't wait. Online resources can be as private as you want them to be, so you can feel free to ask questions that you think are silly. Nobody has to know that you got up at 1:00 a.m. to look up whether non-fat cottage cheese is allowed on your soft foods diet so that you can sleep better knowing what you're going to have for breakfast in a few hours.

Being Cautious with Online Resources

Online resources can be credible and complete, but they're not always so trustworthy. Anyone can post materials online, and there is no censorship or required level of accuracy for "information" to be placed online. Blogs, company or personal web pages, and all other resources can be accurate or inaccurate. Often, there's no true way to know whether a site has accurate information, and you have to use your judgment. These are some warning signs of sites that probably are not trustworthy:

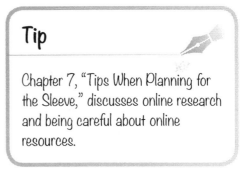

Tip

Chapter 7, "Tips When Planning for the Sleeve," discusses online research and being careful about online resources.

- Lots of distracting ads that direct you away from the site
- Sponsored or hosted by a private clinic or hospital that is clearly trying to recruit new patients
- Contains information that you know is wrong, so you can assume that other information on the site is probably inaccurate too
- Includes a noticeably high number of posts or contributions that are redundant and by a single person. That person might be trying to get you to buy something.
- Has tons of links to an external site. That's a sign that someone is just trying to get you to visit the other site, and that person may be being paid every time you go to that site.

A lot of resources look authentic at first glance, but as you dig deeper, you might start to notice some of the above red flags. You can develop your own set of trusted sites as you continue to use the Internet for your sleeve research. Information from your surgeon and informal advice from social networking sites where you've developed close friendships can be good sources for you to depend on.

Finding One or More Online Communities

You'll run across hundreds, maybe thousands, of discussion boards when you search online. They may be dedicated to weight loss, to bariatric surgery patients in general, or to gastric sleeve patients in particular. They may be sponsored by companies, by surgeons or by individuals.

There's no single "right" board to use. If no single board meets all your needs, you might end up visiting multiple communities regularly. These are some of the criteria to consider when you're test-driving to find one or more good communities:

- Friendly
- Option to remain as anonymous as you want
- Offers mobile apps if this is something you would use
- Policy against selling your information to advertisers
- Additional features, such as live chat rooms and instant messaging

This book has mentioned BariatricPal.com several times. The site is the largest online social network dedicated to the gastric sleeve community. It's for sleeve patients, people who are considering the sleeve, and anyone who is a friend or family member of a sleeve patient.

BariatricPal Weight Loss Surgery Support

BariatricPal is a comprehensive online resource for the weight loss surgery community. It houses four Weight Loss Surgery (WLS) boards, or discussion forums, which together include hundreds of thousands of members. Each major section of the boards is dedicated to a specific type of weight loss surgery.

- LapBandTalk.com, the original WLS Boards community dating back to July of 2003, is for the laparoscopic adjustable gastric band, or lap-band.
- BariatricPal.com, started in February of 2009, is for the vertical sleeve gastrectomy.
- SleevePlicationTalk.com, started in May of 2011, is for the sleeve plication procedure.
- RNYTalk.com, started in July of 2011, is for the Roux-en-Y gastric bypass.

You're welcome to hang out with other sleeve patients in the gastric sleeve board, to hop on over to the other weight loss surgery forums, or to chat in a general section for all weight loss surgery procedures. Together, the boards have more than two million posts per month.

The Story of BariatricPal.com

A unique feature of BariatricPal.com is that it is independent, and not affiliated with a major company or medical care group. Its founder, Alex Brecher, is himself a bariatric surgery patient – and one of the authors of this book. At 5 feet 7 inches tall and 255 pounds, Alex got the lap-band in July of 2003. When he got home from the hospital and looked online for sources of information and support, he was disappointed that he couldn't find a comprehensive source of trustworthy information and friendly encouragement. That's when he started LapBandTalk.com.

Alex didn't forget the trials of obesity and the gift that he feels bariatric surgery gave him. When he saw that patients of other types of weight loss surgery needed information, he started the other communities within BariatricPal, or what was then known as the (weight loss surgery) WLS Boards network.

With over 200,000 members, BariatricPal is the largest online discussion network dedicated exclusively to bariatric surgery, and thousands of VSG patients regularly participate on BariatricPal. Alex and his team work daily to keep the boards up and running, to update the news items, and to monitor the discussions to make sure that they're friendly and never rude. BariatricPal.com continues to serve anyone who is part of the sleeve community, since full membership is free. Alex truly hopes and believes that the boards can play a role in your own VSG success.

And how does Alex's own bariatric story end up? He's doing great! Since hitting his goal weight of 155 pounds, Alex has maintained his 100-pound weight loss for over seven years now. When Alex isn't working on BariatricPal or related projects to help weight loss surgery patients, he loves to run and spend time with his family.

A Brief Tour of BariatricPal.com

The boards are designed to be user-friendly and well-organized. You can see links to the discussion forums on the home page. You can navigate to other parts of the site, such as your profile, your message center, or the surgeon directory, from the home page or any other page. Courtesy and friendliness are very strictly enforced; negative posts are taken down, and posters can be banned.

There's a lot to discover at BariatricPal.com. Our advice is to start with the basics, such as creating your profile when you sign up and learning how to read and reply to posts. You'll discover new features as you spend more time on the boards. You can get help by posting a question in the general forum, clicking on the "Help" link on each page, or by contacting Alex or another administrator by clicking on "The Moderating Team" from the home page.

Discussion Forums

The discussion forums are the foundation of BariatricPal.com. The nearly 2 million posts include nearly any sleeve-related, somewhat sleeve-related, and not at all sleeve-related topic that you can think of. BariatricPal.com gastric sleeve forums are divided into different categories, each with their own focus. Here are some examples:

- *Introductions:* This is where you'll find out how welcoming the community is. As soon as you post your introduction here, you'll probably get a warm welcome from one or more established members.
- *Pre-Surgery Questions:* In this forum, you can read about and ask questions about preparing for the surgery and what to expect.
- *Post-Surgery Questions*: This forum is geared toward helping you after surgery. Topics might include pain medications, your post-surgery diet progression and how to treat possible side effects.

- *The "Main Forums":* Here you'll find discussions on nutrition, exercise, cosmetic surgery, complications, and everything else that can help you throughout your entire journey.

- *Support Groups:* Whatever your situation is, there's a support group for you. (And if there isn't, you can start your own.) There are groups based on your location, personal interests, when you got the sleeve (or are scheduled to have your surgery), age, religion, special health conditions, and more.

- *The "Community Center":* This is where you can find the most recent news articles on the sleeve, on bariatric surgery, and on obesity; a forum for board suggestions and feedback; and archived newsletters. You can discuss off-topic topics in the Lounge.

BariatricPal.com Grows with You

You will have different needs as your gastric sleeve journey progresses. BariatricPal.com can adapt to continue to meet your needs. You might start out on the boards when you're trying to decide whether to get the sleeve and you want to learn about others' experiences and ask your own questions. The site's surgeon directory and reviews can help you find a surgeon. BariatricPal.com can get you through the surgery and recovery process. You can get answers to your urgent diet questions as you're progressing from a liquid diet to the solid foods diet. As you get into the swing of things with your own weight loss, you'll probably find yourself shifting from always asking for help to occasionally providing advice for others. Throughout the process, BariatricPal.com may become one of your favorite online social hangouts where you can kick back and relax.

Other Features on BariatricPal.com

BariatricPal.com isn't just about the boards. It has a variety of other features that make it unique and attractive. These are a few of them:

- *Newsletters*: You receive an electronic newsletter each month. Newsletters include various features, such as site updates, detailed profiles of BariatricPal members, weight loss tips, and news on the sleeve.

- *Surgeon directory*: The surgeon directory lets you search for surgeons in your area. Surgeons are rated and reviewed by BariatricPal members so you can be more confident in their authenticity than on some other sites.

- *Private messaging*: The private messaging system lets you directly contact a specific member or group of members without posting publicly on the boards.

- *Chat rooms*: Live chat rooms let you "talk" in real-time with anyone else who happens to be hanging out in the room.

- *WLS magazine*: Each WLS ("Weight Loss Surgery") magazine, available from the main page of the forums, contains articles on information that can be very valuable in your journey. Topics might include diet, social support, plateaus, and family issues that come up as the result of your weight loss. Authors include bariatric patients, dietitians, psychologists, and other professionals with expertise in the sleeve and weight loss.

Mobile Features

BariatricPal.com has been mobile since 2012, when the site celebrated the launch of its new apps for the Apple iPod, iPad, and iPhone, as well as for the Android and the Kindle. The apps are free and fully functional, so they let you take BariatricPal.com with you wherever you go. You can read and post to discussion forum topics, send private messages to your friends, post status updates and photos, and do anything that you can do from a computer on BariatricPal.com.

These apps are great because they let you stay connected with the board at all times. BariatricPal has so many members that you're almost sure to be able to connect with someone when you're having a tough moment and you need advice or just a sympathetic ear.

You can also use BariatricPal.com smartphone apps and the app for the Kindle to get answers to burning questions that come up when you're on the go. For example, you might find yourself at a fast food restaurant with friends, and you want to find out what to order that's best for your meal plan. You can probably find some suggestions on previously posted discussions on BariatricPal.com. The smartphone app makes it possible for you to find the best choice even when you didn't plan ahead.

Your Profile and Options – Making BariatricPal.com Your Own

In this section, we'll talk about getting started on BariatricPal.com and some options for personalizing your experience and making it your own.

Getting Started and Setting Up Your Account

Only members can post on the boards, so the first step is to sign up and create an account. Again, your full-featured account is free. These are the basic steps of creating an account:

- Click on "Register Now" toward the upper right corner of the page and follow the prompts.
  - *Step 1: "Your Account."* Choose a username and password, enter your email address, select your gender, and check the box that states that you agree to the terms of use.
  - *Step 2: "Your Surgery."* Answer the questions in as much detail as you want. You can always come back later and fill in blank answers.
  - *Step 3: "Confirmation."* A confirmation email will come to your inbox.
- Activate your account by following the prompts in the confirmation email that you receive.
- When you're ready, you can set up your account preferences for which notifications you'd like to receive, such as friends' status updates, personal messages, and general messages to the community from BariatricPal.com administrators.
- You can always edit your profile information and account settings later.

Profile

You don't have to complete a full profile, but it helps everyone else know who you are. There's space for you to write your sleeve story; for your beginning, current, and goal weight and BMI; and for identifying your surgeon. You can also put in personal information, such as your location, age, hobbies, and occupation. You have the option of linking your BariatricPal.com account to your Facebook and Twitter accounts.

Everyone loves before and after photos, and there's a place for them on your profile page. You can post additional photos in the "Photo Gallery," which is like a photo album that you get to share with the entire community if you choose.

Stay on Track with Trackers

Lose weight and stay on track when you log and record everything, including your progress. BariatricPal.com *trackers* are basically online mini-logs—you get to track your measurements and see how far you've progressed toward your goals. You can put in your weight and your body measurements. You can also keep a food log using your tracker so that you always have a place to record what you ate.

Mark Your Progress with Tickers

The *tickers* are what you'll see under some members' signatures when they post in the forums. You can set yours to show your BMI, your percent body fat, your body weight, or if you haven't had surgery yet, a countdown of the number of days until your surgery is scheduled. The ticker is sort of a ruler; on the left of the ruler is your starting BMI, percent fat, body weight, or number of days when you started counting down to surgery. At the far right is your goal value or surgery date. A ticker marker moves from left to right as you make progress toward your goal. You get to customize your ticker by choosing from a variety of designs for the ruler and for the ticker marker. If you choose, your ticker marker will be displayed under your post every time you post in the forums.

You don't have to share your tracker if you don't want to. You can set yours to be private so that only you can see it, or you can set it so that only your approved friends on BariatricPal.com can see it. If you like to be held accountable by a lot of people, you can keep your tracker public so that everyone who looks at your profile can see it.

Automatic Updates Are Optional

You can set your account to send updates to your email address or smartphone. Some people like to get emails and push notifications from BariatricPal.com every time there's an update. Some members, on the other extreme, prefer to only rarely receive emails or push notifications; they'd rather only see board updates when they log in.

Most people are somewhere in between—they like the occasional email or phone notification as a reminder to check in to the boards. These reminders can also provide additional inspiration to keep working at your sleeve diet. These are examples of some of the email or smartphone notifications that you can choose to receive if you want. You can always change your settings from your profile page if you change your mind about what email or smartphone updates you want to receive.

- Updates on any discussion thread of your choice so you know when someone's replied to a conversation that you are in or you think is interesting
- Delivery of the board's regular newsletter
- Communications from Alex Brecher, the board's founder, or any of the staff at the boards. These kinds of messages come only a few times a year when there's big news, so we recommend signing up for these.
- Delivery of private messages from other board members.
- Alerts on your friends' status updates and members' replies to your own status updates

If you choose not to receive a notification via email, you can still find the information on BariatricPal.com the next time you log in. You'll see a little icon near your name at the corner of the screen when you log in. It tells you that you have notifications to check out.

Keeping Your Profile Current and Customized

There are plenty of ways to keep your BariatricPal.com information current so that everyone's up to date on your latest news. As with all of your information on BariatricPal.com, you can set your profile information to be as private or public as you choose. Many members choose an intermediate option by allowing only their approved BariatricPal "friends" to see their information.

You can update your profile at any time. This includes features such as tickers, trackers, your gastric sleeve story, and your photo gallery. These are some of the options that BariatricPal. com offers to keep your profile and information personal and current.

Member Blog

BariatricPal.com hosts members' blogs. The blog is automatically linked to your account, and you access it from your profile. You can use it just like any other blog, where you post entries about your life or whatever you want. Some members keep their blogs strictly focused on the gastric sleeve and weight loss, while others include pretty much everything else about their lives—almost as a regular diary or journal.

Personal News Feed

The news feed feature on BariatricPal.com is similar to those on other online social networking sites. The feed shows your social activity on BariatricPal.com. Members can see when you update your profile photo, when you add new friends, and when you make new posts on the discussion boards. The profile feed is a feature that allows you to post short sentences about what you're doing so everyone knows.

Photo Ops

Photos let everyone put a face to your name. There's plenty of space on BariatricPal.com for your photos. Besides posting before and after photos on your member profile page, you can choose a photo—or any image you want—as your profile picture. That's what everyone will see when they read your posts or get private messages from you. You can also take advantage of the photo gallery to post as many photos as you want and let everyone see them!

The Social Side of BariatricPal.com

Come for the information; stay for the friends! You might start going to the boards to gather information about the VSG. Even if this book doesn't inspire you to look for the site, you'll probably find it when you do online searches. BariatricPal.com is so big that it often pops up in searches on the gastric sleeve. When you make your way to BariatricPal.com, you'll probably find not only the answers you needed but more encouragement and positive support than you expected.

In fact, don't be surprised if you come back to the boards because you like the atmosphere and start to meet some people that you really care about—and that really care about you. You might even start to count some members as some of your best friends. Just as you can on other social media sites, you can become board "friends" with other members by inviting them to be your friends or accepting their invitations to be theirs. This lets you see each others' updates faster and send private messages straight from your profile.

Special "Groups" Let You Make Closer Friends

As mentioned above, the group forums are for members with common characteristics or interests. The groups provide ideal opportunities to share experiences with members who may be going through the same struggles and triumphs as you. Just like in the real world where you're more likely to make close friends with people who have a lot in common with you, you might feel a closer bond with BariatricPal.com members who have more in common with you than just the sleeve. They might be your age, have children of the same age, live near you, or share the same religious beliefs or hobbies, for example.

Using BariatricPal.com Daily

Some sleeve members check out the boards daily or even more frequently as they start to depend on it for instant advice, sympathetic listeners, and, finally, close friends. The site gives you a sense of belonging.

Giving Back to the Bariatric Community and BariatricPal.com

Membership to BariatricPal.com, including each of its services and features, is free for everyone. You can set up your account and get instant access to the boards, including to the smartphone and Kindle apps. Alex Brecher, the founder of BariatricPal.com, is committed to helping you throughout your weight loss journey. His mission is to make the community accessible to everyone who needs this resource for their success. A lot of people depend on this free service. Opportunities are available if you're interested in giving back just a little. These are some of the ways you can help out.

Review and Rate Your Surgeon

The Surgeon Directory is invaluable for gastric sleeve patients who are looking for a surgeon. You can help keep the Surgeon Directory complete by writing a review of your own surgeon and rating him or her. You might be more motivated to write an honest, detailed review when you remember how difficult it was for you to find a surgeon and how much you appreciated each bit of information that helped you make your decision confidently.

Post Fliers in Your Clinic

BariatricPal.com depends on growth and is always eager to welcome new members. You can help spread the word and attract new members by posting promotional BariatricPal.com fliers in your surgeon's office or waiting room, where your bariatric surgery group support meetings are held or anywhere else that bariatric surgery patients are likely to gather and see the posters. The fliers are already prepared and are available from BariatricPal.com, so you just have to print them out and post them.

Be a Good Community Member

You can also help simply by being proactive on the boards. The BariatricPal.com community is based on a foundation of positive energy and member participation. One of the ways you can help out is to keep an eye out for inappropriate posts, such as negative posts, off-topic posts, or spam posters who are obviously there to promote their own interests. Alex and his team work daily to prevent these situations, but extra eyes can always help.

Another way that you help out the community is to provide support for other members. In the beginning, your support might be more geared toward encouragement. You can also play a role in welcoming new members. As you lose weight, you'll be gaining more knowledge. You will soon be an expert at knowing what works and what doesn't with the sleeve. This experience enables you to provide more advice and answers to specific questions.

Other Online Resources

BariatricPal.com is the biggest discussion forum and support system on the web, but it's not your only possible source of support and information. Additional sources include other online discussion forums and social networks, bariatric surgery clinic sites, and government-provided information.

Sources of Information

Government resources, such as Medline Plus and the Weight Information Network, are considered trustworthy sources of information. They're both provided and maintained by the National Institutes of Health within the Department of Health and Human Services. Many bariatric centers at large hospitals and universities have relatively extensive sites. They often provide a good deal of practical information about the sleeve, such as how the gastrectomy procedure works, how to prepare, and your post-surgery diet. For friendly encouragement and sympathetic support, the options are unlimited, starting with BariatricPal.com.

Select the Resources That You Prefer

Which resources to use are completely up to you. You might be the type of person who trusts only what your doctor says and stays far away from online information and social networking. That's okay as long as you are sure to get the information and support you need from real-life sources, such as family, close friends, coworkers, and other members of your support group meeting. If you're an Internet junkie, you will probably be online constantly, looking at every possible resource. You'll probably end up using a few different sites regularly. You might, for example, have a favorite hospital site for when you need to look up basic rules on your sleeve diet, plus one or two social networking sites to keep you motivated and on your toes.

✎ **Summary**

☛ Preparation, without a doubt, increases your chances of success with the vertical sleeve gastrectomy. No matter how well you prepare, though, you can't possibly know every answer to every question all the time. Luckily, the Internet makes it easier for you to get the answers you're looking for and the support you need. This chapter encouraged you to explore the Internet as a valuable resource and provided advice on making the most out what you find.

☛ Reading this book puts you far ahead of most other sleeve patients in terms of knowledge, preparation, and what to expect. You have literally learned about every step of the way, from the possible risks of obesity, to whether the vertical sleeve gastrectomy is for you, to how to get through surgery, to what kind of lifestyle you'll be leading (or are already leading if you already got the sleeve). You're more prepared than someone who jumps in blindly, and this gives you a better chance of success with the sleeve.

☛ Hopefully by now you are confident that you can and should track down information to help you stay on track and make the right decisions when you're not sure what to do. Just as the sleeve is a tool to help you lose weight, this book is a tool to learn what you need to know to lose weight with the sleeve. It's a good starting point, and now you can find out anything you want about the sleeve and connect with others who won't let you down.

Your Turn: Keeping Your Appointments Straight

This book covers a wide range of topics, but there's no way it could cover everything you need to know. What is something that you still need to find out?

Example: I still don't know which cuts of beef are healthiest.

1. ....
....

2. ....
....

3. ....
....

What questions do you think will come up later as you make progress toward your weight loss goal and eventually hit your goal?

Example: I'll probably start to wonder how I can meet new exercise buddies as I get in better shape.

1. ....
....

2. ....
....

3. ....
....

Conclusion

This is the end of *The Big Book on the Gastric Sleeve: Everything You Need to Know to Lose Weight and Live Well with the Vertical Sleeve Gastrectomy.* We've taken you from the beginning of your weight loss journey through surgery to your new, everyday lifestyle with the sleeve. The book was designed to be a complete guide to enable you to take control of your weight, health, and life.

The book covered the effects and challenges of obesity, how the sleeve is a permanent tool to help you lose weight, and what kind of weight loss to expect after the procedure. You know the possible side effects and complications from getting the sleeve, how to try to prevent them, and how to recognize and treat them. You know all about choosing a surgeon, preparing for surgery, and recovering from the procedure. The book discusses the importance of exercise and gives some tips and tricks to get you started and turn an active lifestyle into a long-term habit. And, you've worked on building your support system to keep you motivated.

The VSG diet is among the most important factors in your weight loss success. From the post-surgery dietary progression to your weight loss diet, you're practically an expert on nutrition and the sleeve diet. You know which foods to choose, which foods to avoid, and what to do if you have a reaction to a food. You even know how to create a daily menu that has the nutrients you need and which nutritional supplements may be necessary to stay healthy.

We know that your gastric sleeve journey doesn't stop here. You will continue to have new questions, try new recipes, overcome, and share happy moments with your friends and family that might not have happened if you hadn't gotten weight loss surgery.

We sincerely hope that this book has been and will continue to be an excellent resource for you. We suggest that you keep it handy as one of your valuable references so you can look things up when you have questions. You can use it to look up facts about the sleeve, refresh your memory on basic nutrition, and design a meal plan based on the food phase you're in. Chapter 16 is always there for you, too, for whenever you feel ready to get started with an exercise program or you need some strategies to motivate yourself to continue your program.

We also recommend, if you haven't already, signing up for BariatricPal.com, the world's premier online social network dedicated to the weight loss community. It's a source of information and support, and it'll grow with you. No matter where you are in your weight loss journey or how many new questions and experiences you have, you'll be able to find someone to sympathize, offer advice, or point you in the right direction. You'll probably also make a few very close friends on BariatricPal.com. Your account is free and takes only minutes to set up, so there's no reason not to try it out. We think you'll be glad you did!

We'd like to thank you for letting this book be a part of your gastric sleeve journey. Regardless of where you are in your weight loss journey, whether or not you choose to get the sleeve, or whether you read the book so that you could offer support to a loved one with the sleeve, we hope that this book has met your needs. Our goal was to provide honest and complete information to allow you to make the best decisions for yourself, and we truly hope we have succeeded.

We wish you the best of luck in your sleeve future.

Glossary of Terms

Abdominoplasty (also panniculectomy) – This is also known as a "tummy tuck." It's when your cosmetic surgeon removes the excess skin and fat that are left in your stomach after you lose a lot of weight, such as hitting your goal weight after getting the sleeve. The surgeon might also tighten up the abdominal muscles too.

Adjustable gastric band (AGB) – Also known as the lap-band or the band, it's a band that goes around the upper part of your stomach to create a smaller upper pouch, called a stoma. The larger part of your stomach remains below the band, which slows the flow of food from the stoma to the lower part of the stomach. The gastric band restricts your food intake to help you lose weight because your stoma fills up quickly and you feel full. The tightness of the gastric band can be adjusted by filling it with saline solution to make it more restrictive. An unfill, or removing saline solution, loosens the band, or makes it less restrictive.

Adverse events – These are harmful side effects or complications that are associated with a specific medication or medical procedure, such as the gastrectomy. A low rate of mild adverse events means that the procedure is pretty safe, while a high rate of severe adverse events means that the procedure is pretty risky.

Bariatric surgery (weight loss surgery) – This is any surgery that is designed to help you lose weight. The more common types in the United States are the gastric sleeve, or vertical gastrectomy, the roux-en-Y gastric bypass, the adjustable laparoscopic gastric band, or lap-band, and the sleeve plication surgery. Bariatric surgery itself does not cause weight loss. Instead, it is a tool that helps you eat less and/or absorb fewer nutrients so that you can lose weight.

Biliopancreatic Diversion with Duodenal Switch (BPD-DS) – This bariatric procedure is restrictive because it removes most of the stomach, and it is malabsorptive because it redirects some digestive juices and food to the large intestine for elimination from the body. The BPD-DS is considered too high-risk for very morbidly obese patients, so the VSG is required as a preliminary surgery. Patients can get the second part of the BPD-DS surgery after losing some weight with the sleeve.

BMI (body mass index) – This is a calculation that is used to indicate whether you are at a healthy weight or whether you should lose weight. The formula to calculate BMI considers your height and weight. You can calculate your BMI and determine whether you are at a normal weight or if you are overweight, obese, or morbidly obese.

BMR (basal metabolic rate) – This is also known as your metabolism. It is the number of calories you burn per day just to stay alive. Your body uses calories, even while resting and sleeping, for things like keeping your heart beating, your blood flowing, and your lungs breathing. Your BMR is higher if you are a man, you are a younger rather than an older adult. and if you are heavier.

Brachioplasty – This procedure, also known as an arm lift, is cosmetic surgery to get rid of your "bat wings," or the skin that hangs down from your arms after you lose a lot of weight.

Calorie balance – Also known as "energy balance," this is a comparison of the calories you consume, or take in, versus the calories you burn off, or expend. You consume calories by eating; you expend calories with your basal metabolic (see "BMR"), from digesting food, and from physical activity. You are in calorie balance when you are eating the same number of calories that you are expending. Your weight will not change when you are in energy balance.

Calorie deficit – Also known as a "negative calorie balance," this is when you are expending, or using, more calories than you are consuming, or eating. A calorie deficit leads to weight loss. A deficit of 3,500 calories leads to one pound of weight loss, so you need to average a deficit of 500 calories per day if you want to lose one pound per week. You can create a deficit by eating fewer calories or increasing your physical activity.

Calorie surplus – This is also known as a "positive calorie balance." It happens when you consume more calories than you expend. Basically, if you eat more than you burn off, you will gain weight.

Cholesterol, total – Your total cholesterol is measured with a simple blood test, usually as part of a lipid panel. Your doctor or the laboratory can let you know whether you need to be fasting. High cholesterol is a risk factor for heart disease. A normal cholesterol level is under 200 milligrams per deciliter (200 mg/dL or 5.2 mmol/L); borderline high cholesterol is 200 to 239 mg/dL (5.2 to 6.2 mmol/L); high cholesterol is 240 mg/dL (6.2 mmol/L) or above. You can lower your cholesterol by losing extra body weight and eating more fiber, which is in fruits, vegetables, beans, nuts, and whole grains products. (See Chapter 9, Pre-Surgery Preparations, for more information).

Cholecystokinin (CCK) – A gut hormone that may help reduce food intake by promoting satiety. Levels of CCK decrease after getting the sleeve, so that's another way the sleeve may help you lose weight.

Cholesterol, HDL – High-density lipoprotein cholesterol, or HDL cholesterol, is known as the "good" cholesterol. Like total cholesterol, you'll get your HDL measured in a blood test as part of a lipid panel. A high value of HDL cholesterol means that you have a lower risk for heart disease. Women naturally have higher HDL cholesterol than men. A desirable value for HDL cholesterol is above 60 milligrams per dL (60 mg/dL; over 1.5 mmol/L). HDL cholesterol under 40 mg/dL (1 mmol/L) for men and below 50 mg/dl (1.3 mmol/L) for women is a risk factor for heart disease. Increasing your physical activity increases your HDL cholesterol levels.

Cholesterol, LDL – Low-density lipoprotein cholesterol, or LDL cholesterol, is known as the "bad" cholesterol because a high value increases your risk of heart disease. Your doctor might recommend keeping your LDL under 70 milligrams per deciliter (70 mg/dL, or 1.8 mmol/L) if you have a high risk for heart disease; otherwise, the general goal for your LDL cholesterol is under 100 mg/dL. LDL cholesterol from 160 to 189 mg/dL (4.1 to 4.9 mmol/L) is high, and over 190 mg/dL is considered very high. You can lower your LDL cholesterol by losing excess weight and reducing your intake of saturated fat, such as from fatty meats, dark-meat poultry, butter, dairy products, and palm oil.

Comorbidity – This is a disorder related to the primary disease; in this case, the primary disease is obesity, and common comorbidities include obesity-related diseases, such as type 2 diabetes, hypertension, and osteoarthritis.

Contraindications – These are reasons to refuse to provide a certain medical service or procedure. Some of the contraindications for the vertical sleeve gastrectomy, or reasons why you would not be a good candidate for the VSG, are inflammatory bowel disease, Barrett's esophagus, drug addiction, and lack of understanding of how the sleeve works.

Copay – This is a flat fee, rather than a percentage, that your insurance company makes you pay each time you see a healthcare provider. In most cases, your copay amount is not affected by the services you end up getting at the appointment. An example of a copayment might be $30 each time you see a physician within your health coverage plan.

Deductible – This is the amount you need to pay, usually annually, before your insurance plan actually starts to cover your expenses. The "better" your insurance plan is, the lower your deductible rate; that is, your insurance plan pays for services before you have paid very much out of your own pocket. Let's take an example. Let's say that your insurance plan covers 80 percent of your expense and that your deductible is $1,000 annually. You, yourself, are responsible for paying the first $1,000 in medical bills in each year. Your insurance will only start to pay 80 percent of your bills for the rest of the year after you —have already gotten—and paid for by yourself$1,000-worth of services.

Dehiscence – This is a complication of surgery that is the splitting of the scar site where the stitches are. It can happen after vertical sleeve surgery, such as in your abdomen where the surgeon inserted the laparoscopic tools, or after body recontouring surgery. It's more likely to happen if you do not follow your surgeon's instructions to take care of yourself after surgery.

Diabetes (type 2 diabetes) – This is the type of diabetes that is often known as adult-onset diabetes. It is most commonly linked to obesity, unlike type 1 diabetes, which usually occurs in childhood or adolescence. Diabetes occurs when your blood sugar levels are out of control. Complications include kidney disease, blindness, amputations, infections, and heart disease. (See also gestational diabetes).

Dietitian – A dietitian, or registered dietitian, has taken a variety of nutrition classes, practiced clinical skills in an internship, and passed the national dietetics examination. Dietitians help you plan meals, work through food challenges, choose healthier foods, and improve your recipes. You can recognize a dietitian by the "RD" credential. A nutritionist is not necessarily a dietitian, although many nutritionists are just as highly qualified. They might have an MS or PhD in nutrition.

Dumping Syndrome – A side effect of malabsorptive procedures that leads to diarrhea, nausea, weakness, and fatigue after you eat. It happens when undigested food gets into your large intestine and is worse for high-sugar and high-fat foods. Dumping syndrome is less common with VSG than with gastric bypass or BPD-DS.

Dyslipidemia – This is a condition when your blood lipids, or total cholesterol, LDL cholesterol, HDL cholesterol, and/or triglycerides, are not at normal levels. Dyslipidemia is a risk factor for heart disease, and it is often caused by obesity.

Empty calories – These are calories or high-calorie foods that do not provide many essential nutrients, such as vitamins and minerals. Examples include sugar, sweets, French fries, doughnuts, and bacon.

Excess Weight Lost (EWL) – This is usually expressed in a percentage as the amount of weight lost divided by the amount of excess weight that you started with. To calculate your starting excess weight, take your starting body weight and subtract your ideal body weight.

Fully-insured plan – This is a health insurance plan that you or your employer pays for.

Gastric band – This is the key part of the lap-band that helps you lose weight. It's literally a band that goes around your stomach (the gastric tissue) to create a smaller stoma above ad the larger stomach portion below. The gastric band is cushioned and has room for saline solution. A fuller gastric band makes you feel more restriction to lose weight faster; a less full band makes you feel less restriction.

Gastric bypass – This is a type of weight loss surgery that divides your stomach into a smaller upper pouch and smaller lower pouch. The intestine connects to both. The procedure is restrictive, like the lap-band, but unlike the lap-band, gastric bypass is also malabsorptive, so the amount of nutrients that you absorb decreases. The most common kind of gastric bypass is Roux-en-Y, in which the upper part of the small intestine is divided to connect to a smaller upper stomach pouch and a larger lower stomach remnant. It is reversible but only through a difficult procedure.

Gastric sleeve (see vertical sleeve gastrectomy)

Gestational diabetes (GDM) – This is a type of glucose intolerance, or lack of blood sugar control, that occurs during pregnancy. It often goes away after you give birth, but you are at higher risk of developing type 2 diabetes if you had GDM during one or more pregnancies. Obesity increases your risk of developing GDM.

Ghrelin – Sometimes called the hunger hormone, it is produced by your stomach and pancreas, and it makes you feel hungry. You have higher levels before meals and lower levels after meals. Gastric sleeve patients have lower levels of ghrelin after surgery than before, so this hormonal change may play a role in helping you lose weight.

Glucagon-like peptide-1 (GLP-1) – This is a gut hormone whose levels are lower between meals and higher after meals. It tends to make you eat less. Obese individuals have lower levels of GLP-1 than normal-weight individuals. The VSG leads to lower GLP-1 levels, which might help you lose weight.

Glucose – This is the type of sugar that is in your blood. It provides energy to most of the cells in your body, but very high or uncontrolled levels of blood glucose cause pre-diabetes or type 2 diabetes. Your glucose levels go up as you start to develop insulin resistance.

Glucose tolerance test (or oral glucose tolerance test, or OGTT) – This is a test of how well you are able to control your blood glucose levels. You drink a very sweet sugar solution, and the laboratory technician draws your blood periodically for a couple of hours after that to monitor the changes in your blood sugar levels. You may have diabetes if a glucose tolerance test causes your blood glucose levels to spike high and fast.

Ghrelin – Also known as the hunger hormone, this hormone is produced and secreted by the fundus cells in your stomach. Levels of ghrelin circulating in your bloodstream increase before meals and decrease after meals. High levels of ghrelin make you feel hungry, and low levels make you feel full. Patients with the VSG have lower levels of ghrelin because of the removal of the stomach. This may help you lose weight by making you less hungry.

Health maintenance organization (HMO) – This is a type of health insurance plan that helps cover expenses for doctor visits, medical services, and prescription drugs. Your HMO might cover a certain percentage of most services.

Hypertension (high blood pressure) – This is when the force of your blood beating against your blood vessels is higher than it should be. You get your blood measured, probably at most doctor's visits, when a nurse puts a cuff around your upper arm, inflates the cuff, and slowly lets the air out. Hypertension means your heart is working harder than it should, and it also puts a strain on your kidneys. High blood pressure increases your risk for heart disease, kidney disease, and stroke. If you're obese, losing weight can probably lower high blood pressure.

Ideal body weight – This is a theoretical value that's considered to be the healthiest body weight at your height. It's often set at a BMI of 22.

Ileal brake – Combined effect of peptide-YY and glucagon-like peptide-1 to make you feel full when food reaches the far end of your small intestine—the ileum.

Indications – These are characteristics that make you a potential candidate for a medical treatment. Some indications for getting the vertical sleeve, for example, are having morbid obesity or having a BMI of at least 35 and a comorbidity, such as a chronic disease.

Inpatient – This is often defined as an overnight hospital stay or a stay that lasts at least 24 hours. Many insurance companies require your vertical sleeve surgery to be an inpatient procedure in order to get your costs covered.

Insulin – This is a hormone that is necessary for regulating your blood sugar levels. It's produced by a kind of cell, called beta cells, which are in your pancreas. Type 2 diabetes occurs when you develop insulin resistance and your body can no longer control your blood glucose levels.

Insulin resistance – This describes what happens when the cells in your body are no longer as responsive (or as sensitive) to the effects of insulin. The result is that high levels of glucose stay in your blood. Severe insulin resistance leads to pre-diabetes and then type 2 diabetes.

LAP-BAND® or adjustable gastric banding system (AGBS) – This is the brand name for the adjustable laparoscopic band made by the company Allergan, Inc. It consists of a gastric band, thin connection tubing, and an access port. The system comes in two sizes and is designed to be adjustable and reversible so that you can reduce your risk of health complications with the surgery and afterward.

Laparoscopic surgery – This is also known as minimally invasive surgery, or MIS. Laparoscopic surgery requires smaller incisions than regular surgery. Instead of actually opening up your body and controlling the instruments with his or her hands, the surgeon uses a camera to visualize the patient's interior and controls the instruments with robotic systems.

Laparotomy – This is an open surgery that your surgeon might choose to do if unable to perform the laparosopic surgery on you. The laparotomy involves a single deep cut in your abdomen to give the surgeon access to your abdomen. Recovery time is longer after the laparotomy, and you have a higher risk for infections, but you might need it if your heart and lungs cannot handle the pneumoperitoneum required in laparoscopic surgery.

Leak – This is a complication of VSG in which the staple line of your sleeve is no longer tight. Food and bacteria from your gastrointestinal tract can get into your abdominal cavity and lead to peritonitis. A leak may require a stent or another surgery to fix the leak or revise the surgery to a bypass.

Leptin – Leptin is a hormone that is involved in appetite control. Leptin may reduce appetite, but obese individuals have higher leptin levels than normal weight individuals. That may mean that obese individuals respond differently to leptin. The sleeve may improve the effects of leptin on your appetite, but the research results aren't yet clear.

Lipid panel – Also known as a lipid profile, this is a standard set of tests that your doctor uses to help determine your risk for heart disease. It includes your total cholesterol, LDL cholesterol, HDL cholesterol, and triglycerides. It's a simple blood test, and you'll often get your blood glucose, which is a test for diabetes, tested at the same time. You'll need to fast for a complete lipid panel.

Managed care – This is a general term for health care programs that are designed to reduce total costs to you and the system. Private examples include HMOs and PPOs; public examples of managed care programs include Medicare, for older adults, and Medicaid, for low-income children and disabled adults.

Magenstrasse and Mill – This is an early version of the vertical sleeve gastrectomy developed in the United Kingdom. The surgeon removes the majority of the stomach and makes a long tube out of the lesser curvature of the stomach that goes from the esophagus to the antral mill, where food grinding occurs. The procedure is simple, does not require foreign implants, and retains regular digestion of food to prevent dumping syndrome.

Malabsorptive procedure – This is a bariatric surgery procedure that interferes with regular nutrient absorption. This helps with weight loss because you absorb fewer calories from your food, but it puts you at higher risk for nutrient deficiencies because you are not absorbing all of the vitamins and minerals that you eat. Another side effect is dumping syndrome. Gastric bypass and biliopancreatic diversion with duodenal switch (BPD-DS) are examples of malabsorptive procedures; the sleeve is not malabsorptive.

Maximum out-of-pocket – This is the highest total amount of money that you yourself will need to pay in a specific time period, such as a year, before your insurance company will pay for absolutely all the rest of your medical costs. Having a maximum out-of-pocket protects you against catastrophic financial results in case you end up needing unexpected and expensive emergency care or a long hospital stay.

Medicaid – This is the government-run health insurance program for low-income individuals. It's run partly by the federal government and partly by the state government, so there are lots of variations between states in their Medicaid programs. You might have to do a bit of quick research to find the specific name of the Medicaid program in your state.

Medical tourism – This is when you go to a foreign nation to get your medical procedure done. Mexico is a popular destination country for bariatric surgeries, including the VSG. Some Americans go to Canada, India, or other nations to get their sleeve done. Medical tourism can be cheaper than staying in the U.S. for patients whose insurance won't cover it, and you can usually get package deals with transportation, accommodations, and medical care included.

Medicare – This is the national health care insurance program for adults over age 65 years. It's a managed care program. Hospital services are covered in Part A of Medicare, and outpatient services are covered in Part B.

Metabolism (see BMR)

Morbid obesity – This is when your BMI is 40 or above. It's a level of obesity that is associated with a very high risk of chronic diseases, such as heart disease, stroke, and type 2 diabetes. If you have morbid obesity, you may qualify for the VSG, even if you don't have any other health conditions, because you are at such a high risk for developing them soon.

Non-Steroidal Anti-Inflammatory Drug (NSAID) – These are common painkillers that also fight inflammation. Many, such as ibuprofen and aspirin, are over-the-counter and familiar. Ketorolac is a prescription NSAID that is common after the VSG. Using NSAIDs can reduce the amount of narcotic painkillers that you need.

Nutrient-dense – These kinds of foods provide a lot of essential and beneficial nutrients such as dietary fiber, healthy fats, vitamins, or minerals. Examples include fat-free yogurt, tuna, skinless chicken breast, fruit, vegetables, and beans. Most nutrient-dense foods are fairly low in calories, but some, such as nuts and avocados, are high in calories because they are full of healthy fats.

Obese – You are considered obese if your BMI is at least 30. Obesity is considered a risk factor for a variety of chronic conditions, including heart disease, stroke, high blood pressure, some cancers, sleep apnea, asthma, and osteoarthritis. You may be eligible to get the VSG if your BMI is greater than 35 and you have a chronic condition that puts your health at risk.

Osteoporosis – This is a chronic condition with low bone mineral density, so you are at high risk for bone fractures. The disease takes years to develop, and you may not know you have it until you break a bone. Sleeve patients need to be sure to get enough calcium and vitamin D to avoid a higher risk for osteoporosis; this can be challenging with the limited food intake on the sleeve diet.

Outpatient – This refers to any procedure that does not require an overnight stay in the clinic or hospital. Sometimes "outpatient" is defined as any hospital visit that takes less than 24 hours. The VSG is often an outpatient procedure, but many insurance plans require an overnight stay before you get reimbursed for the surgery. You'll have to check your plan and discuss the requirements with your surgeon.

Overweight – You are considered overweight if your BMI is between 25 and 30. You may not have visible health effects from being overweight (but you might), but you are at higher risk for becoming obese than if you were at a normal weight.

Panniculectomy (see abdominoplasty)

Peptide YY (PYY) – This gut hormone forms part of the "ileal brake" with glucagon-like peptide-1. PYY increases your feelings of fullness after a meal. Levels are higher in obese individuals than normal-weight people, and they tend to decrease after getting the sleeve — which may contribute to your weight loss.

Pneumoperitoneum – Inflation of the wall of your abdominal cavity, created by pumping in carbon dioxide gas, that allows your surgeon access to your stomach to be able to perform the laparoscopic surgery. It is a strain for your heart and lungs and may cause shoulder or neck pain after your surgery.

Post-anesthesia care unit (PACU) – This is where you're likely to wake up after your vertical sleeve surgery. It's a room where patients who just had surgery and are still under the effects of anesthesia can recover. The benefit of having a single PACU, instead of sending you off to an isolated hospital room, is that the PACU nurses continually check on you to make sure that everything is going smoothly. Smaller clinics might not have a PACU, but the staff there will still take care of you.

Preferred provider organization (PPO) – This is a type of health insurance plan that charges based on a fee-for-service. That means that you pay for each service that you receive, but the amounts that you are charged are lower than for someone who is not in the PPO.

Pre-diabetes (impaired fasting glucose; IFG) – This is when your blood glucose levels are higher than normal but not high enough to put in category of being diabetic. Your doctor can diagnose pre-diabetes using a fasting blood glucose test, which you can get in any medical laboratory. Pre-diabetes puts you at very high risk of developing diabetes. If you are overweight or obese, losing weight can often put your blood glucose levels back to normal so that you are no longer pre-diabetic.

Quality of life – Also known as QoL, this is an overall indicator of how good your life is. It considers your physical health plus other factors, such as your social connections, how happy you are, and how well you are able to move around and do the things you want to do. A variety of different tests are available to measure QoL. The sleeve may help improve QoL.

Restrictive procedure – A restrictive procedure is a bariatric procedure that limits the amount of food you are able to eat, and therefore helps you lose weight. This describes the vertical sleeve gastrectomy, which leaves a sleeve that has only 20 percent of the capacity of your original stomach. The small sleeve helps you feel full sooner so you eat less.

Self-insured plan – This is a plan that your employer purchases; it may have specific benefits or exclusions that your employer has chosen as part of an individualized package.

Sleeve gastrectomy (see vertical sleeve gastrectomy)

Stent – This is a small tube that's often used to treat leaks in the sleeve. It may contain a sticky substance designed to slowly seal up the leak.

Stomach stapling (see vertical banded gastroplasty)

Summary of benefits (SOB) or certificate of coverage – This is a critical piece of paper (or online document) that tells you your insurance policy if you are in a fully-insured plan. It tells you which services are covered under your plan. You might have to call the insurance company to have them send you the summary of benefits if you cannot locate it yourself.

Summary Plan Description (SPD): This is a critical piece of paper (or online document) that tells you your insurance policy if you are in a self-insured plan. It tells you which services are covered under your plan. You might have to call your employer's human resources department or the insurance company to have them send you the summary of benefits if you cannot locate it yourself.

Triglycerides – These are a specific kind of fat that float around in your blood stream. Very high levels increase your risk for heart disease. Normal triglyceride levels are under 150 milligrams per deciliter (150 mg/dL, or 1.7 mmol/L). Your triglycerides are high if they are between 200 and 500 mg/dL (2.3 to 5.6 mmol/L) and very high if they are over 500 mg/dL (more than 5.6 mmol/L). You can lower high triglycerides by losing excess weight, exercising regularly, and reducing your intake of sugar and saturated fat.

Type 2 diabetes (see diabetes)

Vertical banded gastroplasty (VBG) – Also known as stomach stapling, this bariatric procedure involves partitioning the stomach with staples and a band to block off the majority of the stomach. The VBG has a similar principle as the VSG, but the stomach is only folded away, not removed, in the VBG. Because of the high rate of weight regain and complications, such as staples coming loose and gastroesophageal reflux (GERD), the VBG is rare in the U.S. today.

Vertical sleeve gastrectomy – This is also known as the gastric sleeve, gastrectomy, greater curvature gastrectomy and simply the sleeve. It's an irreversible procedure that can help you lose weight because it helps to restrict your food intake. The surgeon removes approximately 85 percent of your stomach, leaving only the upper 15 percent. The smaller stomach pouch is then attached to the small intestine.

Weight loss surgery (see bariatric surgery)

New Terms

There are always more words to learn about your sleeve gastrectomy. For easy reference, just add them to the glossary. Use this table to add new terms and their definitions. Also, make note of where you came across the term so you can go back and look it up if necessary.

Term	Where You Found It	Definition

Made in the USA
Monee, IL
14 March 2024

55005245R00260